Primal Estate

The Candidate Species

By

Samuel H. Franklin

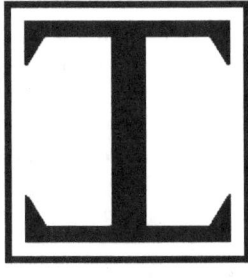

Ithaca

Published by Ithaca Publications
Fredericksburg, Virginia

ISBN:-10: 1496134737
ISBN-13: 978-1496134738

About the cover:

This particular skull was painted using a Cro-Magnon skull as the model. It has the distinctive features of the Cro-Magnon with its high forehead and somewhat square eye sockets.

The blades bordering the skull (see both sides of the book) are the blades of the Provenger gauntlets. The blades represent danger as well as prison bars. The stars of space and eternity exist outside the bars while there is a void within. The theme of captivity is intended to suggest the sometimes limited choices we have, and the potentially negative consequences of being imprisoned by an incorrect paradigm. But those bars that are far enough apart to allow the skull to pass through can typically allow the entire body to also slip through to freedom, if the body is appropriately nourished.

In the left eye socket is a stalk of wheat. The left eye in ancient Egypt was associated with the god Horus, the sky god, usually depicted as a falcon. He symbolizes healing, restoration, and protection. In hieroglyphics the left eye represents action or protection. It means "one who does". The wheat stalk in the left eye socket of the ancient human therefore indicates both what has been taken and what must be realized, what must be done. One must identify or see a problem to be capable of acting against it.

DEDICATION

This book is dedicated to those that suffer day in and day out from autoimmune and chronic disorders that most doctors and other health care practitioners fail to understand, diagnose, or treat properly. You have suffered long enough. No one knows better than you how bad our current situation is. We live in a dark age of medicine where science is advanced enough to know better, but the veil of ignorance has not yet been lifted. You put your trust in a system that demands it and you suffer as a result. Few understand. You must be heard.

Samuel H. Franklin

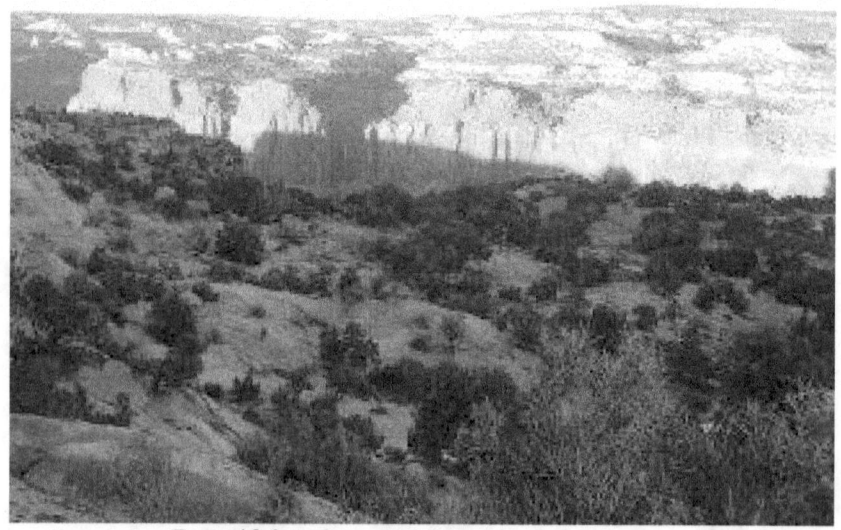

Beautiful and rugged canyon country

ACKNOWLEDGMENTS

I would like to thank my family and friends whose support, patience, and encouragement have made all the difference. I would also like to thank the following individuals, definitely for their friendship, but especially for either their council, assistance, patience, or provocation, good people all: Gary, and Craig, who were there helping me the moment I realized and embarked on the correct path of healing; Kimton, with whom a conversation led to this book; Tim Runk and Wendy Ramer for their help with editing; fellow authors Wendy Ramer, and T.C.F, for their guidance; pisan John S. (You don't even know what you don't know!) and L.S., R.C. and A.C.

I would also like to acknowledge the immeasurable assistance provided by the following researchers, enlightened physicians and authors for their contributions to the concepts in this novel: Dr. William Davis, Robb Wolf, Dr. Loren Cordain, Jared Diamond, Gary Taubes, Nora T. Gedgaudas, Dr. Terry L. Wahls, Dr. Stephanie Seneff, Dr. David Clark of Durham, NC.

David Scott-Donelan, the skill of tracking transcends the physical; its techniques apply to all things.

Marlo Cota, dear friend and mentor, "the unscripted adventure" is indeed the only true adventure.

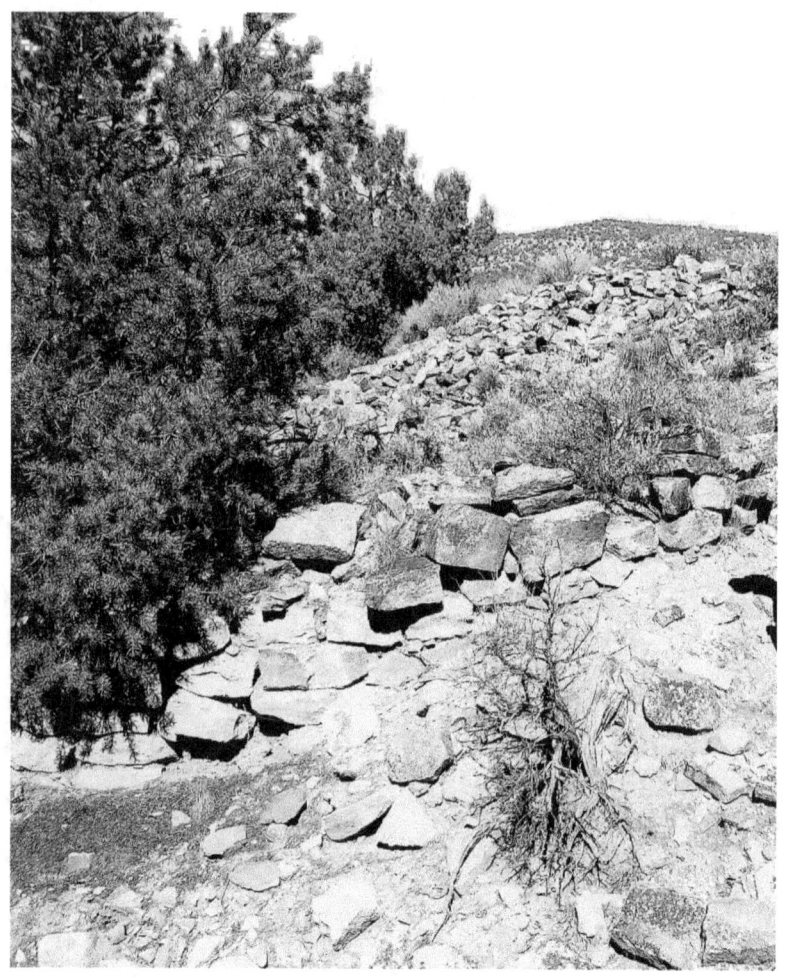

Ancient surface dwelling remains in Ruin Canyon

Preface

This novel was born of the struggle I have personally had with chronic illness. During the search for a solution to my sudden onset of an autoimmune condition, I learned that the conventional approach to such health issues is archaic. It is the progeny of the early alchemists who tried to alter systems they didn't understand with preparations and elixirs.

I also learned that the information people need to overcome much, if not all, of their chronic illness currently exists. It merely needs to be accessed and applied effectively by the sufferer. The main problem is that a paradigm endures that demands we look to doctors, our modern alchemists, for healing, instead of relying on logic and our knowledge of natural history. The fact is as humans we consume a set of foods that were not meant to be food for our species. There is little most doctors can do for autoimmune and inflammatory conditions resulting from this cause. The root of the problem, the environment we create within our bodies, must be addressed. Anything else is patching over rot.

The story of man's development of agriculture is unique and fascinating, almost a complete aberration in natural history. We are certainly navigating uncharted territory with our exploration of this resource and, apparently, spend much of our time wandering. As a consequence, the tragedy of the effect on health is grossly underappreciated. This understanding is key to the solution of our current chronic illness epidemic.

The physical effects meted upon mankind as a result of this drama fit so neatly into the realm of conspiracy. This story demands to be written. Though I have wracked my brain, I can think of no better way to dramatically increase a population while simultaneously making them plump and harmless. The same effects of agriculture that multiply and fatten populations can simultaneously make them succumb to the productivity draining symptoms of chronic disease in later life, when they should be most technically skilled and likely to drive technological advancement from a lifetime of learning. This last effect would be a vital component to serve the interests of the conspirators desiring their victims to be concurrently numerous, fattened, and harmless; the dream of every carnivore.

All movements have their heroes, all causes have their myths. These icons capture our imagination, the inner reaches of the mind and spirit that guide the individual. During my own struggle, I began to perceive the problem of my chronic illness as a villain, the solution as a hero. I gave a face to the monster and an evil purpose to the culinary fraud we live. With a view of this grand tragedy of deteriorating human health as being orchestrated with an evil design, instead of the product of random fate, there materializes a call to battle. We are not simply involved in the question of why we continually feel so fat, tired, or sick. We are involved in an epic struggle to discover the primal estate, the place to which we belong in nature, the right we have to be human and healthy.

My goal is nothing short of promoting the new paradigm, where the infirmed are driven to resolve causes, not mask symptoms, where we recognize that humans, just like all other animals, exist by eating certain things but are unable to thrive on others, no matter how enticing they might seem. We need to realize that our genes are not flawed. We do not commonly have predisposition to suffer disease, but we do commonly force our genes to endure environments that were not intended by nature. The results are evident.

This drama of human suffering makes victims of us all. The descriptions of deleterious effects and physiological processes contained in this story are not fiction. They are genuine and have the potential to operate in your body at any moment with every morsel you eat. The great irony of this book is that I may be the first author to admit both that my book is science fiction and about nutrition. Only in that respect does it join the vast field of other books that are also nutritional science fiction.

It is easy to utter, "You gotta die of something," until you are lying in your own sweat and feces in a bed that offers no rest, trapped in a body that brings only pain. This was not meant to be our destiny and this was not my plan. I made it otherwise. So can you.

This book has an appendix, the inclusion of which is meant to both inform and entertain. It contains a section called "Preparations for Contact, Transcribed Record". This portion was originally included in the story. Its intent is to fully describe the effects of a wheat based diet and how it is used by the Provenger to control their "resource project". It was removed from the body of the story as its length and detail detracted from the flow of the story line. It is still an important part of the novel and the message, but its content is now summarized in the second chapter so as not to further impede the average reader in their enjoyment of the story. For those who suffer from chronic illness, you will both recognize its relevance and hopefully benefit from the perspective it provides.

If I were to be forced to fight a bull and could speak to only one person beforehand, I would want to speak to the bull fighter rather than the biologist who has read all relevant books and conducted studies on the subject. Seek advice of those who have healed themselves of our horrible chronic diseases. They do exist. Then use your judgment to determine if their method is correct for you. If you are smart enough, you are worthy in the eyes of nature. And you will heal. There should be one simple test that determines how a human should live. What way of acting and eating protects or heals us, long term, from the effects of the diseases of affluence?

It is easier to destroy than to create. Destruction requires only neglect and ignorance. Destruction of the body can take a lifetime. Are we to think the preservation of our health takes any less? The new paradigm needs to be acknowledged.

Ladies and gentlemen, I give you your conspiracy. So let's have some fun; it is, after all, science fiction. Or is it?

Samuel H. Franklin

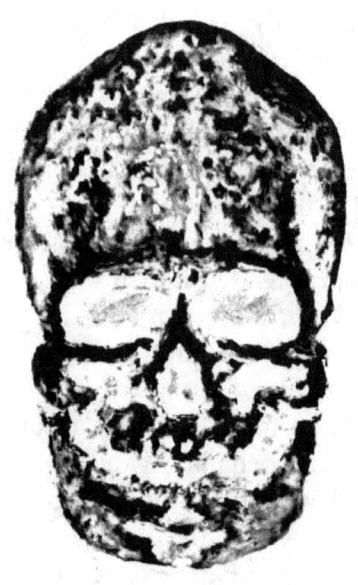

Primal Estate

The Candidate Species

By

Samuel H. Franklin

Is there a place for the hopeless sinner,
Who has hurt all mankind just to save his own beliefs?
Have pity on those whose chances grow thinner,
There ain't no hiding place from the Father of Creation.

Bob Marley

Introduction

In the vacuum of space, too cold and dark to provide solace, too barren of life to allow sustenance, there is a race that lives well. In their past, every planet was to them a reservoir of resources in the vast desert of space. They were the hunter-gatherers of the galaxy. When the pillaged planets could no longer supply their burgeoning population, they began to question their purpose in the universe. When the situation became critical and demands of the masses became unmanageable, their governments turned to the one resource that is never exhausted; war.

Their advanced technology allowed for very effective application of this device. With populations depleted and ideals forgotten in the grief that follows tragedy, there was a new purpose, a new possibility. Emerging from the conflict was a society dedicated to a practical goal, vowed to enable sustainability. They used their technology and their laws to ensure for themselves and their heirs that they consumed only what they created. So they could always provide for their kind, they would never again lay waste to the universe.

Though they had been citizens of space and time for as long as their society had records, they realized that the planets and the plants and animals that sustained life were a special gift, a gift that when properly maintained, would give forever. They leveraged their technology to nurture, they endeavored to manage, and they learned to harvest sustainably.

In nature there are neither rewards nor punishments, there are consequences.

Robert G. Ingersoll

Chapter 1

The intrigue and the sample

12,893 years in the past

"I'll lift you up, and you look to see what's in there," Qayen instructed his little brother.

"I'm not sticking my head in that thing," Ablu replied. "It looks dark in there. I can't even see anything from down here." Annoyed with his brother, he challenged, "You go first. You're the oldest." Ablu paused before issuing the ultimate challenge. "Or are you scared?"

"I'm not scared," Qayen replied, leaning his three long flexible spears up against a bush. He searched for something to poke in the hole before he looked in. His spears and his throwing stick were too valuable to probe into an unknown place. He would need them later for the wounded aurochs. The area was unusually empty of sticks he could use, but he quickly spied a stand of tall grass, pulled up a few long stalks, and motioned for Ablu to help him up.

Putting a foot in his younger brother's interlaced fingers, Qayen was lifted for a better view. He clutched the entrance rim with his left hand and peered in. It was black as night, right before his eyes, like a deep pool of dark water with no reflection. He stuck the grass stalks in and they were gone. The darkness seemed to consume the stalks as soon as they entered. It scared him, and Qayen recoiled violently back from the hole in fright and caught himself, hoping it didn't show to his brother below.

Qayen cast his eyes toward the heavens to ask his spirit for courage. He saw that the sky was filled with billowing clouds, and yet the air around him was still. For a moment, he wondered at the brightness of the day, even though there was not a single patch of blue sky to be seen. The heavens were obscured from his view, and yet he felt that his spirit had answered.

The massive wheel-shaped spacecraft slipped into solar orbit near the planet, and the six satellite scanners immediately deployed to get a comprehensive assessment of the surface biome. "Complete scan of life forms for physiologic baseline," Synster spoke aloud. The scanners voice-matched and registered his official approval. They raced away from the ship on courses to position themselves around the planet.

The Provenger Nation Ship phased into its presence in the star system; it didn't simply arrive. Five days prior, when the ship was appearing in local time-space, it was simultaneously there and not there, and time measured two hundred years earlier on the planet surface. With considerable expenditure of energy resources, the Provenger sent probes outside of their time-space bubble for specimen collection. And the decades raced by.

Ryvil couldn't get the invasive images out of his mind as he waited in the shadows for the probe to be sent. Whenever he had to be patient or quiet, the frights came. He was a nervous Provenger. He had good cause.

At over two hundred years old physical age, he'd been through too much to come out unscathed. Many thin lines crisscrossed his scalp, face, and body, remnants of severe wounds that had been expertly repaired to appear as mere blemishes. But the psychological scars were deeper, largely unseen, and couldn't be repaired.

A former martial instructor at an academy that no longer existed, from a time much more remote than his contemporaries knew or his physical age indicated, Ryvil needed to conceal his former allegiance. He'd been on the losing side, and he still served his old master.

Ryvil had managed to avoid the outer perimeter of security that regulated access to the Species Collection Port. It was a massive bay containing multitudes of devices. Fortunately for Ryvil, the security was not tight. The Provenger didn't have any known enemies, so precautions were minimal and designed to keep out the merely curious to prevent contamination.

He now stood crammed among the variously engineered apparatus. They were all traps and containment vessels designed to collect specific species throughout the galaxy. Ryvil was watching a large black sphere that would hold the carnate sample, the Subject Species that he needed to access before it was fully examined. It must be contaminated. The sphere was scheduled to phase at any moment. It would be transported to the planet surface, trap its species, and return.

Since time was still moving very rapidly outside the Provenger Nation Ship, it would appear to leave and reappear with its sample, instantaneously, even if it spent twenty years on the surface waiting for its quarry.

The delay was brief but seemed endless, as the repercussions of being caught plied through Ryvil's mind. If his presence was detected, he had an excuse in place, but it could expose him to suspicion. Detection needed to be avoided at all cost.

The confined space where he concealed himself was flaying his nerves. He suppressed a tremor, closed his eyes briefly, and began to sweat. He thought of open spaces and the pleasant prospect of ending his days on the planet surface.

The transport of the black sphere initiated with the telltale low-toned vibration of air pressure modulating and the brief condensation and immediate evaporation of moisture in the air. It emitted fuzzy light and formed a brief, hazy white barrier around the space containing the probe.

On the planet surface, two carnate brothers were out hunting a lone young aurochs that their cousin had seen from a distance the day before. It had appeared injured, and he told the brothers about it, hoping to help them. As young adults of the tribe, they still had not killed one by themselves. The brothers set out, hopeful that their first aurochs hunt would provide for their tribe and increase their status for future marriage negotiations.

At about midday, they were in the described location for only a short time when they came across a large and strange boulder. All the others of its size in the area were settled into the ground, and they were gray and hard. This one was black and textured with even bumps across its entire surface. What first drew their attention to this rock was its color, its uniformity, and absolute distinctiveness. It sat lightly on the surface of the soil, as though it had just been placed there. It was massive and noticeable. They were familiar with the area and had never seen anything like it. It must have arrived from somewhere, they thought. It was so perfectly round. They approached it carefully, and when they touched it and finally knocked on it, it sounded hollow.

Ablu and Qayen considered the possibility that this large rock, significantly higher than their hands held above their heads, had been sent by a god. They were anxious to get back to their tribe to tell everyone what they found, but they felt they needed to investigate first. They couldn't climb it because the shape and texture provided no handholds. They walked around it and discovered, on the far side, a large round hole. It was too high to get to alone, and it was a size that would allow them to crawl in. They stepped back from the boulder, trying to see further into the hole, and considered their options. They decided they should investigate.

After snapping back in fright, Qayen stuck the stalks in again and twirled them in circles, as though he were clearing unseen cobwebs. Nothing. He pulled them out and sniffed at the hole, thinking it might smell damp or rotting. "Ablu," he called down, "it smells a little sweet, like honey. Maybe there's a hive with no bees. I don't see or hear any."

"Let me smell," Ablu said, withering under the weight of his bigger brother.

"Yes," Qayen replied, getting down. "But don't stick your head in. It's so dark I can't see these when I put them in," Qayen said, casting the stalks to the ground.

"Help me up," Ablu insisted. "I want to smell it."

Qayen interlaced his fingers and helped his brother up to the level of the hole. Ablu had a rabbit hanging from his belt that he'd killed along the way and thought that if there were snakes inside, or anything else, he'd rather sacrifice the rabbit than a hand. He unhooked it and held it out for Qayen to see. "I'm going to hold this in first and see what happens."

Ablu slowly put the rabbit into the hole. It was as dark as his brother had said. Darker, he thought. The moment it was in, he couldn't see it. His hand disappeared with it. Ablu put his nose near the edge of the hole to take a sniff, but he never got the chance to breathe in.

Qayen, helping his brother from below, felt a strong tug at first, and then a sustained attempt to pull his brother in. All that he heard from Ablu was a low moan just as his head would have been entering. Qayen instinctively tried to pull back, but whatever was drawing them in was so strong his efforts amounted to only a slight hesitation in his brother's slip into the darkness. Struggling for the one leg he'd been holding, Qayen was lifted toward the opening. The tremendous force was nothing he could match. As he was pulled up toward the hole, he instinctively knew he must let go or be dragged in himself. As he released his brother's disappearing foot, he screamed with fear and grief at what horrible beast must be inside.

As Qayen fell to the ground, he saw Ablu's blood on his hands and chest. He looked up at the black opening in panic, and the entire rock began to move. It lifted a small distance above the ground and disappeared in a sphere of white light.

Qayen knew his brother was dead. He would never see him again. He waited the rest of the afternoon and evening under a nearby tree until the sun fell low on the horizon. He held out a futile hope that if he just stayed, the boulder would return and he might discover his brother's fate.

As the sun disappeared into the distant trees, Qayen knew he would have to return home alone. He would have to tell his parents and his tribe how he had lost his brother, how they would never see him again. They would insist on coming out to search. They wouldn't believe him. He could lie and say a lion had eaten Ablu, but he knew there were no prints or blood trails to support such a story. He decided to tell the truth. They would believe what they wanted. And Qayen would forever suffer from poor Ablu's fate, both for the loss of his brother and the link of his name to evil.

The black sphere's white haze dissipated and Ryvil knew it was back, a little dustier for the trip. The trap had been successful, and what Ryvil needed was onboard. He approached the sphere quickly, accessed the com-port, and pressed the outside edge of his gauntlet to make contact. His mission was accomplished. He had made a subtle change in the sample. Now, to escape without notice, he thought.

Inside the sphere, contained in a suspension fluid in complete darkness, was a living carnate male named Ablu, and a dead rabbit. Ablu was conscious and unharmed, save for a bleeding shin and a heart that was racing from the panic of being trapped. He was unable to breathe in a black fluid that had the slimy thickness of blood. As minutes passed and his lungs filled with it, Ablu wondered why he did not suffocate, and he began to calm. If he had known what lay in his near future, he would have wished instead to be mauled by a wild animal.

Outside the sphere, Ryvil strode away with purpose, amazed, yet again, how the Algorithm had correctly predicted the preceding events. Despite the fact that it was simply a conscious entity existing only within the confines of the Provenger computer networks, Ryvil considered the Algorithm his friend. It was able to process infinite variables simultaneously, consider every element of a known system, and accurately determine future outcomes. It had told Ryvil, in its usual dispassionate and secret report, exactly what was needed to achieve his plan. It was one of his few allies and fellow conspirators.

When the sphere arrived, a signal had been sent to the main science deck where Provenger began to respond, initiating systems that would make use of the new sample. As automated equipment came to life and began approaching the sphere, Ryvil had reached the main exit. As he passed out of the threshold cloak and looked up, Project Minister Cybuls and two security aids were standing an arm's length away, looking at him with surprise.

"What were you doing in there, and how did you get in?" the Minister questioned, balancing a tone of suspicion with the due respect that Ryvil's position warranted. As the Director Designee of the Managed Collectivization strategy, Ryvil could become a very important Provenger if the current program failed, and this was not lost on the Minister.

"I was looking for you," Ryvil snapped back. "Aren't you supposed to be here for the arrival of all probes? And how was I able to just walk in here without any kind of security warning? What kind of a program are you managing here?" Ryvil accused.

Minister Cybuls was immediately defensive but still respectful. "Well, I *am* here, and I don't know how you were able to walk in. I suppose the cloak shield must be malfunctioning. They are checked regularly and I don't…"

"Well, check them again," Ryvil interrupted. "We can't have any Provenger just wandering anywhere they want. What if samples become contaminated?" Ryvil moved on before giving Cybuls time to think. "Now, I need you to reschedule the Planning Committee Vote later today. I need it about three rinsects earlier. That should give me enough time. My team needs to review both the incoming samples and produce a rebuttal to Synster's plan within the day. There just won't be time otherwise. There's been more data than we thought. He already has the majority of his projections, and I doubt he'll have any problem getting his vote. For my team, it's just a matter of following the law. We need to get our rebuttal filed in time. Can you do that? Or will you be too busy double-checking your broken security systems?" Ryvil asked with a sarcasm that pushed the limits of his authority.

"Ryvil, I don't appreciate your tone. You know very well I have the authority to alter meeting schedules, but I really should check with Synster first," Cybuls replied, defending himself.

"Well, get it done then. We all know this project should never need Managed Collectivization, but if it does, I would hate to have to review the need for a new Project Minister." Before Cybuls could respond, Ryvil excused himself and walked through them, terminating the encounter on his own terms.

Cybuls turned to watch him go, irritated that his authority had been questioned and concerned about his future should Ryvil ever become the Project Director. Would Ryvil question his abilities? Cybuls touched his collar, activating his com-monitor. "All 3-237 Perpetuant Cycle Project principals, Planning Committee meeting has been moved earlier by four rinsects." Cybuls didn't want to give Ryvil any reason to question his nerve or commitment. Synster would just have to be flexible.

Chapter 2

His project

Synster, Director of the Natural Proliferation strategy of the current Project, needed the final scan on the subject species sample that had just arrived. With this information, he could conduct final modifications on the genetics of the candidate species to fit their needs, and he'd be ready to implement. With the scans fully automated, he'd have just enough time for a quick lunch with his son.

Synster stepped out of his shuttle and into his home. The cloak shield on the main threshold sputtered as he walked in. Then it blinked out momentarily, allowing everyone outside a view directly into his great-room. He grew annoyed. Vwannan had one of the best apartments on the ship, and yet strangers moving by could stare in at their family.

"Vwannan, are you here?" He spoke softly as he entered, wanting to tell her immediately about her front cloak.

Vwannan was 115 years old and had taken many children from Synster. She had invited him into her dominion when she was only 33, and their relationship had gone well. The youngest two were currently living with them; the daughter, Nwella, 27, and the son Beyn, 7 years old. Provenger men were considered welcome at the home as long as they behaved. Vwannan had never cast Synster out.

Beyn ran up to Synster as he entered. "Father, I can see the planet. Isn't it exciting?"

"Yes, Beyn. It is. I came home to watch it with you. I can only stay a short time. Then I have to get back to work, so let's get a snack and watch."

They sat at the window and looked out; Synster spoke to his wife as she entered the room. "Vwannan, my love, hello. Is the server working?"

"Yes, Synster. I'll get you what I already made."

"Father," Beyn interrupted, "they said in school that we're going to change this planet. What are we going to do?"

Synster thought about this question for a moment. He wanted to give Beyn an answer that would be a credit to his intelligence, but didn't want to get too involved in the details. Beyn was still a child and hadn't yet been initiated into even second tier social realities.

The Provenger cared very much for their children. They were considered sacred, and a formal system governed their social exposures and education. At various stages in their lives, they were considered prepared to encounter certain realities, intellectually and emotionally. Only the Provenger final tier initiated their young adults into the graphic and violent realities of the universe, as well as the true nature of their resource acquisition.

"The most intelligent species on this planet," Synster explained to Beyn, "what we call the Subject Species, have no way to make their own food. They spend much of their time moving from place to place catching or collecting everything they eat."

"That's what we do!" Beyn interrupted, referring to their movement from planet to planet, collecting or harvesting resources.

"Why…yes, we do." Synster continued. "But they don't have cities or nation ships like we do. And to have them a species needs to be able to settle permanently in one place. They need to be able to establish an environment where things that they eat will grow, and grow enough for all of their members. So we are going to modify some of their plants, what we call the Candidate Species, so that they'll grow them for food, in one place, rather than roaming around looking for it all the time. This way they can live in towns and cities. They will eventually grow smarter with their accumulated knowledge and be able to fully populate the planet with their kind."

"If these plants are already theirs, and they already eat them, why do we need to modify them?" Beyn asked.

"Well the plants already grow on this planet, but they, the carnate, don't really use them for food that much, only a little bit, every once in a while. So we're going to change things so they have enough to eat it all the time," Synster explained.

Beyn thought for a moment, "Father?"

"Yes, Beyn?"

"These animals are going to get sick. Mother said you shouldn't eat the same thing all the time or you're going to become ill. Remember the adventure we had at Celnius Five and all we had to eat was the Groktar fruit. I had diarrhea constantly and even pooped in my pants one night. I hadn't done that for a long, long time, Mother said. Even Nwella got sick, and her face broke out in pimples that had these little white dots on them, and she was anguished because that boy wouldn't talk to her. Father?"

"Yes, Beyn?"

"Did they ask us to do this?"

"Do what?" Synster felt trouble ahead.

"Make these plants that will be food for them," Beyn clarified.

"No."

"So why are we doing it?

There it was, the question Synster was seeking to avoid. "Beyn, would you like some fruit? I promise you it's not Groktar."

"No, thank you. Mother was already making something else."

Synster's com-monitor vibrated, indicating a message. He accessed it with a touch to his shoulder. The meeting had been rescheduled to an earlier time. The scanners information would be back by then, but it would give him much less time to process the information collected.

"So, Father," Beyn pulled on his father's thick, muscled forearm. Synster wanted to avoid the last question, but it seemed Beyn had moved on. "Will the planet look the same?"

"Yes, from here it will look exactly the same."

Vwannan walked up, leaned down, and put a plate on the table. In the center was a pile of roasted meat and four strips of gelatin-encased, air-fried fat on layers of green leaves. Surrounding the center, heaped around the edge, were blueberries and small, young Shinsta root with a curry sauce. Beyn began to eat.

Synster could still see in his wife the twenty-year-old he'd literally run into one day while in a rush to get to work. She'd been wearing her public gown and was coming down some stairs. He'd been facing away, trying to escape from an acquaintance who kept talking. He turned around quickly and took a step as she came down behind him. He planted his face right into her chest, between her bare breasts, in the exact manner of the marriage ceremony. They immediately laughed. Then both became embarrassed as they realized they were making a scene, and they went about their business. Every time after that when they made eye contact, they knew there were feelings between them. It took a considerable amount of time before Vwannan approached him and allowed him to identify himself.

She now had her home clothing on. Her skin tone was perfectly peachy-bronzed, glowing through the thin, white cloth, and a long, wide sash she wore around her slim waist barely covered her lean muscular legs. The sheer cloth draped over her chest and back caressed her as she moved. Synster was in awe of her physical beauty. Provenger bodies did not grow hair, and Synster admired the smooth surfaces of her skull, flawlessly shaped. Not all males were so lucky, he thought. Vwannan smiled to him with her dark brown eyes as she walked behind where he was sitting, draped her arms over his shoulders, and let her soft hands lay down over his bare chest. She sighed and looked out toward the new planet.

"I have to go sooner than I thought," Synster told her.

"I thought that would happen," Vwannan muttered.

Synster returned to the science deck. They had already been in orbit long enough for the scanners to begin sending data back. They were not in silence mode as there were no advanced civilizations to detect them. From all current analysis, it seemed little had changed on the planet surface. Nevertheless, the Algorithm would need to process all information prior to the vote. It seemed there would be just enough time. The massive amount of data was currently coming in and was being catalogued by the Algorithm. The full assessment couldn't be made until it was complete. That would take a little more time.

Synster excused himself to his office. Once inside he glanced out his window at the planet. He felt as if everything was going well, but now, with the meeting being moved up and the data from the scans flowing in, he wondered if anything else would change.

He looked in the mirror on his wall and focused on his own eyes. If he looked deeply he could see the age. He was aged 153 Earth years. That sounded old, he thought. He was middle aged for a Provenger and still in excellent condition. His tenacity compensated for his slightly smaller than average stature. But at six two Earth measurement, he was only a little short of average, with enough muscle on him to make up for any deficiencies in height.

Synster made a mental note to find out why the meeting had been moved up. He suspected Ryvil had something to do with it. They were all working toward the same goal, yet Synster had never done anything for Ryvil, therefore Ryvil had no allegiance to him whatsoever. It was remarkable, really, how separate their careers had been, Synster thought.

As the scanning was being completed, it became clear there was something wrong with the existing plan. On his screen Synster reviewed some variables that were marked as problems. It seemed the weather patterns were a little too volatile to enable significant sedentary use of coastline by the Subject Species. Early permanent settlements would not be established in many productive coastal areas due both to this weather and the erratic tides in these locations. Weather or tides individually would not be a problem, but every half dozen years or so, seasonal weather trends and tidal patterns would conspire to develop into especially violent floods at certain coastal areas.

The Algorithm showed that this would periodically result in the near, or complete destruction of any early settlements at critical locations. The result would be no permanent settlements. These locations were vital to the Perpetuant Cycle's success. Coastal trade was vital to the development, exploration, and propagation of the carnate to new productive areas. Something would need to be done and the answer was right in front of Synster. The Algorithm never identified a problem without providing an answer. The smaller of the two moons would have to be removed.

Synster couldn't believe it. They'd never attempted anything this big to influence a biological system. How could the initial survey team have missed this, he wondered? For something this big, he'd need the specific approval of the Committee as well as assistance from the Tactical Director of the ship. Normally this authority would not be his, but fortunately the Union was wise enough to put the Tactical Director under Synster's authority only for decisions being made for the purposes of the Project.

Streyn was first at the meeting, well before Synster arrived. It was his job to get a feel for the members' mood and give Synster warning if anything had changed. The meeting needed to go well otherwise Ryvil might have an inroad to taking over the Project. If Natural Proliferation was not going to work, to meet their quotas in the time required, Ryvil would take over. Nobody really wanted Managed Collectivization, but it was required by their mandate. The planet surface would be completely molded to the will of the project requirements, and nothing would exist but that which furthered the project; an extremely intensive, expensive, and invasive prospect.

Streyn spoke to the major players in the courtyard to get their feel for the coming vote, then spoke with some of those most resistant to Synster's plans. There weren't many, and they were the ones who didn't understand most of the science. He was well versed on Synster's reasons and logic for what he had planned, and knew that no arguments against it could prevail.

Later that evening, after the Planning Committee vote…

Vwannan stepped into Synster's office, impatient to discover the course of the project and, therefore, the course of their lives.

"My proposals were approved. The transcript from the meeting is there on the desk," Synster pointed. "It's the typical dry pitch you've been hearing all along, so you don't really need to read it all unless, of course, you're interested in the details about the deleterious effects on the subject species."

Vwannan glared at him critically, head cocked to one side. "I want to know about everything that effects my life." And she began to read.

****

Preparations for Contact
TRANSCRIBED RECORD

Meeting of the
3-237 Perpetuant Cycle Project
Planning Committee-
Vote for the Approval
Candidate Species: Yngorn
Subject Species: Carnate

Project Minister:

Listen and be heard, this twenty-fourth meeting of the 3-237 Perpetuant Cycle Project Planning Committee, all who have Interest be here withheld of all selfish undoing, and maintain the good of the Nation for all and forever.

Science Director Synster:

As you've already been informed of in your brief, our objective of populating this planet through the advancement of their agricultural technology has been fully vetted by the Algorithm. A delicate balance of both the subject species population growth and technological impairment must be maintained to provide us with a maximum population increase over time without their posing a technological threat upon our return. As has been well established, any intelligent organism, provided with the efficiencies of agriculture, will have the time and the incentive to develop and accumulate technology. A hunting-gathering society, on the other hand, has the time but not necessarily the incentive or means to do the same.

If we merely provide the carnate with a wholesome, reliable, and nutrient rich source of food to generate the population numbers we need, the Algorithm has calculated that they will reach a technological advancement comparable to ours within a period of approximately five thousand years. We will be absent from this planet well beyond this time as the Union schedule demands. There is every indicator that we would return to a superior society technologically capable of defending itself. This would obviously be counterproductive. We are therefore compelled to include various progressive deleterious effects to our agricultural product introduction. These qualities are designed to obstruct health and productivity in their post-harvest years.

Our goal is that they be reasonably healthy and of proper carcass mass index during harvest age, without being advanced enough to defend themselves against us. Our return to this planet is scheduled for nine years, eight months, our time. Allowing for Accelerated Gravitational Time Dilation, we will return in approximately twelve thousand, eight hundred and ninety-three years planet time. We have the charter to proceed as necessary to generate a viable product. We must be aggressive. Let's just say, any enemies we make now, won't be around to trouble us later.

General Reaction:
Laughter, Agreement, scale 6.5 out of 10

Synster:
Prior experience has shown that it is imprudent to rely on a single mechanism to achieve our ends, and we are best rewarded by implementing multiple strategies. We are fortunate in regard to this planet as we have a grass that grows throughout a great variety of regions that is highly receptive to genetic modification. We can amend its qualities to suit our needs. This enables us to implement not a single, but a multi-pronged approach with this one species to achieve our goals. There is other vegetation that offers potential, and will also be made available for agricultural development. But it is only this one grass that produces a grain, largely poisonous, and unpalatable to the carnate population, which we will modify to enhance its beneficial properties for the purposes of achieving production goals.

This grain, Yngorn, a subgroup of the broader wheat group, and named after the Provenger that discovered it, is currently of minor use to the subject species population, particularly in its non-germinated form, due to a great variety of deleterious effects it inflicts on carnate physiology. When these populations do find it in quantities that allow for its collection, they are only able to make use of its limited nourishment through soaking it long enough to sprout or have it ferment. In its un-sprouted grain form, it is hard on their teeth, dry in their mouths and almost void of flavor. It requires significant effort to access and collect, and considerable processing to be consumed. It is the last thing the subject species would perceive as food.

Despite these efforts, it is still detrimental as food, as it is small and course, imbued with toxins and proteins damaging to their digestive systems, and relatively deficient in nutrients even when processed. We will introduce strains that will eliminate the high degree of these negative aspects. The resulting plant will retain certain elements of its poisonous characteristics. These effects are by design. They bring us numerous benefits to help meet our goals. These benefits involve the deterioration of subject species health at a measured rate, with the majority of degenerative effects occurring after the subject species' reproductive and harvest age. This will reduce individuals' contributions to their society later in life when they are most knowledgeable and experienced, ensuring slow technological progress while simultaneously maintaining the level of civilization necessary for perpetuated population growth. We can count on this grain to provide general nutrient scarcity, impaired nutrient absorption, innate and adaptive immune system responses, and addictive tendencies.

PAUSE

Let me elaborate...

****

"Where's the rest of it?" Vwannan asked.

"You'll have to link to the appendix. The rest is there, in its entirety. I explain all of the deleterious effects in detail," Synster replied quickly, eager for her input. "It's quite thorough and..."

"Please stop. I can't go on right now," Vwannan said impatiently. "You are the herald of recombinant coma!"

"I try to give complete information."

"I'll read the rest later when I'm trying to fall asleep. Why don't you just say that they'll tolerate it until they don't tolerate it anymore? Then they'll get sick and die early, like we want them to."

"I said that eventually, in so many words."

"In too many words. Because this would have put me to sleep. You really need to engage your audience more," Vwannan continued.

"Well, it was a vote on the issues. That's all. It wasn't like we needed to discuss anything. We had a question and answer period," Synster explained.

"Sure, for those who were still awake," Vwannan criticized.

"I had very little time to prepare. I had to make the decision about elimination of the moon. But they accepted my judgment. It is best this way, less wasted time, lower costs. I chose not to mention that the Algorithm predicted the removal was likely to cause various immediate but temporary extreme weather issues, possible minor earthquakes, and a polar ice sheet to break in half, flooding, extended global cooling and a drying period of the atmosphere for many centuries after the fact!" Synster sucked in a deep breath after his long and significant list as he rolled his eyes at the magnitude of it all.

"But I wasn't required to divulge this, and no one asked. Besides, they are mostly fools on that committee. If I bring something new to the Project, it is their job to ask. It's my job to make things work, to act, to get the job done. That's why the charter is written as it is. I will not be delayed. Delay is right next to failure on these projects, and that is one of my main responsibilities." Three days to the Contact Protocol, he was getting impatient; he had much work to do. "Do you think everything looks right?"

"I'm unsure." She moved to take a step and after almost a century of marriage, he knew pacing meant she was about to get critical. "I think the deleterious effects are too aggressive, and this new spectral energy reading we have yet to fully qualify is disconcerting."

Streyn arrived at his office cloak and entered. He immediately saw that Vwannan was in the room and extended his greeting. "Peace between us," he said while moving toward her. She walked in front of him and as he leaned forward, extended her palms where he momentarily laid his right cheek, in the standard formal greeting of a married woman of her rank in the presence of her husband.

Streyn looked up as her hands retracted and she stepped back. "Ryvil was the one who moved up the meeting. Claimed he had a scheduling conflict and convinced the Project Minister that we already knew all the issues, so there was no reason to delay."

"Did you check to see if he really had a conflict?" Synster asked.

"Yes, he did," Streyn replied.

"He's participating in preparations for the Contact. I hope he doesn't have any more scheduling conflicts. Is there anything else?"

"No Synster."

"Leave." Synster responded.

Streyn did so quickly. Vwannan always made him nervous.

Looking at Vwannan, Synster inquired, "Please explain."

"The deleterious effects are too greedy." Vwannan resumed her pacing. "You're trying to get everything you want with maximum efficiency. We know, regardless of what the Algorithm says, nature has its secrets. It has its ways of making this more difficult, or more efficient. It operates on its own agenda and circumvents our motives in ways that we cannot see. It is mystery. Providing a grain that gives them easy energy should be enough. We should determine another way to slow their technological growth. You don't have to leave in proteins that force their genetics to express themselves in grotesque ways.

"For instance we could use the lead poisoning option. The deleterious effects are very nearly the same. The lead substitutes itself for vital minerals and creates aberrant genetic expression and immune system problems, almost exactly like the symptoms of wheat phytates sequestering minerals. We can easily put the end product through the biofilter before marketing, and it's something they are likely to discover and correct for themselves just prior to our arrival, assuming their technology is properly tuned."

"We can't use lead. The biofilter treatment was unacceptable to the Union. They demand an organic product."

"Still, the wheat grain should be cleared of these effects, much as the rice candidate is. I don't believe the Algorithm can account for all the factors involved. You have added uncertainty, not efficiency. I don't think they will ever reach a level of advancement that could threaten our eventual harvest."

"But the Algorithm suggested these effects, it was not my decision." Synster responded, looking at her and waiting. "And the unexplained energy readings, the spectral scan? What is your opinion there?"

Vwannan suddenly became thoughtful. "We really have no idea what these energy readings are. We've never seen them in living beings and that alone brings me caution. We have known ferocity in beings from other systems but never seen an energy reading for it. In my reasoning then, ferocity can only be associated with it, but is not its source." She stopped her pacing, moved toward him looking more serious and lowered her tone. "We do not see all that it entails. The reading's root source may be from something very different. We have reason to believe that there are other traits that this energy influences. The spectral reading is foreign to us." Vwannan glared at him for a moment. "Synster, we have the Algorithm. Nothing is foreign to us. Doesn't that concern you?"

"It does."

"It should," Vwannan insisted. "Of all the life forms we've encountered, this is the only planet where the spectral readings exist. There's got to be something important we're missing."

"I agree," replied Synster, "but until we figure it out, we need to move forward."

"On top of all this, you are going to remove a moon from a planet. Certainly we've done this before but never with a living planet."

"I've looked at all variables through the Algorithm and relatively little life will be destroyed. And that which would be is not in any area critical to our objec..."

"You are killing the moon of a living planet! What if life important to our requirements uses this moon for something... biological cycles, navigation, anything?" Vwannan raised her voice at him. "What if the spectral scan readings have a relationship to this moon?"

"There is no other option," Synster could tell that her opinion was final but knew he could not change what had already been presented. "The plan has been approved. You know that."

"And why didn't you tell me the cloak on the front threshold wasn't working? I couldn't tell from the inside and I've been home all day with pedestrians walking by. We can't let Provenger think we've opened our home to anyone who would like to wander in."

"I meant to but I got distracted with Beyn. Vwannan, I need to go through with this plan. It's a matter of protocol. The issues that have been decided cannot be changed."

The project proceeded as planned with great hope through the Provenger Nation that their harvest would prove productive and profitable. Once the ground teams were established as gods among the carnate, the Provenger ship began its phase sequence to depart. As Provenger time incrementally slowed due to accelerated gravitational time dilation, time on the planet surface began to speed by.

After decades had passed on the planet and only minutes onboard ship, there were some problems on the planet surface. This was to be expected. The Provenger made their agricultural introductions in numerous locations, knowing that some could fail. But this particular failure was very unusual.

One location was lost due to a rebellion of the carnate. This possibility had not been anticipated by the Algorithm. It led to significant apprehension among the Provenger. At the expense of much energy and at great individual risk, a rescue team was sent. Nothing could be done to save the ground team, and there were no survivors. All was lost.

In the confusion that followed, all Provenger technology that had been used at that location was either destroyed or reclaimed, accompanied by one carnate that was mistakenly transported to the Provenger Nation ship. The cause of the carnate rebellion was never discovered. Little did the Provenger know the cause was among them.

When the required gravitational supercriticality was obtained around the Provenger Nation ship, and thousands of years had passed on the planet surface, their phase completed, and the ship appeared across the galaxy at the rendezvous point with their own race. Only ten years would pass for the Provenger before their return. Over twelve thousand would pass on the planet surface.

Chapter 3

Earth, Ruin Canyon

12,893 years later
Our near future

Life brings the bold a continuous stream of surprises; this day was no different. Discovery of Indian ruins and lion attacks were not on his mind that morning as Rick Thompson parked his old Jeep Wrangler in the dark at the top of the desert mesa. Light was just barely threatening with a glow on the horizon and, even though it was not his plan to be in place before sunrise, he still wanted to get there as early as possible. He was at the eastern edge of Ruin Canyon, an aptly named gouge in the earth about 25 miles northwest of the southwestern Colorado town of Cortez. This area was known for its links to the ancient Anasazi, its ruggedness, its outlaws, and its secrets.

He wanted to make absolutely sure he had everything he'd need. He was already in the middle of nowhere and was about to go even further in. Rick reached up and disabled the interior's dome light, opened the door, and got out of the driver's side. He left that door open and, able to see only shades from black to gray, opened the back door to access his gear.

He didn't want to bring too much as he had an area of cliffs to negotiate, then an even deeper descent on a slope to the bottom of the canyon. It was still dark and starting down the cliff now might be dangerous, he thought. It wasn't really a lighting issue, though; it was a frost issue. Even though it didn't seem that cold, especially for November, the night had brought a frost, and Rick knew from experience that almost every foot placement and handhold all the way down ran the risk of being on top of a thin layer of frost, between him and the smooth stone, every tiny crystal conspiring against his safety. Seeing it first was always helpful.

Rick had carefully packed everything the night before: water, a couple cold cooked sweet potatoes, a compass, a small first aid kit, knife, large black plastic garbage bag, a couple extra clothing layers, wool cap, a lighter, an extra magazine. Hanging around his neck, underneath his jacket, were his issued binoculars. They were much better than anything he could afford to buy on his own. He had experience with this type of thing and knew what he needed.

He put the backpack down outside the car, unzipped it, took out a sweatshirt, and considered it for a moment. It'll probably get much warmer today. He threw it in the Jeep. One less thing to carry. He might need the extra space in his pack if he brought anything back. Next, he grabbed his rifle case, unzipped it on the back seat, and removed a full gray steel magazine from an internal pouch.

Rick picked up his rifle, an M-4 he'd had for decades, checked the selector with his thumb, and used the charging handle to let the bolt forward slowly and quietly on an empty chamber. He then clicked the magazine in place and put the rifle on his pack outside the car. He didn't want to chamber a round before going down the cliff, and he had a method of doing it quietly along the way if he had to. He never liked climbing with a loaded weapon flopping around on his pack. If anything bad were to happen to him, he knew there wouldn't be any help. This kind of thing was risky enough without inviting catastrophe.

Rick conducted a final personal check. He had his keys, wallet, pistol, binos, and his call was in his front left pocket. Good to go, he thought. Rick carefully and quietly closed the back passenger door. Before closing the front door, he checked for his keys in his pocket a second time and locked all the doors from the inside of the driver door and closed it quietly. He picked up his rifle and pack and moved to the cliff's edge. It was still half dark, but his eyes had adjusted well for a fifty year old man. The sun had not yet broken the horizon. Perfect. No matter what he was doing, Rick never liked to silhouette himself at the top of a mesa against a sunlit sky.

Rick spied a medium sized rock under a bushy juniper tree

and walked up beside it, just close enough so he could reach in. Without changing his footing Rick took his car keys out of his pocket, bent down, reached in, and placed them under the rock. He then made sure it didn't look dislodged. Any impression in this desert dust could be interpreted by those who knew how, revealing the secrets of their creator's attempts at stealth. Now, with the keys hidden, if he for some reason were to come back having lost all his gear, he'd still be able to access his keys and drive away. In addition to that, keys that aren't with him can't jingle and can't be lost. Everything else on his gear was properly silenced. Being thorough and thoughtful came from his training. Taking easy precautions during potentially dangerous activities was in his nature. He was frugal with danger.

Rick looked out at the rough desert canyon and thought, this is where I belong. He was happy with his life. It was pleasant and simple. Everything just seemed to be falling into place. His only worry was his son, Carson, but he was certain he'd get better; he'd already shown signs of it.

The morning was cold with a promise of midday warmth. There was the slightest breeze coming from the south end of the canyon. Its smell was of virgin desert, piney, earthy, with the slightest fresh, musky scent of small things trying to grow on the very edge of nature's meager desert allowance. Rick had a feeling about today. If all this maintained, he thought, hunting would be good. "Predator hunting predator, the unscripted adventure starts now," Rick muttered to himself.

He picked his way down the cliff-side as the light of day slowly came to his aid. He worked to avoid a slip or a knock of his rifle on a rock as it shifted on his back. Reaching the gradual slope at the bottom without incident, Rick had to load. He carefully pulled the charging handle of his old M-4 all the way to the rear, then slowly let it move forward. Rick watched it pick up the top round in the magazine and guide it forward. A short distance more and the round was in the chamber. He tapped the forward assist to assure it was chambered. Barely a sound was made.

Rick picked his way down the slope toward a location where he knew of some deciduous trees growing in a ravine, an indication there might be water there. He'd seen them from a distance the last time he'd been in the canyon but hadn't had time to thoroughly explore. He knew the general direction but would still have to feel his way as distance vision in the thick growth of pinion pine and juniper was impossible, and the light was just beginning to beat its way down the canyon walls.

Along the way, there were periodic clearings, and these enabled Rick to get his bearings and even spot the trees. They were either cottonwoods or some other kind of poplar; he wasn't sure. Before he made it to those trees, he came across an area in a small clearing that was littered with broken pottery. It was the design painted pottery refuse from an ancient Indian dump, thrown there perhaps a thousand years before. And now it was an old garbage dump protected from plunder by federal law. Still, when Rick saw an exceptionally pretty piece with an unusual zigzag design, he picked it up and put it in his pocket. Since these dumps were usually downhill of ruins he headed back uphill at a diagonal from where he'd been.

He pressed through more trees and was confronted with the ruins of a considerable settlement. He walked up the slope and around them. Before him was possibly a half acre of stone, all moved there for the purpose of creating buildings for some society that existed long ago. Rick had read about these people. They probably hunted and farmed. Then at some point the area grew too dry, the crops failed year after year, and people either starved or left. Then their buildings fell down.

Rick had heard stories from a local that, almost a hundred years ago before the 1950's, boys would go out to the area at or near Hovenweep National Monument, now a preserved ruin site nearby, and have a little fun by knocking down the towers and walls of the ancient Indian dwellings with their trucks.

Rick wondered if these in front of him had been knocked down by vandals. The way the stone walls seemed to have flopped on their side and sunken deep in the earth, he doubted they'd been pushed over any time in the last couple hundred years. Maybe the vandals that destroyed these walls were the people that came to eat the people who lived here.

Rick had read that there was evidence of surface dwellers, like the ones who would have lived here. They eventually moved away to live in the cliffs, now also a national park at Mesa Verde, for protection as people resorted to cannibalism. "Food chain reorganizations can really motivate a people," Rick muttered quietly.

He stood still for a moment and looked around. There were possibly a dozen very large pits in this one area. They were all full of and surrounded by the stone that had been the structures' walls. Rick thought about how they must have never imagined, while their little village was humming along, that it would ever have reverted to this.

Rick thought how silly all cultures are. They conduct themselves as if they will always exist. Humans always seem to think things will get better. But that has never been a natural law, only a hope. The hope of improvement is the luxury of civilization that distracts us from the simple survival that confronts most animals on a daily basis.

From the clearing of the ruins, Rick could see he was very close to the trees he was trying to reach. This makes sense, he thought, as a settlement this large would have been established close to a good source of water. There must be water at those trees.

He continued downhill and came to a steep ravine on his left with a slight trickle of water. He continued down the drainage and came to a small, deep pool of crystal clear water, no larger than a few bathtubs, shrouded by the plant life it supported. What a gem in this barren place! He saw in his imagination Indian children getting in trouble for peeing upstream when their parents sent them to fill their jugs. He saw teenagers of the past who were in love sneaking a skinny dip and having a splash fight in an attempt to accidentally touch each other. And now there was nothing here but an almost silent trickle, overgrowth, and a lonely 50-year-old man looking for something to kill. This is a good place to remember, he told himself.

Rick moved on quickly. As long as his feet fell on stone or sand he could be almost completely silent. And he made sure he was. He reached the bottom of the canyon, traversed the dry creek bed that thick foliage hid, and worked his way up the west side of the drainage, back uphill toward a rocky, sparsely-treed slope full of ledges and small boulders.

Rick found a small ledge facing south east. Right in front of the ledge was a thick juniper tree, whose branches filled out all the way down to the ground with just enough room for him to wriggle his way in.

It was a great spot. He needed protection from the rear, which the ledge and the trunk and branches of the tree provided, and a good view to the front, which he had sitting with his back to the trunk. The branches filled out the space around him, but not enough to obscure his view. The breeze was in his face, guaranteeing he was downwind of anything that heard his call. The brighter it got during the course of the day, the more he would be sitting in relative darkness of shade under the tree. His full camouflage completed the package and made him virtually invisible. Rick pulled up a mesh hood that covered just the left eye and settled in.

Having protection from the rear was important as Rick was predator hunting. This is a relatively sophisticated type of hunting where the human predator produces the call of a wounded animal that makes the non-human predator think that lunch is about to be served. The non-human predator quietly, slowly, sneaks up on what it believes a ready meal. Meanwhile, the human predator remains that meal until he can see and kill his rival. In this country, the non-human predator could be quite a variety of animals. Today it was coyote that Rick had in mind. Fox, bobcat, and mountain lion were always an option, but the chances were slim. Out here coyote were common.

Rick recalled a friend that once told him of a bobcat that jumped down from the ledge he had his back to, and landed right on his head. Marc had been in full camouflage and the bobcat, looking down from above, had no visual cues to identify the source of the sound. The bobcat, not knowing what or where that sound must be coming from, but knowing with all certainty that if he jumped in its general direction, with fangs and claws deployed, a meal would produce itself from somewhere. Marc was justifiably startled, as was the bobcat. The mutual rush of realization, with the startled movement of Marc from the sensation of claws on his head, the smell of human suddenly coursing through the nostrils of the cat, both, needless to say, for that moment, wanted to be rid of the other. The bobcat jumped off Marc's head and ran before he could rally with an accurate shot.

Rick wondered at how amusing it was that the hunter wanted to call in the cat as close as possible, and ended up wearing, for however briefly, the feline on his head. And yet nothing seemed to go right…that unscripted adventure, again.

Rick felt right beneath his tree and began to call. The green plastic cylinder previously in his pocket now sounded like an anguished rodent singing its death song. Rick started slowly. The first call was very weak, almost silent. If there was already something in close, Rick didn't want to crack the silence so suddenly as to scare it away. He called, then waited five minutes, called again and waited two, called again and waited ten minutes. His next series was a little louder.

On the first call of this series, a good three hundred yards away to Rick's front and left, a stealthy beast, headed in the direction of the water hole, had stopped to sniff a deer print in the sand. Unconsciously the animal's left ear moved from forward to straight up, and yet the nose continued to sniff. On the second call, the head rose from the ground and lifted to its full height, both ears up.

Two miles north up the same canyon lay Carson, Rick's son. He had been dropped off in the dark prior to Rick reaching his parking spot. His dad had shown him a good location earlier that week and suggested it would be an interesting place to use his new binoculars to glass the canyon for something moving through and, maybe, call a bit.

The canyon wasn't as deep there nor edged with cliffs, and might provide a good long range shot. More than anything, Rick just wanted Carson to be out early and get some fresh air. Carson knew this and complained a little, but ultimately enjoyed it. He was pretty accommodating for a sixteen-year-old. Plus, he had a lot of things on his mind and this gave him a chance to really think about them. He'd gone a long time living without his dad, and participating in these early morning shenanigans made them both feel close, even though they were not hunting together.

As usual, his dad had gotten up way too early, fed the dogs, made his shirtless sprint down to the mailbox, then back, and then cranked out as many pull ups as he could on the bar by the garage before coming in. He did this all the time, regardless of temperature. The colder it was, the faster he ran to the mailbox. He skipped icy days to avoid injury.

Carson had gotten up just in time to watch him run back up the driveway. Seeing the old guy in shorts, bare chested, with prematurely gray hair and beard, running the 200 yards from the mailbox made Carson chuckle. It was 29 degrees outside. Dad thought he was pretty hard core.

Carson had lived with his mom for eleven years and moved in with his father just about a year ago. The change had been good for him. It was tough at first. Not only were there the issues between his divorced parents that he had to deal with, but there was a dramatic change in lifestyle. His mom lived in Denver, and now he lived in the sticks. Most of the people around Cortez worked as either cattle ranchers, bean and hay farmers, or in the tourism or service industry. There wasn't much else. He'd been having some health issues in Denver and that, along with the neglect by his alcoholic mother, prompted the courts to grant his dad's demand for custody.

That's when the real changes started: exercise, fresh air, a new diet. His dad wouldn't let him eat anything unless he'd killed it or it grew at some organic vegetable farm. No candy, chewing gum, soda, nothing any normal kid enjoys. Occasionally Carson would cheat and eat something he wasn't supposed to, but only when he was away from the house. For the first few weeks, Carson's favorite word was "Auschwitz". Even though he was getting plenty of food, he always seemed to feel empty inside. His dad told him it was all in his brain and that he had to come down from all the "crap" that industry had him addicted to.

Carson's cancer had been diagnosed about eighteen months ago, and Rick's lawyer had made a pretty good case that his mother's condition was contributing to an unhealthy environment. Now Rick had to endure almost constant complaining from his ex, Sarah, about Carson not getting the proper care, the right doctors, or enough medication. It was starting to get on Rick's nerves, but he still loved having Carson live with him. It was victory in a battle that had cost him eleven years and half his net worth.

Carson was very aware that his dad was thankful that this change happened right when it did. Dad thought he could help him live a healthier life, and quite possibly, Carson thought, he could. His last checkup showed that his tumor had stopped growing and maybe even shrunk a little. But the doctor said that he'd also lost about ten pounds, and it may have been a result of that. Carson didn't know, but he did feel better. The doctor questioned his father about the weight loss, concerned that he might not be getting proper nutrition. Rick almost flipped but then got control of himself. He turned to Carson, right there in front of the doctor and asked, "Son, how many pull-ups could you do when you started living with me?"

"Two," answered Carson, with a slight rolling of the eyes that only a teenager can perfect.

"How many now?"

"Eleven."

Rick looked at the doctor with a glare only a man who knows he's right can perfect. "See ya next month."

Rick was required by the government to bring Carson every month to get checked. They were waiting for the mandatory appointment to see a surgeon about removing the tumor, but the surgeon was backlogged and Rick wasn't allowed to go elsewhere; otherwise, he risked being fined and charged more for Carson's coverage. There was also a matter of the drugs they were trying to force him to take. They made Carson sick and weak. Rick had researched the drugs and threw them out. He swore Carson to secrecy, and both insisted that Carson had been taking them on his weekly questionnaire. If Rick's wife found out about it, he'd lose his son.

Carson looked out at the canyon and somehow knew he'd get better. He had his back to a big rock that was at just the right angle, and he had soft sand under his seat. He felt like he was in a recliner. He put his small pack behind his head. The canyon spread out before him. It was getting warmer and the winter sun was on his face. It felt good. Knowing he had hours to wait in that location with plenty of time to glass it or make use of his new call, Carson gave in to his drowsiness and drifted off to sleep on his comfortable stone easy chair.

From eons of genetic experience, this lion knew that if she had the slightest sensation that something had been heard, then there was something out there. Why would her ears move if there hadn't been a sound? She was a system of infinite perfection for her environment, tuned to seek, catch and eat, and the faintest hint of a signal had just been detected. Her only option was to seek. But only part of the system, her ears, had been put on alert. And though hearing was important, that wasn't enough to satisfy her feline curiosity. The process of the hunt was an intricate package, and, instinctively, a more complete picture of the situation was required.

She stood listening for a moment in an attempt to identify the sound as living or non-living. This first filter would potentially eliminate wasted effort. Before she could determine this, her legs began moving her slowly, quietly, toward the sound. She didn't think about this movement at all. The sound must be of the living; otherwise, why would her legs move her there? The wind, the walls of the canyon, and an infinite number of other variables competed for her attention. But the supercomputer that was her brain made calculations of the variables so quickly that she was soon zeroed in on the general direction that was correct. She quickly realized that she would not be able to scent this noise maker, as the wind was at her back. This would have to be corrected before contact was to be made. With all the care expected of any feline in sneaky mode, she made her way through the brush, around the boulders, and over the prickly pear.

Then it came again. The sound flashed images through her mind of past kills and her consciousness settled on jackrabbit. If one of those was injured and couldn't run, this would be an easy snack. Then the more lucrative possibilities imposed themselves over the image of jackrabbit. A coyote distracted while eating a jackrabbit stuck in her mind and things suddenly got more interesting. Then instinctively, caution kicked in and more intricate images came. A coyote stalking an injured jackrabbit, a hawk sitting on a branch above an injured jackrabbit, teaching its offspring to hunt, or a fox dragging it to its young. The possibilities quickly multiplied and would only be limited again with further information. All this occurred to the lion as she crept slowly but continually toward the sound, monitoring its distance, assessing its tone, and compiling a visual image of the source, continually readying a response to every situational variable in her imagination.

Four hundred yards directly to Rick's front and right, a pointy muzzle probed the breeze. The sound of a meal was piercing the air, but there was nothing to sniff. Thoughts raced at the coyote. Gotta close. Too far out…move fast…nothing else can beat me…must be first…will fight for it…would rather not though…must take direct route…must make time…the others are gonna love this…

The coyote made haste to cover ground, his nose continually scanning for the scent of prey or competition. His salivary glands started producing, which moistened his mouth and nose, making his scenting even better. His excitement was nurtured as the sound grew louder. Occasionally, when he hadn't heard it for a while, he stopped. If it was moving, he didn't want to blunder into it. So he listened each time and moved in that direction quickly and carefully until he thought he might have gotten disoriented in the brush, then waited to listen again. Making his way as best he could, he closed the distance to a full belly.

Rick had been sitting cross legged, calling for about an hour, and was starting to get stiff. He was thinking about changing his position but instead flexed the muscles in his legs. This changed the pressure points on his body. That'll buy me another half hour, he thought.

He looked over the desert by moving only his eyeballs; he saw no living thing except some birds flying over the mesa to his right. His blue eyes were pretty good for distance. On the gun range on a good day, he could see .223 caliber hits on paper targets at fifty yards. Lately, though, he was beginning to wonder how long this would last. He had to strain more and more.

It was starting to warm as the sun rose higher. Rick set a goal. If nothing showed in the next half hour, he'd take literally a minute to slowly put down his rifle and a couple minutes to shed a layer. He knew from experience that whether he was fishing or hunting, making himself unprepared seemed to make something happen. If he was fishing and took a sandwich out of the cooler, he'd get a hit. If he was hunting from a stand and closed his eyes for a wink or two, some animal would appear…always seemed to work that way.

Rick kept with his calling cycles, mixing the sounds and the timing into what he thought sounded like the agonizing drama of a jackrabbit being trapped, then scared, then wounded, then stuck, then threatened, then lonely, and on and on. It was a wild theatrical auditory masterpiece of carnivorous horror being orchestrated by a poor, defenseless, fat, juicy, make-believe rabbit.

The lioness knew she was close and purposely diverted to the right of where she thought the sound emitted. A more complete picture was needed, and that required scent. She must know exactly what was happening. Boulders were all around her. She saw only with her ears as the brush and boulders rendered her vision useless. She must have scent. Was there blood, intestines, feces, of what animals, in what condition? She was too pure a huntress to let anything slip. She purposely put the boulders between herself and the sound maker whenever she could. The slight breeze at her back generated a picture in her mind of a scent cone blowing, spreading downwind of her own body and of a second cone from the noise maker's body. Her scent cone could not intersect with the prey's cone. The first part of her body to reach the prey's cone must be her nose, and she must reach that cone before she was discovered. With the realization she was passing the sound maker to her left, she began to circle in the same direction, scanning scent. It must be here soon. Crouching lower and lower she moved forward.

The coyote could now see to his front, beyond boulders and sagebrush, a large juniper tree with a small ledge behind it, a few leaps away. It seemed that the sound was coming from the ledge. His prey would be trapped. He knew he was almost there. He slowed a little and sniffed a little more. Nothing. Looking up toward the ledge, the sound…

The lioness had reached the top of the ledge from directly behind the noise source. The branches of the juniper tree hid her meal, and she shifted her head from side to side trying to get a better view. It must be there. She wanted this meal. It was right in front of her, but she could see nothing.

The hair on his back stood erect in a moment as every pad on his four paws immediately launched him straight into the air as if the ground was on fire. Ambush! Lion! With the flexibility of an Olympic diver his body contorted in mid-air, facing him in the opposite direction, and he began convulsing his legs trying to gain traction to run while still three feet off the ground. He was dark for a coyote and for the brief moment that Rick saw him, only fifteen yards to his front, he almost looked like a wolf. Rick's surprise left him completely unable to shoot or even move for that matter; everything happened so fast.

The body of the coyote rose into the air above the portion of branches that were directly in front of her face at the top of the ledge. The lioness instantly knew she'd been seen. Coyote flying, twisting to escape. Too far to catch. Injured jackrabbit just below…flashed in her mind as she simultaneously entered the downwind scent cone that just then had managed to crawl up and around the ledge on the light breeze…Human! Fear struck her soul as she realized that the cunning of the human had brought her in closer than ever before. Her whiskers froze, and adrenaline flooded her brain as she silently whirled away from the top of the ledge and jumped from boulder to boulder in a panicked effort to reach distance and concealment at once. She forgot completely about her hunger and wanted only to become again the ghost that was her kind, always unseen, always unapproachable.

Two airborne predators were bounding away from the human who hadn't even known they were there. Never in the history of the Southwest had so many top predators been so close, so hopeful, so fooled, so surprised, so panicked, and so disappointed all within the space of a few leaps and a few seconds.

"What the hell…" Rick muttered, unable to control the announcement. He hadn't moved, sniffed, snorted, anything. The breeze was still in his face and he was in full camouflage sitting in the black shade of this tree under the full solar glare of the open desert. How the hell did that coyote see me?! He scanned the distance, then called a little more hoping to bring the coyote back.

Finally, curiosity overwhelmed him and he decided he'd rather figure this out than continue hunting. He slowly emerged from his hide and crept in the direction of the coyote's last position. As he moved slowly, he thought quickly and discounted the possibility that he had been seen, smelled, or heard. It must have been something else. Everything happens for a reason, and out here in the desert, unless that reason flew in and flew out, Rick would find evidence of it on the earth. Tracking was one thing he was very good at.

Rick soon located the spot where the coyote had executed its aerial half gainer with a running re-entry. He chose to follow the incoming tracks rather than the outbound as this would give him insight into the behavior and methods of the approaching animal. He already knew its motivation and method for the outbound tracks: fear and speed.

Rick turned around to look back at the place where he'd hidden. It was a great spot. The underside of the tree was pitch black in the brilliant glare of the late morning sun. There was just no way! Something else had spooked the coyote. He backtracked the inbound coyote prints for about 25 yards and then broke off to the left with the intent of conducting a 360 around his position to see if anything else had been in the area. It didn't take him long before he found them.

The mountain lion tracks were large compared to the coyote, with the telltale spread pads of a feline instead of the two aligned front toes and visible nails of the canine. Rick looked back toward his hide. They were headed slightly to the right of that spot. "All we need to do now is see how close she got," he muttered under his breath. He always thought of cats in the feminine. It just seemed right.

Rick followed the tracks through brush and around boulders as they weaved their way through the terrain. It was remarkable how the path maintained concealment, almost as if the cat didn't want to be able to see anything. That makes total sense, thought Rick. One of the general rules of a gunfight is that if you can shoot them, they can shoot you. To be seen is to be exposed to a threat. To be seen is to be naked before the enemy. To be unseen, you must not be able to see. To be invisible you must be blind yourself.

The tracks passed his former position, proceeded up the boulder-strewn slope, and curled around to the top of the ledge. Sly old girl, Rick mused. They disappeared on the ledge, just above his hide position, on the exposed rock. Rick turned and looked northwest, downwind, lifted binos to his eyes and glassed the area in the hope of seeing her. Silly, he thought of himself.

She is long gone. He walked to the edge of the ledge and looked down at the spot where he'd hidden, then out to the spot where the coyote had made its abrupt retreat, and shook his head. The only thing that saved him was that the cat was surprised by the smell of a human. His being tucked into the tree didn't hurt either. Rick wondered, how can an animal such as man, concealed, with advanced weaponry, optics, planning and intelligence be nearly caught by the very animal he was trying to hunt? How can the apparently superior be beaten at a game of his own making by the inferior? Rick knew the answer. Out here, despite all my advantages, she was not inferior. "But she didn't get me, did she? I'll remember this one," he said aloud.

Not having many opportunities to track fresh lion spoor, Rick looked for prints all around the cat's presumed escape route. He found nothing. These cats are thought of as ghosts, he reminded himself. No wonder. She must have made her hasty departure over rocks. It was as if she had disappeared, leaving no trace. What's the spoor left by a ghost? Rick questioned. He'd found his answer listening to the dead quite of the advancing morning. It was silence.

Rick looked at his watch. There were procedures for recovering the track, but they were time consuming and time was up. He didn't want to leave Carson alone any longer. People hunting alone for big or dangerous game was a relatively modern phenomenon, made possible by advanced weapons. Not all the animals necessarily got that memo.

Rick turned in the direction of his truck, up on top of the mesa a couple kilometers away, and started walking. "Three hunters walk into a bar," he spoke aloud in a conversational voice, "a mountain lion, a coyote and a human. The human is looking for a coyote, the coyote is looking for a rabbit, and the lion is looking for..." Rick couldn't think of that part of his new joke composition, so he skipped it and continued, "So the bartender asks the human, 'What's your poison?' The lion looks at the coyote and says..." Rick realized his joke wasn't taking him anywhere. He'd had his little adventure today and was getting curious about what Carson had been up to. He had a little over an hour to get back to the Jeep, then to pick up Carson. He lengthened his stride, still making sure to step on either sand or rock. No sticks allowed. The entire distance he kept the M4 in his shoulder, thumb on the selector, ready to shoot should he encounter a target. Nevertheless, in his mind the hunting day was over, and he needed to get his head in gear for his real life back in the world.

The dark green SUV crept down the mesa-top trail. It made its way unseen from the canyon below as the lonely road was closely trimmed by scrub pinions and cedar. Ahead of it was Rick Thompson's Jeep. The SUV approached slowly from a distance down the thin dirt trail and then stopped while still one hundred meters away, but within view of the Jeep. It remained there for a minute or two and then backed out, as there was no place to turn around. The one lane trail made it difficult for the driver to back up easily, and the pine trees crowding each side of the vehicle periodically scraped down the side of the new paint. After about fifty meters, the single lane opened up, and the SUV turned around, making haste to leave the area. The driver had seen what he was looking for. No need to hang around.

Rick reached the top of the mesa, a considerable distance from his Jeep. As was his habit he never doubled back over the path he'd previously taken. His reason could have been for all kinds of stealthy, high-speed, low-drag tactics. But it wasn't. He simply found that if he went a different way every time, he'd learn more about an area, see new things, and make occasional interesting discoveries. His path back had led him to a particularly difficult area of climbing up that cliff on the top edge of the mesa and he'd been forced to divert in the opposite direction from his vehicle.

Once he reached the mesa top, for a considerable distance he had to walk down the road he'd driven in on. He noticed another vehicle had come in while he was away as some tire tracks were covering his own. They'd come in then left, it appeared. He wondered if whoever it was had messed with his Jeep, until he came across the spot where the vehicle had made a three point turn after backing up a distance. Since they'd backed up, they must not have gone all the way to where he parked, as it was open enough there for them to turn around. Maybe another hunter looking for an unoccupied spot saw that he was there, backed up, and left?

Rick crouched and examined the tracks. They had a design that reminded him of a reptile, an alligator to be exact. He tried to take a mental picture of the pattern of knobs on the tread. Had he been seriously tracking someone he would have drawn a quick sketch of it, scraping it on his arm with a stick to make a picture with welts if necessary. But today was not that day. Rick named the pattern something that would describe it, as his training had taught him. "Gator" seemed appropriate. He looked away and visualized "Gator", then looked back at it again. "Gator" was now his for as long as he cared to remember it.

Rick continued further toward his Jeep, retrieving his keys from under the rock only after scanning a quick 360 to see if anyone was around who might be watching him. He smiled to himself as he approached his vehicle. So much great training, courtesy the American taxpayer. Had they gotten their money's worth? Rick didn't think so.

As he pulled the Jeep away from his little hunting adventure, the lioness in the canyon below listened to the distant engine noise. She looked up at the mesa top and the image and smell of a vehicle invaded her thoughts. She'd seen them a few times before and didn't like them. Sometimes dogs came out of them. This was very bad. After today, she would have an even closer association than she had before between vehicle sounds and humans in her territory. A controlled rage at her previous lapse in vigilance arose in her that magnified her hunger. Energy overtook her as her ears and eyes and nose soaked in the desert, and all the things living in it. She turned and moved slowly, calmly, and carefully away.

Rick pulled up to the location where he'd left Carson, which he had memorized by a unique cedar broken and bent over. He'd nicknamed it "arm bar" so he'd remember it. He pulled to the side of the single lane, got out, and located the boy's prints in the dirt. Five minutes later Rick walked up to his position. Carson was wedged into a crevasse in a ledge and was making a reasonably good effort at making squeaks on his call. He heard his dad coming, knowing he was making noise on purpose to announce his arrival.

Carson looked in the direction of the approaching sound and sighed in relief. He'd just woken from sleeping for a good three hours. He'd been more fatigued than he'd thought. Like most boys his age, he couldn't always get a good night sleep and last night hadn't been any different. It took him a good twenty, thirty minutes to get fully awake, and he was surprised how soundly he could sleep in the sand. The rising sun had kept him warmer as the day progressed, even as his body cooled with deeper sleep. It felt just perfect. He had dreamed the most fantastic things but couldn't quite remember them. When he looked at his watch to see the hours he'd missed, he crawled between two rocks, got out his call, blew a couple squeaks, and heard his father coming.

Rick sat near him and smiled, saying nothing.

"Any luck?" Carson asked.

"Nope. You?"

"No, but I enjoyed it," Carson replied, feeling better rested than he could remember.

"Ready to go?"

"Yeah."

They got up and started walking back to the Jeep. Rick looked at him and said, "A lion almost got me, so I guess I did have some luck." Carson looked at him as if to scream, Tell me! Rick related the adventure on the way home.

Chapter 4

On the Provenger ship,
RecentlY returned to the solar sYstem

Over the years, his anxiety and excitement regarding his
fights with these beasts had faded into apathy and calm. He didn't
really care about winning anymore. His record was about even;
he'd won as much as he'd lost, consistently through the last ten
years. But whereas in his early years he exerted a full effort, he
now only went through the motions. What the Provenger didn't
know was that in the last few years he'd purposely thrown half of
his fights. He could beat them now, always, but he didn't want
them to know it. As he had learned to move with their speed,
anticipate their actions, watch their eyes, and see their center, he'd
begun to taper off his efforts. He had become so adept at reading
them that when the fights became a grapple, he could even get
cues from their scent.

He'd made a study of how to beat them, and when he'd
learned all he could from victory, he'd made a study of how to
lose to them. Learning the markers of their emerging confidence
and arrogance, he gained knowledge of when and where they
would let down their guard. He'd learned what they would do in a
moment of confidence, the traps they would set, and he would
deliver himself to them, for fun, to see what they would do. Yootu
could even manipulate their reactions after achieving a victory.

He realized all this gave him even more insight into who they
were. He obtained a sense of the engineering of their minds. They
seemed to him as machines made of flesh, complex yet
predictable, passionate yet soulless. Despite their superior
technology, size, and strength, he was planning for the day that he
doubted would happen, a day that he would need his skills to

exact revenge. Yootu feared the day would never come. But if it did, he knew they would never see it approaching. Their hubris would be their downfall.

Just as they knew nothing of his physical abilities, he also wisely hid from them his true intellect. For reasons Yootu didn't completely understand, he had always been able to speak with strangers in their own tongue very quickly. He could communicate with animals in their own way; he understood them. And when he was abducted, he quickly learned the Provenger language, and he remembered all that he heard. He was, in fact, brilliant.

Yootu slipped on the level two sparring gauntlets that served as his weapons, securing one on each forearm. As he touched it to his skin, the intelligent fabric almost integrated with his alien flesh, for he was human, and it was made for Provenger.

The gauntlets were almost exactly like the ones the Provenger wore for real fighting and hunting except for two major differences. They had no embedded technology, and the two long, ridged blades which extended out along the back of each hand were made of moderately hard, but only slightly sharp polymer. They were formulated to break if used to stab, and if used to slash, which was its standard use, to be of minimal effectiveness. It was just enough to let the opponent know they'd been sliced. The level one sparring gauntlet that was normally used for these bouts had soft polymer blades with dye markers on the end. Wherever an opponent was hit, it would leave only a line of pigment.

Today Layrd, the first Provenger Yootu had ever fought and a particularly powerful opponent, was paying Yootu's keeper extra for the use of the level two. Yootu knew he could not only beat Layrd, but that he could kill him if he wanted. And he wanted to, for it was Layrd that had brought this curse of bondage upon him many years before. Layrd had taken him from his tribe on Earth during the rebellion and fight that caused the death of Youtu's father, Romus.

No, Yootu thought, I will lose again today, and tomorrow and the next. I will make them think that I am getting old and slow. They will see me as tame. I will no longer be dangerous to them. And we will see if I can improve any of my opportunities. I have nothing else to do.

Standing over six feet tall, hulking, and ripped with lean muscle, in his breechcloth and bare chested, scars replete across his arms and chest from previous battles lost and won, Yootu was an imposing figure. To the Provenger he was a wild man with alien blue eyes, long reddish brown hair and beard. They perceived him as simpleminded, even if he happened to spar especially well. They joked about how he'd never improved, and thought him incapable of learning much. Despite this, he felt dangerous to them because, unlike sparring with each other, they always sensed the anger in him and imagined that quality of a real fight, where the rules of etiquette and technique immediately became irrelevant, and the struggle for life emerged as the only arbiter of success. It infused a thrill to their sparring that they could not get otherwise. And they paid well for the opportunity.

Yootu and Layrd assessed each other from across the ring, a large circular pit twelve feet deep, all white, with a highly textured floor and walls to enhance traction while one was covered with sweat, blood, or vomit. Toward the center of the ring were six graduated columns in a circle, wide enough at the top to be mounted by a single fighter and only so far apart that he would be within reach of the fighter on the adjacent columns. Yootu had learned long ago that taking the fight to the top of the columns rarely, if ever, provided a fighter with any advantage. The tops were merely pedestals that allowed the prideful to display themselves to onlookers. The best place to fight was on a surface that offered itself any time the foot sought its security and aided in a variety of stances.

Their fight would continue until one was injured, exhausted, or yielded to the other. Yootu had practiced his fighting skills while acting like he'd been beaten; he practiced his humility in the form of yielding when he knew he could win.

Layrd started talking to Yootu in his own ancient tongue, as the Provenger were also masters at language. "Well, my old friend, how have you been?"

"I'm alright," Yootu droned, as they both walked toward each other, to one side of the columns, testing the fit of their gauntlets.

"I hope you don't mind using the level twos today, but I'm looking for a little more excitement than usual," Layrd said especially loud so that his friend and the few Provenger milling about in the ring's auditorium could hear.

Because you'll get a thrill out of cutting me up, Yootu thought as they slowly circled each other. "No, that's okay," Yootu replied. Maybe I'll give him just a little surprise if he wants some excitement. I just want to see the look on his face. Then I'll let him win.

Layrd began speaking to Yootu, this time in perfect English. "Have you made the most of your five minutes prep time? You'd better, my big idiot. You've got a beating ahead of you."

Yootu faked a quizzical look. Now you're definitely getting a surprise, you sadistic prick, Yootu thought.

"Does the new language still sound strange to you?" Layrd continued, this time in Russian. "It shouldn't. It is of your own planet. You know we are now back in your solar system, now subject to its language protocols. You are breaking our law if you refuse to speak it," Layrd said with a smile.

Yootu faked another curious look.

"Or are you too stupid to understand?" Layrd asked in French.

Now I really want to crack your skull. Yootu slowly backed away from Layrd as they circled each other, three times was the requisite before they could engage. Yootu had used this trick only twice before in the last five years. He was saving it for a special occasion and figured now would be as good as any. Layrd was special to him.

As Yootu backed, Layrd sensed apprehension in his opponent, perhaps because they were using the level twos today. Layrd inched closer as they completed their third circle. As their center shifted closer to the columns, they completed their third circle. Yootu had timed his rotation perfectly to align his back to the column. As this happened he moved slightly toward Layrd, relaxed his guard and shifted to a flatfooted stance. Layrd immediately saw the opening and with blinding speed lunged at Yootu, positioning his left gauntlet high to block anything incoming and swiped, mid-level, with his right.

Under normal circumstances, this would have been a devastating blow, but it happened to be exactly what Yootu had arranged. In a move that could only be accomplished with complete anticipation, Yootu sidestepped to his right then in toward his opponent. He hooked under Layrd's blocking arm with his left, slashed across Layrd's back with his right gauntlet, and used his knee and Layrd's momentum to enhance his flight head first into the column that had been at Yootu's back. Simultaneously, a slight sweep to Layrd's foot had him almost air born when he hit. And, in a moment of brilliance that was in Yootu's nature, he used the foot sweep to fake a trip and launched himself flying into the floor in the opposite direction.

He'd learned to go to the ground when besting a Provenger. It calmed their pride a little while they were recovering. Yootu would make some faces, express some pain, massage a shoulder, and think about what fools they were.

Yootu was worried for a moment when, lying on his stomach, he looked back at Layrd. First, there was no movement, then some, then a groan. Yootu had gone a little too far. Perhaps he wanted it too much? If Layrd is unconscious, I'll just stay down so he sees me get up with him, Yootu thought.

In a moment, Layrd stirred and brought himself to a sitting position as Yootu forged a moan and rolled onto his back, feeling a bit childish with his acting. "We both got the worst of that one," Yootu muttered, loud enough for Layrd to hear. Layrd sat up and a trickle of blood ran down the side of his head. Yootu was worried. If he was injured too badly there would be an inquest, normally restricted recordings of the fight could be reviewed and Yootu might be discovered. His fights had been reviewed in the past, and only their confidence in Yootu's limited intelligence had saved him.

They both stood, recovered their bearing, and resumed the fight. Yootu was impressed with Layrd's recovery. Damn he is tough, Yootu thought. Now I will get beaten, badly. I'll have to make it look good after that stunt I just pulled.

To the Provenger, Yootu was a guest/slave on their interstellar ship, kept under tight security and continual observation by both his keepers and school children on field trips. He was a forty-five year old man who, they thought they could tell, was beginning to show the effects of his species' age.

As a Paleolithic member of the early Homo sapiens, with a brain capacity slightly larger than the modern human, the Cro-Magnon was of a dense and powerful build. He was the progenitor of the smaller modern man, scourge of the mammoth that he would hunt to oblivion, and executioner of the Neanderthal. They were masters of the elements and the sole survivors of climactic changes and harsh environments that administered to the extinction of all their related species.

Yootu was an exceptional example of this race. To his ancient tribe, he was known to be fathered by the sun. He was keeper of the red moon spirit, a hunter, warrior and their supreme shaman. To the current humans of Earth, Yootu was now a twelve thousand, eight-hundred and ninety-two year old Cro-Magnon stranger.

Since their first arrival on Earth, the Provenger had picked a fight with the human race. As a child, Yootu's first feeling for them was contempt. In adulthood, it became a spiritual hatred. Yootu was determined to avenge his father's death, the destruction of the Earth's small red moon, and free his people from the slavery they endured--big plans for an over-the-hill idiot.

Meanwhile, somewhere else on the ship...

Nwella was by any standard a beautiful creature, one of multitudes of a species that held physical beauty, youth, and health as some of their premier individual and collective values. Thought of as barely an adult by her long-lived kind, at thirty-seven she was ready to start her own household, but had found neither a partner nor domestic space. Her father's position in the Perpetuant Cycle Project had delayed her progress. Potential suitors were skeptical over her father's prospects at success and therefore cautious about her. Lodgings suitable for a young female even of her social stature were extremely limited due to the maturity of the Provenger Nation Ship. The population was packed into every available cell of this massive intergalactic voyager.

Nwella didn't hate her father for these converging circumstances, but there was resentment; for what, she was not sure. If only she could have been born at another time or in another ship, before the last war that marked the culmination of the Provenger golden age. She always felt she belonged in that era.

They had just arrived in this system, adjacent to a massive gaseous planet with colorful rings of dust, stone, and ice circling it. The indigenous called it Saturn. They named it after a god from one of their ancient societies, a god who presided over agriculture, among other things. How appropriate, she thought.

Provenger always took a few weeks to learn the languages of the systems they visited and use them while they were there, as long as they could form their sounds. The Provenger mastered so many languages that they had to mandate times for speaking only their own, lest it get lost to them. These humans, being very similar anatomically, were easy to imitate. She learned their dominant languages ten years ago during their first visit, and since that time well over twelve thousand years had passed on Earth. She now had to learn the new ones.

Alone in her room, Nwella looked at the viewer and admired the planet with its orbiting ribbons and moons. She remembered the last time she was here in this system when she and her father went to a light green ocean. They swam in the warm water and he promised they would be back some day. He'd been horribly injured by a wild animal during a hunt, and it had cut their adventure short.

Nwella was anxious to see the success of her father and his project bring them into a new era when resources would be more plentiful. She could start her own dominion and have innumerable adventures available to her.

If he failed, they, as a family, would drop into obscurity. This had always been a risk. It was the nature of their opportunity, as her father put it.

Nwella knew she was expected in the common room to celebrate their arrival. She didn't feel like going, but it was required of her position. She was looking her best. She had just completed a few minutes standing in the health light, had thoroughly oiled her hairless body, and had a vibrant glow across her skin. Provenger prized the tone of their skin as an indication of internal health, which it was, just as they tended to consider the roundness of their bald heads as an indication of their intelligence, which they knew it was not.

Though she was thirty-seven, Nwella looked about seventeen years old due to the Recombinant technology that kept them young. Their walks through this wonder of science applied their wave technology to filter their DNA of errors. It made them young. It made Nwella who she was. She had deep brown eyes that dominated her surrounding delicate bone structure, and light features that concealed a volatile nature. She had a drive to possess something extraordinary, and an impulse to shock the structure in which she lived. She didn't have many close friends and didn't really know why. She felt she should have many, given her beauty, intelligence, and humility.

She quickly finished dressing in her best public gown, a special one she had selected just for this occasion. It was even more revealing than the traditional type and would display the curves of her body well--her attempt to shock in a way that was allowed.

It was incumbent upon a female of her position to exhibit her form, and she would not disappoint. As typical with the unmarried female's public gown, her neckline began with a high, stiff collar decorated with blue and gold beads that, at the shoulders, plunged outside the breasts to below the navel, exposing her entire chest and flat stomach. Her long muscular legs were completely exposed on the right side to the waist while the gown dropped almost to the floor on the left. On formal or recreational occasions Provenger wore no shoes. Footwear was seen as an obstacle to the grounding of their body to the structure of the ship and to the foundation of their posture, both from an electrical and structural standpoint.

Nwella assumed a pose and gave the verbal command, "freeze." She then stepped away and looked back, making one last examination of her holographic image. There she was in perfect detail, her body and attire from all sides. She reached out her hand with a wave motion to spin the image and view it from all angles. She was satisfied. She left a few minutes late and walked out the door to the waiting shuttle. "Grand Common Room," she said clearly, and the shuttle sped off down a massive corridor, filled with hundreds of vehicles and levels of walkways where Provenger lived, worked, strolled, and shopped.

In the Grand Common Room there would be suitors lining the wall when she arrived--males on the right, females on the left. She would walk the right side, on her toes to make her calves look their best. They would all be focused on her, and whether she liked them or not, she would have to cheek the males. They would reach out to greet her, purposely brushing their arms across her exposed nipples, presuming to be oblivious of the fact. When she continued down the line, each would check to see if their touch had made them rigid and puckered. It was part of the game. Then they would walk away, concerned about being too close to her. The females would ignore her, and she would feel alone again.

Chapter 5

TuesdAy morning, Cortez, ColorAdo

Rick was up early, as usual, going through his morning routine: feed Barnes and Nobelle, his two German Shepherds, do his "20 and 80" (twenty pull ups and eighty sit ups, Marine Corps style), sprint to the mailbox about two hundred yards down the driveway, get the mail, sprint back, and then do pushups. He did all this in the cold November morning wearing only shorts and boots.

Rick's home in Cortez was typical for a civil servant toward the end of his career. If it was seen as quality, it was due to his ability to make the most out of a modest but sufficient salary. If it was wanting in certain quality it would be due to the expenses of attorneys necessary for the many legal disputes of divorce. To someone driving by, it could be perceived as a sprawling adobe style ranch house on some beautiful high desert acreage with extensive views of the surrounding countryside.

The general uphill slope to the north of the town of Cortez provided most homes, randomly situated, a sometimes outstanding view. Rick's three bedroom, three bath, ranch house on twelve acres provided that luxury. On that general slope, Rick's house sat atop a prominence providing slight downhill slopes on all sides. From his back patio and its adjacent small patch of struggling lawn, one could take in, with a casual scan to the southeast, Mesa Verde National Park and Sleeping Ute Mountain to the south, with the Four Corners nestled somewhere between them in the distance. Further to the right, to the southwest, was the gentle rise of a plateau hiding in its desiccated drainages some of the roughest desert canyon areas of Colorado, trailing further west into Utah. The house lived among the usual pinion pine and juniper cedar high desert forest that held a surprising number of mule deer, coyote, and jack rabbit, with the occasional mountain lion and bear. The privacy of his place was complete with much of his property surrounded by some irrigated fields and undeveloped land with only the occasional neighbor.

Rick took advantage of the size and position of his land to shoot a variety of weapons to practice marksmanship, but he never took any game there. It was a kind of pact he had with the wildlife. He would live there in peace, and so would they. It provided him with the additional benefit of being able to simply observe their behavior.

Rick was unusually well provisioned on his government salary, but only due to his frugal nature. He had a great collection of guns, one for every occasion. He had a wood shop adjacent to the house, a three-car garage complete with his old jeep, a newer Dodge Charger, and a pickup truck. Under a carport outside was his 17-foot fishing boat that served every purpose he could think of, from the nearby McPhee Reservoir to Utah's Lake Powel, where he frequently camped. He had a John Deere tractor with a front end loader and a backhoe. And he had his health. He had seen to that. He had a short time to retirement with his work for the NSA and was intent on spending the rest of his life helping Carson get a good start. His free time would be spent fading into the mountains and desert wastes. The end.

He was in the kitchen heating some venison stew left over from the night before, just starting to break a sweat from his quick workout and the warmer indoor temperature of his house, when Carson finally rolled out of bed and shuffled into the kitchen.

"Morning, Dad."

"Morning, Carson, how'd you sleep?"

"Okay, but I've been having the craziest dreams." Carson rubbed his eyes, finding a seed in the left one. He tried to rub it out of the tear duct. "I can remember them when I first wake up, but then I fall back to sleep and I forget."

"Put a pad and pencil by your bed and write it down as soon as you wake up. Then if you go back to sleep..." Rick trailed off. "You want some stew?"

"Yes, please." Carson sat at the table as Barnes walked up, nosed him, and gave him a small lick on the elbow. Nobelle circled him and watched. "The funny thing is when I dream, it's not like I'm imagining something, it's like I'm remembering it. Does that make sense?"

"I think I know what you mean. Maybe its genetic knowledge you're becoming aware of." Rick glared at his son, slowly cocking his head with raised eyebrows and whistling the Twilight Zone theme. Rick put a bowl of stew in front of him and stuck a raw carrot in it. "You ready for your test today? You weren't up very late last night."

Carson began to eat. "I'm ready, more ready than anyone else in my class, if I can judge by all the texts I got last night. For some reason, everyone was after me with questions."

"They needed your help. You're a smart kid. Take after your dad, no doubt." Rick sat down across from him and stared.

"Are you going to eat?" Carson asked.

"Nah. I ate yesterday," Rick replied with a smile, "I'm just not hungry. Maybe dinner tonight with you. Today's my fast day."

"So, I was talking yesterday with the guys at school." Carson began randomly, "How many evil toddlers do you think you could take on, like in a fight?"

Rick liked this kind of "what if" question, and he and Carson would often have fun with them. Rick looked at him as seriously as he could. "Toddlers, eh? Do I have a weapon?"

"No weapons."

"Do they keep coming at me or do I have a rest period?"

"They keep coming at you."

"Do I kill them or do I just throw them off of me?"

"It's a fight to the death, so do anything you need to."

"How fast are they? Normal toddler speed?"

"Yeah."

"Can I move around … run from them?"

"Not really. Let's say they're just everywhere, an unlimited number of evil toddlers all coming at you without letting up. How many could you take?"

"Let's see. Not knowing how quickly I could dispatch a single toddler, having never done it before, and considering that all the other toddlers would be coming at me simultaneously, I think I could answer the question better by estimating how long I could last from this toddler onslaught, rather than how many I could take." Rick continued slowly. "For instance, no doubt a pile would accumulate around me, a kind of protective barrier of unconscious or..." he nodded knowingly at Carson, "expired malicious toddlers."

Rick cleared his throat. "This could limit my mobility and affect my footing. But now that I think of it, their footing would be even worse, given those tiny legs. Of course, this developing mound of toddlers would no doubt create a kind of wall, somewhat akin to the 1415 Battle of Agincourt, limiting their access to me."

Carson chuckled.

"This could provide some time to rest, giving me a distinct advantage." His dad continued. "If I could rest, and depending on how long it took the toddlers to climb the resulting barrier of decommissioned tots and how high I could throw them to the top of the pile, though toddlers are pretty good climbers, that could provide me with some precious time."

Rick stood and began to pace around the table as Carson ate and watched him. "A knight of the realm in good physical condition could swing his sword for no more than about fifteen minutes before having to be replaced by the knight behind him. So, with only my hands," Rick held them out and looked at them, "and dealing with toddlers, I think I could last twenty minutes, maybe twenty-two." Rick paused and leaned in, close to Carson's face. "Do they bite?"

Carson laughed and slurped down the rest of his stew.

"Carson, I've gotta spread some winter wheat on the primal estate during lunch. How about helping me load the truck?"

"Yeah, no problem," Carson replied, still smiling from his dad's monologue.

Rick had a fifty acre plot on the west side of town that he'd bought two years ago. It came with ten shares of irrigation, which is to say roughly ten acres could be irrigated, which in that desert country meant you could coax something out of the ground. Rick didn't plant all of it, but he did like to seed as much as he could. It attracted wildlife, particularly mule deer. In the winter, elk would arrive from somewhere. Rick wasn't sure if it was the nearby San Juan Range or from the canyons, maybe both. For the cost of a few dozen bags of winter wheat and alfalfa, he could be assured of attracting and perpetuating the populations of the game he loved the most. It was an easy choice. Some people bought their grain-fattened meat at the store. He attracted and killed his forage-fed game from the field. He felt it was his right as a human, his right as a born predatory animal. He called this right and the land, his primal estate.

For Rick, diet went further than preference. With past health issues, the type of foods he consumed made all the difference, and it would with Carson. Rick considered Carson's cancer an issue of diet. It was a disease of affluence. It must come from the abundance of continual and misappropriated foods of affluence.

Carson had been diagnosed two years before and they had been battling with the healthcare process ever since. The current government system required certain drugs which Rick didn't agree with. He'd read the literature. He'd familiarized himself with all the studies relevant to Carson's type of cancer and knew what the government required wasn't the correct way to treat it.

Many doctors agreed with him, but they weren't the ones with the government who made the decisions. What Rick had researched wasn't important to administrators. Only the government protocol was acceptable, and if he didn't comply within six months, he would be required to pay twice the amount for both Carson's insurance policy and his own, since he was the legal guardian now.

It was an impossible decision. He could continue to treat Carson as he knew, intellectually, was the proper treatment, and lie about complying with the government's treatment so he could keep his current insurance coverage, and if discovered, lose all coverage for himself and Carson. Or, he could outwardly abandon the government's required treatment and pay twice the amount for anything that might be needed in the future. And he would give Sarah an opening to take Carson back. He felt like he was being blackmailed.

So far, Carson was responding to his diet change. But whatever had started his cancer had been a long time coming. It would take a while to get him out of it. The question is, would the government bureaucrats allow them the time.

Rick was determined. He had Carson on a wild game and

vegetable only diet, restricting his carbohydrates to vegetables only, with rice very rarely as an occasional treat. His son was in a ketogenic state that provided little blood glucose, the cancer's favorite food. With his body able to use fats and ketones as energy and the cancer being starved, his tumor had been reduced in size over a period of six months while they waited for the mandatory operation followed by chemotherapy, if they chose to cooperate. The only good thing about socialized medicine was that the lousy treatments the government required arrived at the end of a long waiting period. Meanwhile, Rick's ex-wife knew of his real plan for Carson's health and tried to derail it at every juncture.

As Carson and his dad finished getting the bags and the spreader in the truck, the sun began to show on the horizon. "You'd better get ready for school."

Rick would drive out to his land during lunch and spread the seed. That was one of the advantages of working for the government in a small town in the remote southwest. He could take an extra-long lunch, especially if he wasn't eating it, to do some of the things he wanted to do. But this morning he was intent on taking another look at something he'd noticed Monday evening, just before he'd left for home.

Rick worked for the National Security Agency; as he saw it, hopefully the last step in an undistinguished career with the federal government. It had all started with the Marine Corps, then the Defense Intelligence Agency, then the NSA. All he wanted now was to retire. He was four years away and just hoped to serve his time in this quiet little town and be done.

Lately, Rick believed he was either paranoid or someone was following him, though he knew it was probably both. He'd gotten this feeling only rarely, but he'd never been wrong about it. Rick did operate at a covert offsite and his front for the office was that he worked as a computer networking consultant. Actually, that's what he really did, except it was for the government regarding satellite communications, mostly of the heavily encoded foreign type that were picked up by some radio telescopes in that Four Corners area. Rick shared his office with two others who assisted with their work, both good people. He could have done his work anywhere in the southwest, but he'd chosen that area for its diverse natural habitat, archeology, and culture. Nowhere, so far as he was concerned, offered a better mix. Now he seemed to be looking over his shoulder a lot.

Monday had been like any other, except for one thing. A transmission came in that was very strange. He'd seen it before when space garbage slowly passed between an orbiting satellite and the terrestrial radio telescope receiving its signal. The data signal had the look of something passing in front of the satellite. Rick checked all other sources to see if a spy satellite or something else he wasn't aware of was in that area, and he found nothing. As a test and a precaution, he'd programmed signals to run all night long to that satellite and others along a predicted trajectory to check if he could capture a similar signature. He knew the chances he would see the phenomenon again were slim, but he wanted to try.

This morning he would take a look at the results. He doubted he'd discovered anything, but it had been bugging him all night. Rick spent all morning checking the results of the program he'd filed, but found nothing. He knew it wasn't nothing. Something is never nothing. He was smart enough to know that.

After four hours Tuesday morning, he'd had enough and decided to spend his lunch hour seeding his land. It was only a ten-minute drive and he arrived in a contemplative state. His mind was still working on that phenomenon.

Rick unloaded his push spreader and half the bags of seed. It was too late in the year to do this and he knew it, but he'd been busy completing a big project. He already had the seed, so he'd try to make it work since it had been an unusually warm autumn.

The seed needed time to sprout before it got killed by frost and, chances were, it would be killed. He'd get some exercise and see. The ten acres that were clear enough for him to spread seed had been an alfalfa field once, and the rest of the land was covered with the typical scrub juniper and pinion pine. The rest of the plot ran down to a ravine which ended on the edge of a canyon. It was a great hunting area, full of jackrabbits and coyote in addition to the deer and elk. But aside from taking a few jackrabbit every once in a while, Rick reserved his hunting there mostly to big game. Unless he was going to put a hundred pounds of meat in the freezer, he didn't want to heat up the area.

Rick spent about an hour walking his land, spreading the

seed, knowing it would probably come to nothing. He packed up his truck and headed back toward town. Driving over the next hill, he was immediately confronted by an SUV pulled over on the other side of the road. A man was changing his tire and Rick figured he'd stop to help. He unconsciously unzipped his jacket, giving him easier access to his sidearm, as he pulled to the SUV's side of the road, nosed in to its front grill. He left the truck running, unplugged his cell phone from the charger, punched in the password to activate it, and put it in his pocket. He stepped out the door, leaving it open. The man looked up from his work on the front left tire. "How ya doin'?" Rick greeted him, thinking he might be a nearby land owner.

"Oh, could be better," said the stranger as he crouched to pick up the spare.

Rick checked out the vehicle as he approached. He idly pressed his hand onto the front left quarter panel. It was this year's model SUV Cadillac. He didn't see many of these around.

Rick thought it strange the man didn't stand to offer his hand for a shake. "Need any help?"

"Nah, making pretty good progress," he said as he picked up the spare and wrestled it in place.

"Nice truck," commented Rick.

"Thanks. Runs okay when it's got four tires," he responded while wrestling the tire into place.

"Do you have land down this way by any chance?" Rick examined the man. He was about mid to late thirties, well dressed, black hair. He was kneeling but he looked tall. He smelled of money. Well-funded.

"No, I'm just out for a drive," the man said as he looked up at Rick and scratched his cheek with a black hand full of road dirt.

Bad liar, Rick thought and smiled. "You just got dirt all over your face when you scratched it like that." Rick's way of telling him that he knew he'd just been lied to. The man went back to tightening nuts. Rick looked at the tire lying in front of him. Gator!

He immediately became much more alert and scanned around the vehicle, his eyes landing on the paint job of the new SUV. There were numerous light scrapes down the side of the door; in fact, they were down the entire length of the vehicle. Rick had the same scrapes down the side of his Jeep. They came from the trees on the narrow back roads. Rick smiled to himself with satisfaction. "You must have been out on these back trails. Looks like you've got some pretty nasty scrapes here. Too bad, but they do buff out." Rick knew he was being a little too friendly now, maybe to the point of being obvious. But this was a challenge for him, to see where this would go. If he denies it then he must be following me, Rick thought.

"No, I'm not sure how that happened."

Rick parted his jacket and unconsciously put his hand on his belt, just in front of his pistol. "I'm Rick Thompson. I was just out for a drive, too." Rick put out his hand. "Sure you don't need any help?" Rick thought, let's see what this asshole does now.

"Tony Carrian." He shook Rick's hand after wiping it on his pants. "Nice to meet you, and, no, but thanks for stopping."

"See you around then." Rick walked back to his truck while keeping the corner of his eye on Tony and listening for movement when his back was momentarily turned. He memorized the license plate as he pulled away and wrote it down the first chance he got. Why has that asshole been following me?

Chapter 6

Yootu Restricted to his cell

Yootu put his fish on the heat plate and surrounded it with the green stalks of some new kind of plant that they'd recently brought him. In the customs of his people, he would cook the plant, eat a small bite, and wait for hours to see how he felt. The fish was his favorite. He didn't eat any red meat because he knew it might be human.

He missed sharing his customs with the people of his tribe. But he was wise. And he had learned patience. He sat on a simple stool next to his sizzling food and watched the steam rise. Yootu missed his dogs. He'd had many of them. They were his greatest company when people had been scared of him.

He glanced up at the school-aged Provenger watching him from behind the large window. He smiled while thinking that someday he would like to kill them all. Because, someday, they would grow into adult Provenger.

Emotionally, Yootu was feeling his age. He'd been a prisoner since he'd been taken during a battle which, to him, seemed to have happened many lifetimes ago.

Without their knowing, he had managed to learn their language. From that day on, anything they said, he remembered. His excellent memory kept every detail, every word, and he made it his own. He had the unique ability to remember what one of them had said, even without knowing the word or language they used. When he later learned the word or language they had spoken, he then had the knowledge of what they'd said. He did all this while acting the animal that they expected him to be. He never let on any understanding. Even during his captivity, except for communicating a few meager preferences to make his lodgings a little more bearable, he maintained the image of an idiot.

Despite the stress he'd endured, he was in excellent physical condition. The Provenger saw to it. He had nothing but the best nutrition and physical care. Yootu was an imposing human specimen. He was allowed access to a vast array of strengthening equipment and made good use of it. Though he was covered with scars from the sparring bouts that went a little too far, any injuries of significance were carefully repaired by the excellent Provenger surgeons. Yootu wore his light hair long and preferred his beard short. His alert, bright blue eyes, unique among humans from his time, seemed to challenge the Provenger males and delight their females.

Provenger males would take him to the rings where they would fight him. This was the only reason they kept him. When he was abducted, he had been fighting Layrd, a powerful Provenger, and had very nearly gotten the best of him, with the help of his father. Since that time, the stories of him had circulated aboard the ship. Since Provenger males loved to fight, they kept him as an alternative to their usual methods of sparring. He provided them with something different.

Slowly, over his ten years of captivity, Yootu had accumulated a vast knowledge of the Provenger merely from listening to their conversation. When he first started learning their secrets, he imagined that one day, when the time was right, he would blurt out, in their own language, what he knew and lay out for them their stupidity and arrogance in allowing him to become so informed. But the more he learned, the more he began to realize that he may have a purpose.

It had been a similar situation with his tribe. As he'd grown from a boy, he noticed that he was different. He eventually realized his purpose. It had been to free his people from the Provenger. When this same process of realization had happened after his abduction during the rebellion, he recognized the pattern.

It was now his purpose to remain the idiot in the eyes of the Provenger, allow them to speak of all their activities, their science, and their abilities. He would accumulate as much of their knowledge as possible and wait for the day he would be given the opportunity to destroy them. He would take his final revenge for his father, his mother, his entire tribe, and the life he could never have. This was his sole focus.

It was remarkable, he thought, what Provenger would reveal in his presence when they thought he couldn't understand them. The males were not his only source of information. The Provenger females were a passionate group, he learned. Apparently a small percentage of their many millions were deviant enough that they obtained great satisfaction from sleeping with him. Sex with a "sub-Provenger" seemed to offer them a sexual charge and psychological boost they couldn't get otherwise. He'd even figured out ways to maximize the information he could get from them. Since many Provenger had learned his tribal language for the introduction Contact Protocol and never forgotten it, speaking with him was merely a mental exercise for them to maintain these skills. For Yootu, it was a free flow of information that he took full advantage of. They loved to impress him with their knowledge and enjoyed sounding smart. And he would give them every opportunity. He grew adept at acting dumb, but then it was easy to give someone what they expected.

He was known among the Provenger as the good-fighting imbecile. But they really had no idea who he was. If they had bothered to inform themselves, they would have found he was considered almost a god among his people.

Yootu spent ten years fighting the males and almost as many laying the women. In a strange way, he realized he was already getting his revenge, but he yearned for their total destruction. Perhaps, he felt, their arrival at this planet called "Earth", which he knew to be his own, would bring him an opportunity. Since they were learning many of Earth's new languages, they often spoke them in his presence. So far he'd identified and started to learn three of them, understanding they were called English, Arabic, and Mandarin. But he had not heard his own language, and this caused him great concern.

Yootu was worried. Despite all his company, he was getting lonely. He didn't know how much longer he could last. The Provenger, masters of physiology, had recognized this and were interested in the effects it had on his health. They were concerned for two reasons. First, he was in demand for sparring, which paid his costs, and he would not be in peak condition if he was allowed to deteriorate. Secondly, having been abducted and held for a purpose other than a harvest, he was subject to guest protocols. He could not be simply killed or discarded. The Provenger had to provide for him.

Guests were guaranteed quarters, sustenance, and care. But the provisions for guests did not necessarily include freedom. The Provenger could not, by law, simply dispose of their guests. They had their law and it needed to be followed. As long as he had to be maintained, it was to his keeper's benefit to have him producing revenue in the sparring ring.

Yootu turned his fish over and recalled the days of his youth on his green land filled with animals. Even though many had been taken by the Provenger, his family hunted every third or fourth day, as needed. Some years they followed the large herds for much of the summer and fall, as they had before the Provenger arrived. Then they returned to their tribe and caught fish in the river during the annual spring runs. Small animals were especially plentiful in the lowlands, by the river for which he was named.

Legend had it that his mother, Noanan, was kidnaped and impregnated by the sun god. This god turned himself into the river so that he wouldn't burn her. Yootu was therefore named after this river. But the story his mother told him was different. She said that she had been making love to a boy she had met and was taken to a Provenger temple and healed of her wounds after being horribly burned when the Provenger arrived.

From his birth, he was considered special, and his people revered him. Stories of his ability to understand foreigners and animals became legend. Fortunately for Yootu, the Provenger were focused mainly on the successful development and spread of agriculture. Therefore, when he was grown they used him as their emissary. He wanted to roam and hunt. Since he was very capable, he managed to survive the many dangers of travel away from his tribe, and he always returned. The Provenger gave him wheat and told him to share it with distant tribes. When he returned Yootu managed to convince them that he had.

Yootu's power and fame grew among all people in the surrounding territories, and he saw how they lived from the bounty of the land, following the herds. He saw many of his people growing fat and drunk from the constant use of the Provenger grain and determined he could wait no longer. Yootu led a revolt against the Provenger and stole a bolt from a battle gauntlet that provided its power. He gave it to his mother, who hid it with the help of her cousin, Shainan.

Yootu was accidentally transported to the Provenger ship while he was holding technology that the Provenger needed to take with them. He never saw his people again.

Yootu's keeper, Bryock, didn't like the way things were developing. The quality of sparring matches had deteriorated considerably, and the patronage of the program had fallen off as a result. Bryock knew it was due to his fighter's mood. Instead of having many months' backlog of reserved matches, they were now being scheduled on a daily basis; no reservations required. Yootu was getting too easy to beat, and word was getting around. It could soon reach a point where fighting him wasn't considered a bold activity. In his prime, he'd been able to stand his ground and even beat a Provenger now and then, but not anymore.

Bryock made a deal with the keeper of Shainan, the female human they had taken ten years ago from the same Anatolian location. She was spared from being carnate for the ritual banquet because she walked in her sleep. The Provenger Psychiatric Unit insisted that she be kept for study. The duration of the studies now subjected her to Guest Protocols.

Bryock's deal was to allow Yootu visits with her. He had to try something to motivate Yootu. At the rate things were going, Bryock would have the responsibility and costs to care for Yootu the rest of his life without the benefit of the income from the sparring matches. And school visits and gratuities from Provenger females would not cover his costs. Certainly, as Yootu got older and his abilities in the ring waned, the females would also be less interested. And a one-animal zoo wasn't a viable solution.

To that end, Shainan found herself standing outside the threshold of Yootu's apartment cell, waiting. To reduce stress levels, they had both been told the day before that they would be meeting. Even though they'd both lived on the Provenger Nation Ship for the last ten years, they had not seen each other. It was a big ship and their movement was under constant control by their keepers.

They had been told they would be able to see each other in person, that this would be a part of a regular visitation program but that they would not be allowed to copulate. Shainan's keeper didn't want another generation of carnate to feed and maintain under the Guest Protocol. They would be allowed to talk for a limited amount of time once per day.

Shainan was very nervous. She had seen Yootu only once during her brief return to Earth at the time of her tribe's revolt against the Provenger. That was when she learned he was the son of Noanan, her cousin, and Noanan had told her that Yootu had great abilities. In fact, Shainan had seen him begin a fight with a Provenger, and when she returned, the Provenger was gone, and Yootu was still alive. He must have great powers, she thought, to have survived.

Shainan was also worried about her age. She was fifteen seasons when the Provenger took her, and was told by her handler that ten seasons had since passed. At twenty-five, she was well beyond the age for an opportunity with a strong hunter, and yet she had always thought she would bear many children. It had been foretold by their tribal Shaman. He said she would have many and they would be great leaders. She had never given up on this hope. At times, some Provenger had tried to take her, but she made it so unpleasant for them that none had ever returned for a second try.

Now was her opportunity. She must somehow get to Yootu, despite the tag on her arm, a band designed to inflict pain in response to disobedience. She must have his child. The cloak phased out, and they could see each other through the threshold. She walked in slowly and he stood still. Their thorough briefing regarding permitted behavior had left them overly cautious. Also, they weren't alone. School children and various adults watched from Yootu's audience window.

They both sensed a growing sorrow as they slowly walked into each other's arms. Tears flowed silently down their cheeks, tears for the ones they missed, tears for their common plight. They had not seen another human in ten years. They had believed they were alone on the Provenger ship and that they might never see another as long as they lived. Now, they were back with their tribe, for it took only two. They were overcome, all at once, by the realization of their loneliness for another, the need for the presence of another human, the communion of man. They forgot their briefing and their tags as they stood together. They held each other and cried. Their current existence dissolved around them as they became their tribe. Warm nights with big fires, the smells of meat cooking in ash, the laughter, and the songs all came back to their minds with the simple touch of another human, their distinct smell, the feel of tears on cheeks.

The Provenger applauded, and the children laughed. Nwella, sitting in a back row, alone, watched with great interest. She sincerely wanted to understand what was going on between these two. She understood they were from the same group of people, the same tribe. She understood that tears were a reaction to both joy and grief. Nwella could understand that circumstances that create both joy and grief could occur simultaneously, but she didn't understand why the human wouldn't decide on one or the other. They must decide on one, she thought. Their tears seemed to come from holding each other, so the tears must be joy. And yet their facial expressions indicated grief. Nwella was perplexed.

As they embraced, Shainan whispered quietly in Yootu's ear, "Who are you?" She had seen him only once. He'd not yet been born when the Provenger had taken her to be food for their banquet, but then she was retained for study due to her sleepwalking. On her return to Earth during the revolt, the Provenger had hoped to use her to influence her people. That is when she saw him, he was by then a man. But now she had lost her recollection of what he had looked like. She wanted him to say it.

"Yootu," he whispered back. "I remember your face. I can see the resemblance to my mother. I know you are her cousin."

Shainan burst into a new round of tears, more violent this time, as the reality that she was with one of her own overcame her. As she held him, she realized the Provenger had control over whether or not they ever saw each other again, and that thought incited intense grief. Ultimately, she knew this reunion would destroy her if she were never permitted to see him again. She'd spent ten seasons building an emotional wall to survive, and it had been utterly destroyed in the last few moments.

They spoke their language in slang, hoping to confuse the

Provenger. They used metaphor to convey meaning; they filled their conversation with references to tribal mythology, their gods, or those they both knew to infer emotions, actions or intent. This was their method of speech while trading with other tribes who knew their language, and though not direct and incapable of describing precise detail, it enabled secrecy that permitted privacy under the eyes of all. Their cryptic speech bored the Provenger that came to watch, and the audience soon shrank to only a few. Among them was Nwella, sometimes watching but always lost in her own thoughts.

When the signal came that their visit would soon end, Shainan and Yootu had been able to communicate a number of important details. Yootu knew that Shainan had been able to hide the weapon he'd stolen during their tribal revolt. Shainan knew that Yootu knew how to use it. They both knew of the other's intense desire to go home, to return to life as normal, and if that was impossible, then to kill the Provenger.

Knowing the ways of the Provenger, they suspected they might not see each other again. They knew that only now was real. They held each other for a long time. Occasionally they whispered a promise, occasionally a vow. They told the other of the wonderful things they would do, the fires they would build, the game they would roast, the stories they would tell, and the children they would have. They cried with each other again. Then they were pulled apart by Bryock and returned to their isolation.

Chapter 7

Crop failurE

Synster's daughter, Nwella, entered his office on the science deck to bring him a meal as Synster was reviewing the recent scans of Earth. He didn't look well. He looked angry or sick. He rarely was sick so he must be angry, she thought. "What's wrong, Father?" Nwella asked.

"Nothing dear, just some complications with this project again." Some complications, he thought. This project had been a nightmare. Just about everything had gone wrong since the Contact Protocol at the site he first supervised. After the deleterious effects of wheat had been recognized by the humans, the rebellion had started. None of the other locations had noticed the effects. Why this one? The evacuation went well as far as the technology was concerned, but they'd lost the entire Provenger ground team. Mobs of humans had surprised and overwhelmed them.

Now he'd arrived on schedule with the expectation of a smooth Harvest Protocol to find the worst nightmare he could possibly imagine. He needed someone to talk to, and, though he didn't want to distress her, he decided to share it with Nwella. She had a right to know, after all, and she always had a way of making him feel better.

"Alright, there is something wrong."

Nwella's expression grew concerned, and she sat at the bench against the wall, half reclining. "Tell me."

"The scans have come in and things are bad. The population we need to sustain a harvest is certainly here, but the quality is not consistent with standards."

"Are they not fat?"

"No, they're plenty fat. Their stupidity is the problem!" Synster raised his voice. "They're not nearly as advanced as we thought they would be. They haven't managed to figure out how to maintain their own bodies. They're full of drugs and toxins they've made for themselves. If anything, the Algorithm theorized that they might eventually discover the deleterious effects of their diet and modify it to sustain optimal health, but they would only do that after we had the population we needed, and they arrived at harvest date without the technology to defend themselves. But what they've done instead is use what technology they've developed and applied the methods of their very first scientists to attempt to manage their health."

"Father, you're not clear. You must be upset. What methods are you talking about?" Nwella asked.

Synster forced his mind to calm and took a deep breath. "When I saw the problems they were having with their health, I quickly reviewed their history over the last five hundred years to see what we're dealing with. It seems the humans' first scientists were motivated by profit, much as we believe ours were. No surprise there. They wanted to find easy ways to make more materials that were valuable to them. Gold is one example. They would start with other less costly materials and add elements or compounds to it, generally manipulate a variety of elements in different ways. They would simply add compounds to a system and expect the sum of that addition to amount to what they wanted! It works, of course, with a few simple things, like mixing colors, or making concrete, but not with anything as complex as their physiology.

"In this manner they would try to do things like change lead into gold. That never worked, but they maintained this method, developing chemistry, where the very simple manipulation of nonliving chemicals showed them they could predict a variety of outcomes. They toyed with this for a few hundred years.

"Then they discovered that there are life forms so small they can't see them, life forms that can infect them and cause disease. They developed treatments that could be added to their physiological systems to kill these infectious diseases, just as we did. That's where the parallel nature of our development ends.

"For any kind of illness other than infectious disease, for instance, the failures of our systems as we age, instead of researching those bodily systems and enhancing their own protective and healing mechanisms, humans thought they could develop single or multiple physiologically unrelated treatments, and add them to the failing system to cure the problem." Synster noticed Nwella was beginning to look at him with a blank stare.

Synster realized he was rambling again and decided to give an example. "Remember two years ago when one of our meal storage units was improperly calibrated and the storage field was causing the destruction of all the food's essential nutrients?"

"Yes," Nwella replied, hoping to understand soon.

"Some Provenger began to have some very mild issues surrounding the ability to concentrate, their children either falling asleep at school or behaving inappropriately."

Nwella understood where he was going. "Obviously due to a micronutrient deficiency that was affecting healthy cellular metabolism, hormone function and synapse firing…"

"Exactly. So the first thing we looked for was the root cause. Getting them the correct nutrients so their bodies can operate as designed. We looked at the source and recalibrated the storage unit. The problem turned out to be with those who were eating more than half their meals sourced from that unit. Problem solved. Do you know what humans do?"

"I have no idea," Nwella replied with the same blank look on her face.

"In the tradition of their first scientists from hundreds of years ago…they called them alchemists, they try to add a compound, a drug, to their bodies, which they think might help the symptoms. Sometimes it helps, sometimes it doesn't,"

Nwella chimed in. "But in the process they don't identify or correct the original problem or deficiency, so it persists."

Synster continued, "Exactly…affecting the other organs that are deficient but not symptomatic, they continue to atrophy while they suffer additional side effects throughout their other systems from this foreign chemical they added to the body."

Synster paused to access some information from the panel on his desk. "Some of the drugs they take don't even actually help the problem they take them for. They may help to mitigate the symptom, but for reasons often unknown to the human. The medications then cause other damage in addition to what they're suffering. And you know what the crazy part is?"

"That's crazy enough; is there more?"

"They know most of this," Synster said, exasperated, his voice rising in pitch.

"Know most of what?" asked Nwella, afraid he was going to say it.

"What I'm telling you, that their drugs don't help the problems they take them for, and may even hurt them. It's all in their own literature."

"If they know it, then why do they keep doing it?" Nwella asked, now believing that her father was somehow misinformed.

"Their own studies clearly state and show proof of these issues, and yet some of the best studies are ignored. It appears they're very slow in changing anything that has to do with diet or medical research. It is very difficult for them. Also, the interpretation of studies is left to humans that the masses consider experts, when those experts are operating from the wrong foundation -- a presumption that chronic disease originates from somewhere other than nutrition and immune system function. Most of their doctors don't even study the effects of nutrients and anti-nutrients on the body. Can you imagine trying to correct a failed system that lives and dies solely by nutrient absorption without studying, or even considering nutrition? That's like trying to solve equipment malfunction without a power source. On top of that, individuals don't pursue the information themselves. They leave it to others."

Nwella looked at him as if he'd gone insane. She couldn't comprehend why beings would ignore their own nutritional responsibilities and instead opt for the addition of a foreign substance, which would react with all systems unpredictably. And they would do this in preference to optimizing their body's own repair systems. Nwella thought she might joke with her father that they'd better not eat their brains because they'd have virtually no nutritional value, but then thought better of it. This issue was too serious. Their very lives were hanging in the balance.

When he continued, she was glad she hadn't joked.

"So when their bodies have a systemic failure, which is

almost always due to a failure of their nutrition, they try to add chemicals to achieve the outcomes they hope to see. They may often achieve a single outcome and reduce symptoms, but their interventions change a multitude of systems in the body that alter outcomes they don't see. Some of these chemicals change the actual qualities of their organs and flesh. They treat physiological failures the same way they treat infectious disease. They think they can use a single or even multiple compounds to kill the problem."

Synster stood from his desk as he became agitated. "Their liver, heart, lungs, all of them are tainted to a degree that they may be useless to us." Synster paced as he spoke. "Their flesh for instance, is corrupted by a drug they use to inhibit their own liver function, known generally to humans as statins, to the point where they are breaking down their own muscle tissue while they still live. This drug promotes the destruction of their liver, kidneys, and brain." Synster hit his fist on his desk. "It's insanity, and they know it." He looked up and realized he was scaring Nwella. She had a horrified look on her face.

"Does this mean we've failed?" she asked. Nwella was fearful for the Project. All the organs he'd just listed were vital to the Provenger and the Union to make the Project viable. Without them, he would be terminated from the Project and effectively everything else. But she was also concerned about her future as well, as the time she may have wasted going through all these socially obscure ceremonies that made her feel both alienated and insecure. All she wanted to do was be free of her parents and start her own life. Even if it was in obscurity, she almost didn't care. It sounded as if their family might be ruined. She rose to her feet.

"Are you telling me there is no harvest?"

"No," Synster said, now aware he'd upset her. "There will be a harvest; it's just going to be a little more complicated. We have to correct some of these issues. Patience is the key. We have the population we require; all we need is to correct these issues."

Nwella started trembling. Synster mistakenly thought she was concerned for the family. She was not. Nwella was enraged over the last ten years of delay, the false hopes about her future, and getting on with her life.

As Synster looked at her, he realized how much he wanted

for her. She was so beautiful, and he was so proud of her. She was the only daughter, probably the last, who had not yet established dominion over a male. She would make a great spouse. Her fitness level was immaculate, her health was perfect, and she was intelligent enough to reach top levels in the science community. His only concern was her love for adventure. She was a risk taker, a rebel, and he knew that this only served her self-image. It wouldn't have much bearing on social or professional achievement. He was determined not to let her down. He took control of himself. "I have a plan for this. Don't be afraid, Nwella."

She studied him and didn't know what to think.

"You need to control yourself better," Synster said as he walked toward her. "This will work itself out. This is a big project and not everything can be expected to go perfectly. Don't be afraid." Synster took her hands and looked at her palms. "Things will be right." He flipped them over and saw her fingers, "You need to do something about these nails. They don't look good."

Nwella nodded and moved to sit back down, "I'll stay while you eat."

"No, go. I need to get some things done first anyway."

Nwella left the room feeling empty. All that she had hoped for seemed to be slowly slipping from her. The Project seemed to have started so well. When they arrived the first time in this system almost ten years before, she had been thrilled. The carnate were delicious and exciting. Nwella recalled the feast which celebrated their departure, to honor those Provenger who would stay permanently and live out the rest of their lives on Earth for the sake of the project.

On the first trip to Earth, before the Provenger Nation Ship departed, a banquet was held for the team remaining on Earth. The carnate collected for the event were treated to remove all parasites, well fed on a diet of grain to fatten and soften their flesh, and scrubbed and washed daily by young Provenger detailed for that purpose. They lived in luxury and comfort for twenty-four days. They thought they were to become gods.

For two days before the banquet, they were given nothing to eat, a fast they were told was to prepare their bodies for the ceremony. They were then led away to a room where they were washed one last time and sedated. Each was lashed to their own circular frame that left their bodies suspended in the center, limbs stretched out to their extremes. These circles were then freed from gravitation and allowed to float freely in the center of the banquet hall, where the carnate once again became fully aware.

They held out hope for some kind of a religious ceremony. When they noticed the knifed gauntlets beneath the Provenger's robes, they all knew what they were really there for but didn't dare to think it. None wanted to scream first, for that would make it all too real. The carnate were silent, except for some crying. The only obvious noise was from the Provenger, talking and laughing, while pointing out features on the carnate, planning for where they would cut first and how they would eat. Some were interested in sucking blood out of their victims whereas others wanted flesh, and still others would make a race for the organs.

Music started and the floating circles began to slowly rotate around the room, displaying the carnate meals. In other locations around the ship, similar banquets were being held for each Provenger that was to be left on Earth. This particular team and their guests had decided to choose their victims at random, although the female Provenger were showing most interest in the male carnate, while the male Provenger were congregating around the female carnate. The music pulsated through the room as the tempo and volume increased. The Provenger could feel the energy building as they grew more excited for events to begin.

Twenty-seven-year-old Nwella stood aside from the various groups, not speaking to anyone, only eavesdropping.

"This is so exciting. We've rarely banqueted on beings so similar. They look like us in almost every way."

"Yes, I know. That came into consideration during the preparation, I heard. Even though we don't prefer eating through hair, they decided not to shave them. Otherwise, they'd look almost exactly like us."

"I think it's creepy"

"I love it. It's so close to deviant behavior without actually being so, it's wonderfully consistent with the nature of the festivities."

Nwella walked away, in full agreement. It was exciting. She was certain the banquet would bring her to ecstasy.

Nwella was there as a friend, but she didn't really fit in. Her father was the Director of this project and she had to be invited to one of the banquets. This was the one. Some approached her to ask about her father's accident during a hunt and how he was healing, but otherwise she had no one she cared to speak to.

The change in music was a cue. Nwella knew it was about to begin, and that most Provenger would remain watching and talking even though the time to begin mounting and eating was near. As the moment was close, they all turned to the wall, removed their robes, and hung them on hooks. Tradition held that clothing was bad luck, both for the victim and the Provenger, and unnecessary in a feast of living blood and flesh. It got in the way, could interfere with cuts, become very slippery and cause snags. It could hide wounds if a Provenger was accidentally injured in the melee, and tended to look like the victim's flesh when fully saturated with blood, causing some to mistakenly sink their teeth into a layer of fabric.

Nwella had completed a skin toning treatment and had her nails done for the event. She wanted everyone to admire her. She strutted out in front of all, displaying for the males while trying to make the females jealous. Like all Provenger, she was trim and muscular, her fresh skin bronze with a glowing sheen undeserving of the imminent dowsing of blood. Her long nails were shiny and painted black, and glinted in the bright light. Her head was beautifully shaped from her round dome to her square jaw.

Nwella turned her flashing eyes away from the assembled Provenger and trained them on a particularly attractive carnate male suspended within his circle. He looked back at her with fear in his eyes when he met her gaze. Nwella raised her short, curved knifed gauntlets, the style designed especially for the banquets, her only raiment, and made fists that she positioned before her face. She clinked the blades together as the young man hoped for mercy. Nwella let out an open-mouthed hiss, sourced from the back of her throat, baring her teeth, intending to terrify him. To her disappointment he did not scream but only watched in horror.

The circles were floating freely and each movement of the victims' arms and legs struggling in their restraints changed the course and spin of their circular rack. In a moment, they were floating in every configuration. This would make them a challenge to mount with elegance.

Half the Provenger began to move in on their meals as the signal was given, just a subtle tone shift in the music. Nwella, aiming herself at the young man on the rack in front of her, jumped into the zero gravity field in a single leap. Tears and whimpers gave way to screams. What all the carnate knew and feared most was now real.

Nwella caught him in the side of his rib cage with her right blades first, then pivoted on that stick, swinging to his opposite side, while grabbing him with her legs wrapped about one thigh and finally sticking in her left blades, in a razor-hooked bear hug around his torso. Her contact with him in the zero gravity field sent the frame and its two occupants gyrating, spinning wildly.

With her left fist clenched to get her fingers out of the way she plunged the curved blades deep into the connective tissue between his ribs and twisted, locking the blades in place. With the opposing forces of her left blades sunk in his ribs and her ankles locked into his groin, she removed her right blades from his flesh, raising them up near his neck. She paused. They looked into each other's eyes. Had one seen only that image they would have looked as lovers in the throes of a passionate goodbye. He let out a groan of agony straight from his fear of death, a disbelief of the inevitable, and a sorrow at the realization that such a lovely thing could be so cruel.

As the other carnate secured on their floating frames looked on and screamed, Nwella's victim became quiet, until she crunched her teeth into his lower lip. Violently shaking her head, she bit it off his face and chewed. He emitted the pale cry then the shrill scream of a man quickly learning new definitions of horror. She swallowed. A moment with his head thrashing about, attempting to escape, and she cut his neck at the carotid artery with both blades, careful not to sever the wind pipe, allowing him his continued agonized shrieks.

She took a deep breath and plunged her face into the lower cut, imperfectly sealing her lips on the wound, blood pumping from his heart, down her open throat and into her stomach. Pressurized by his rapid heartbeat, the blood flowed freely from the second cut, and it filled the air around Nwella, floating on zero gravity, liquid bubbles twisting and bowing from the wave action within. When these wafting balls of blood reached the edge of the field, they fell to the floor, soon pooling together beneath the doomed. Nwella managed an inadvertent swallow now and then, as the blood pumping into her slowed. The screams reached an infectious din as other Provenger jumped and clung and ate from their chosen.

Slowly the screams changed to moans and whimpers as the victims watched their own and their neighbors' bodies become torn and disemboweled. It had been bad form for Nwella to cut the artery so quickly and deprive the others of a lively struggling meal. But that is why others didn't like her. Poor table manners aside, she was selfish and always seemed to break the rules.

Given the large amount of meat, organs, and blood to be consumed, the event was surprisingly short. As each had their fill, they released themselves from their victim, pushed away and out of the gravity-free sphere. They dropped to the floor splashing in a puddle of blood. Nwella was among them, naked bodies all, saturated inside and out with the blood and flesh of their victims. As they hit the floor, they stripped off their gauntlets and threw them to the side of the room so that the others who fell would not be cut or impaled. What happened next defies a rational explanation, given the usual sophisticated behavior of the Provenger.

In the smell of the blood and its slippery silk texture, they had driven themselves to a frenzy. Bodies writhing in masses on the floor along with chunks of their victims flesh, covered in blood, most Provenger blinded from it stinging their eyes, they indulged themselves in whatever debauchery occurred to them. This was their custom.

Nwella, with her prancing about, had caught the attention of many of the Provenger, male and female. Her show was a challenge and an invitation to them. They had kept track of her location during the feeding and, though it was now difficult to recognize anyone, they crawled through each other to get to her. Some desired to hurt her for the infraction of a killing cut so early in the feeding, while others were bent on her pleasure. The most any of them got was a part of her, while the whole of her enjoyed it all.

Nwella recalled it all as though it was only yesterday and

yearned for another banquet to indulge her lusts.

With Nwella gone from his office, Synster began to formulate a plan. Before he could report complications to the committee, he must get some samples and see for himself exactly how bad things could be. He called in Layrd to order a harvest of humans from three different locations. He needed samples from locations where the tainted flesh would be the worst. The North American continent would probably be the best source based off of the initial information he had. He made the order.

Layrd informed him there was an additional concern about their scans. "I think we may have been detected but not identified."

"Explain."

"When our probe was orbiting, it passed in front of one of their satellites. It was fully cloaked, but it may have caused a wave shadow. Subsequently, an entire series of signals emanated from multiple locations on Earth. These identical signals seemed to be looking for the phenomenon again, or trying to establish conditions that could simulate it. That we know of, none of their technology is programmed to look for such a phenomenon. So we suspected it was a single human that observed it. Not likely, I know, but it was our most logical conclusion. We followed the signal to its source for the initiation of the series and isolated an identification number that is commonly assigned to individual humans, in this case, a number authorizing these transmissions. We traced it to this human, Richard Thompson. We have this address. Shall we terminate him?"

"Not yet. Was he able to see the scanner?"

"No, it was a chance occurrence. Not likely to happen again; in fact, we will make sure it doesn't."

"Good. Conduct a level four surveillance on Thompson and give me a full report in 48 hours."

Layrd left. Synster sat in his office alone and realized his error. His conversation with his daughter revealed it to him. In his arrogance, he had overlooked a major element in the use of the Algorithm for this project. Just as the humans thought they could add a chemical to their bodies to repair a complex failing system, he thought he could manage deleterious effects of wheat to limit the advancement of technology. But the same effects that caused a myriad of health and psychological problems, caused them to also poison themselves in an attempt to correct it. Certainly, the Algorithm was incredibly complex as well as incredibly thorough. Intellectually, he had no doubt it should work. And yet, it stunk of the same pride the humans displayed in their audacity to think they could even begin to directly control the functional nature of their own physiology, the details and subtleties of which they had only begun to understand.

Synster wondered about the future of the project. Had he been operating under the same audacity, so certain in his intelligence that he believed he could use computing power and algorithms to overcome the inherent uncertainties in all wave systems and predict outcome parameters over centuries and millennia? He was adding agriculture of an unnatural grain to a complex environmental system, just as they were adding drugs to a complex physiological system. Would he be as wrong? He was just as arrogant as they were. How could he be so stupid? There was no going back. He was completely committed.

Chapter 8

Quality Control

Layrd had decided to personally supervise the sample collection. It would be a simple matter. He selected three sites. The first was centered in the North American Continent, political jurisdiction of the United States of America, State of Texas. The second location was in East Asia, political jurisdiction of the People's Republic of China, Guangdong Province. The third was western Asia, the political jurisdiction of Afghanistan, the outskirts of Sangar.

Layrd chose to accompany the team conducting the sample harvest from the Texas location. Each area was chosen for its particular population density, potential drug availability, and level of technological development. Each location also had a natural event in progress that would easily mask the abduction without the notice of authorities. The Provenger were currently ramping up their own natural disaster program for harvest missions but didn't yet have their technologies in place. In Texas there was a tornado, in Guangdong there was a typhoon, and in Sangar there was civil disruption during a dust storm. In each location, five samples were ordered, more or less, with a range of ages from childhood to elderly.

Texas

Forty-eight-year-old Sam Caldwell was just getting the grill heated when his wife, Kerrie, arrived from the kitchen with the burgers and sausage. "Are the buns defrosting?" he called to his wife. She nodded. Sam wanted to try a new Kielbasa with his burger, and their seventeen-year-old son's birthday was the perfect excuse.

Ron, Sam's son, had decided he wanted to celebrate his

birthday outside since the forecast was good, thinking it might be easier to sneak away sooner with his new girlfriend, Laura, who was also there. Aunt Ginny had just arrived, over from Oklahoma with her new friend, Pat, and they were getting the cake and ice cream out of their car. Other family members were on the way.

Sam had just built a new shelter at his place in Bergman, Texas, and when he saw the tornado, he knew, revealing just a little satisfaction, this would be the first time they'd use it. They hadn't heard any warnings on the radio, and the approaching tornado wasn't that big. But they did see it coming in the distance, and it appeared to be heading right for them. It was unfortunate because it was an especially nice day and, though November tornados are rare, they do happen.

Sam and Kerrie covered the food and brought what they could down into the shelter. It was only built for six with a little extra room for storage that hadn't even been claimed yet, so the food had a great place to rest. They went back out, grabbed some drinks, and ushered the others to safety.

From across the yard, Kerrie yelled over the increasing wind. "Sam, I shut the dogs in the house. They were getting into the food."

Sam waved his hand at Kerrie. "They'll be alright. It probably won't hit us." Sam watched the twister as Aunt Ginny and her friend Pat, followed by Ron and Laura, walked down into the shelter. Sam held Kerrie's arm as he helped her down last. He pulled the door closed just as the wind started to pick up. Maybe we will get hit, he thought as he reached up to bolt the door.

At that moment, the door swung open. Sam was startled because he thought the wind was taking it. There was a large man standing there. He was bald and wearing a tight, gray, collarless long-sleeved shirt. Before Sam could speak, he yelled over the wind, "This is an emergency." He gave six thick bracelets to Sam. "We have to get out of here. Give one of these to each carnate!"

"What?" Sam yelled.

"Each person, one to each person."

At first Sam thought they were radios. He quickly obeyed and as he did Sam realized they must be some kind of GPS, in case they were separated. Then he wondered how this man knew there were exactly six of them. As soon as he handed the last one to Laura, the bracelet in his hand moved on its own to his wrist. It clamped down, encircling it, making a distinct latching sound. A feeling of dread overwhelmed him as he heard the same metallic clamp from all the others. Sam's vision quickly dimmed to black.

Provenger Nation Ship, Physiology Unit

Kwinon touched the green circle on the main panel and flooded the chamber with an imperceptible gas that brought the occupants of the "Texas" room awake. Kwinon turned to her coworker, Daytnin. "We'll do the China and Afghanistan room after lunch. A class is observing for those also." Daytnin nodded.

The doors of the vivisection theatre room opened, and a class of sixteen-year-old students quietly filed in and sat in the graduated rows, behind glass, perched above the operating deck. Some looked nervous, others eager. Their teacher came in last and waved to Kwinon. Daytnin rolled out a table with instruments and walked to the first table.

The subjects were all fully awake now. All six had been stripped of their clothes, cleaned, and dried. They were each secured to their own table with straps on their foreheads, necks, wrists, and ankles. The tables had a deep groove all around the edge that terminated with a drain at the foot.

Daytnin approached the first table. This one contained an older man with a prodigious belly. It was truly large, and Daytnin wondered how he could keep his balance while walking.

As the man became fully awake, he started to groan. "No, please, oh God, no…"

The other five, secured to their tables, started begging and screaming, tugging with their arms and legs. "Silence," uttered Daytnin. The tags vibrated on their arms and an excruciating numbness coursed through their brains. They all stopped screaming or making any sound at all, other than that created by the contortions of their limbs attempting to pull free. There was relative quiet. "Full live flesh sample array," Daytnin commanded.

A mobile arm appeared out of the ceiling, lowering itself just above subject number one. Daytnin selected a hose with a narrow metal tube resembling a thick needle at the end and prepared to take samples from this first subject. He would insert the needle, activate the crimp, then start the suction inside the ears, then nose, then mouth, working his way down the body, obtaining flesh samples of the mucosal membrane at various locations around and inside of every body cavity.

In the auditorium above, surrounding the large white room, the teacher narrated in English, as was dictated by the language laws. These laws enforced the use of local language at all times when dealing with indigenous beings, that is, of course, unless the circumstances required secrecy. The Provenger all knew these people weren't going anywhere, so no effort at secrecy was made. The narration was broadcast into the operating room so the technicians could listen to their own progress and hear the students' questions. It boomed and echoed through the flat-walled room.

"Each insertion snips a small amount of flesh off that organ or mucus membrane. Each removal creates a unique sensation, resulting in a message being sent to the rest of the body, and especially the brain. This signal is recorded through the head brace sensors and analyzed. It measures the relative sensitivity of that particular tissue. Since mucosal membranes are our body's interface with the external environment, this information is very important to assess the body's progress in maintaining homeostasis with the external environment. This is why they need to be awake.

"As you know, every organ of a living being communicates with every other organ on a continual basis, both through the nervous system and through many chemical and protein signals.

"You'll notice that the older humans on the table are all obese. We introduced Yngorn wheat agriculture for this species approximately twelve thousand years ago. High in carbohydrates, it was designed to both enable their population growth and improve their fat marbling. Since then, they have modified it through selective breeding and made it their major food source exactly according to our plan. The entire wheat family is now especially nutrient deficient when compared to the nutrient dense foods demanded by the physiology of the human species.

"Humans evolved for over half a million years with a diet primarily of animals that they hunted, caught, or collected, as well as a large variety of minimally-used leafy plants, tart fruits, and roots, since these were accessed while moving to follow protein sources. This was how they were able to populate most areas of Earth. Anywhere animals lived, humans could also, regardless of climate. All the resources they needed to survive, from food to clothing, were provided by wild game. Vegetable food sources, on the other hand, changed region to region, being very sparse in many areas, and varied seasonally, making them unreliable and often nonexistent. Human population densities were necessarily very low due to the factors of predator-prey ratio. The top predators are always fewer than their prey.

"Keep this in mind while you consider the following question. Since each cell in the body absolutely requires certain nutrients to function properly, if those nutrients are absent for that cell, what does the cell do?"

A student stood up. "It dies?"

"Why, yes, eventually, but living cells, just like the larger organism, want to keep living, and they are tenacious. What does the cell do before it dies?"

Another stood, "It calls for the nutrient? It demands it?"

"Exactly, like a sponge craves water. Since any organ is merely a mass of similar cells, you then have that entire organ calling to the rest of the body, especially signaling to the digestive system and the brain, for that nutrient. As we've already stated in our scenario, the nutrient is lacking."

Another student immediately stood and blurted out, "And since we get nutrients from eating, this need causes the brain to tell us to eat more."

"Or it can steal the nutrient from other organs!" another student chimed in.

"Very good. And sometimes, if it is really desperate, it will use some similar nutrient, but not exactly what it needs or prefers. All this, of course, creates problems. It's nice to see that some of you did your reading. I like to see this kind of involvement."

The teacher paused to collect her thoughts. "So, any species that does not eat what it was specifically designed to digest is likely to have nutrient deficiencies. Each living organism has spent millions of years adapting to a specific niche in its environment. We've found that the first major mistake that an emerging intelligent species makes is to think they can eat foods that they weren't designed to eat. They fall into this trap because they develop the technology to prepare the food in a manner that makes it taste good and allows them to digest it. But this still doesn't mean that it is food appropriate for the species. It can still be harmful to the intestinal environment in a number of ways. It also acts as an inferior substitute to what the species should be eating.

"For the long-term health of the organism, the internal environment is much more important than the external. Just as a hostile external environment can kill over the short term, a simple deficiency of the internal environment can kill over the long term. It gradually prevents the body's systems from doing their job.

"You see this here," she said, pointing, "in our first subject. Even omnivores have relatively narrow parameters for food types, as they need to maintain an optimal environment in their digestive system to maintain homeostasis. All ingested material effects the internal intestinal environment. Some foods contribute to nutrient yield, some are neutral, and others are inhibitory. Some fit all categories regarding different nutrients. The foods a species has evolved to eat fall mostly into the contributory and sometimes neutral categories. Disease results to the organism that consumes predominantly the neutral and inhibitory foods for too long of a period.

"Homeostasis is an important concept. It is the body's task to continually maintain its healthy internal environment despite outside conditions. The digestive system can be considered somewhat of an internal outside environment. It is the outside that we have taken within. If those conditions are hostile to the digestive system, failure begins, systemically. Because of their contact with the outside, the intestines provide the source material for all functions as well as act as a gateway to the immune system.

"Imbalance over the course of their lifespan can lead to the majority of their non-infectious disease. And in case you were wondering, we generally harvest before these diseases take their full effect. So please don't leave perfectly good fat and protein on your plate and tell your parents that it is diseased."

The technician working on Sam had almost completed the tissue sampling, and the increasingly bored students were eager for their teacher to stop droning away. They wanted to see the interesting part. The teacher read the expressions on their faces and thought she'd better start getting them refocused.

"After all the tissue samples are taken, the technicians will work their way back up the subject, removing those organs of interest for further, complete compositional analysis, as well as nutritional and flavor assessments. For instance; knee caps, testicles for the male, sections of skin, bladder, uterus and ovaries for the females, intestines, liver, kidneys, pancreas, gallbladder, and stomach are all taken for testing."

The students noticed all the bodies increased their writhing on the tables, testing their restraints, trying to pull free. But not a sound came from them.

"As I understand it," the teacher smiled to Kwinon through the glass, "we are going to see the removal of a heart while it is still beating." Kwinon raised one hand in the air to acknowledge the students' applause. "As each organ is removed, arteries and veins are tied off or cauterized to prevent exsanguination, so that the subject's brain wave readings are still available for measurement."

Daytnin worked up the torso, making a cut starting at the groin and only going so far as to accommodate the removal of each organ. He tied off the veins and arteries first, removed an organ, setting it aside in a special container for that organ on the rolling table next to the subject, then cut further up the torso for the next.

Three professional Provenger tasters enter the room and filed directly toward Sam, stopping next to his slab. Looming over him, they made final adjustments to their headset, inputting their personal identification numbers. The mechanisms created a neural connection directly with their brains and made accurate records of what they were actually tasting. They eliminated the many variable individual factors that influence the enjoyment of food to include whether they were hungry, feeling well that day, or just had an argument with a friend.

The headsets were connected to a long tube, the end of which was affixed with a pincer that would cut off and hold a morsel while simultaneously extracting and preserving a small sample of the material being tasted. This sample would be assessed for nutrients. In this manner, the flavor could be directly related to the nutritional value.

Sam felt more than just the cold of the slab on his back. He saw, out of the corner of his racing eyes, his own body parts and internal organs being placed on the table beside him. He felt the vibrating pain of another cut, like scissors through nylon fabric, up his abdomen. His prodigious belly suddenly sank and became flat, as gobs of yellow fat interlaced with intestines were placed on the table next to him.

The tasters frowned and shook their heads. While the Provenger coveted fat in their diet, their least preferred was this visceral fat of which the Sam subject seemed to have ample quantities. This fat acted as its own gland in his body, producing all kinds of hormones, and while its flavor was not repulsive, it was not considered good. It had the texture of slime and made some Provenger gag. Since there was so much, all three of them would have to taste samples from numerous locations. But they were professionals and would maintain their bearing.

Sam looked up and saw these bald men eating from his organs on the table beside him. His heart raced and then seized with pain. As he died, Sam knew this must be some kind of nightmare from which he would wake. When he did, he would hug his wife and his son, feed his dogs, and try to lose some weight.

Sam never woke.

"…not going to make it to the heart on this one," Daytnin reported aloud. There was a hum of disappointment amongst the students.

Kwinon completed some work at the panel and she rolled out a second table. The next slab held a young female. "Let's get started on you, Laura," she said as she looked at the nameplate and started in with her samples. Again, all the membrane samples were taken, starting at the head and working down the torso. For the females, mammary gland tissue was vital and obtained easily by inserting the needle into the nipple.

Observing Laura's heaving chest, flat belly, and strong heartbeat, Kwinon announced to the class, "I believe we will make it to the heart on this one!" The cuts were started at the groin as Kwinon worked her way up. She would tie off veins and arteries, removing organs one by one.

The tasters, done with the subject Sam, moved next to Laura. This one proved to be more enjoyable. The removal of the intestines created a buzz among the students. They looked so different that the audience couldn't believe they were the same organ as in the obese man. The tasters were relieved.

The teacher chimed in, "As I said, the longer a deficient nutritional environment is maintained, the more the organs suffer. This younger sample does not suffer yet from the chronic effects of carbohydrates."

Laura's heart pounded and her eyes raced around the room, taking in as much as she could see, looking for a way to safety that she knew would not come. The tag on her arm prevented her from screaming, and her panic reached every limb. Contorting to every angle, she vainly attempted to move in any way to stop what was happening. She sensed the release of pressure from her lower abdomen, and a constant dull tension on the insides of her chest, as the pull of gravity and the open cavity allowed her exposed organs to seek level. Laura tried to distract herself, to avoid the sensation of the cutting and pulling inside her, to avoid the smell of her own fluids, to keep from seeing the Provenger eating her organs at the table next to her. But there was no escape from the horror.

With the specimen named Laura, the heart was reached and slowly lifted, intact and pounding wildly. The students grew excited as it was pried up with two cold metal tongs, above the surface of her rib cage, stretching its plumbing. Laura glimpsed her heart in her lower peripheral vision, still connected, still beating. It tried to pump blood through a liver and kidneys and other organs that were no longer there.

Slowly, struggling to breathe as her lungs leaked and flattened, she began to suffocate and lose consciousness. Her strong heart continued beating for some time propped up on the outside of her chest, thrilling the students and giving them a new respect for the resilience of the organ.

And so the technicians continued down the tables that held muted, panicked, and hyperventilating subjects all seeking escape, pulling at the straps holding them down. One by one, the Caldwell family and guests silently waited for their turn, monitoring the progress of the one before them, knowing with undeniable certainty that they were going to be cut apart and eaten while alive. The students watched and learned, asking questions regarding the organs removed and how they would be analyzed.

Chapter 9

Results
Twelve hOurs later…

Sitting at his desk, Synster raised his monitor to speak to the physiology deck technicians. "What have we got from the samples?"

"I'm sending the results now," replied Kwinon.

Synster looked at his monitor and didn't like what he saw. Of the six taken from Texas, four were obese, three of those were on statins, one of which had advanced heart disease, two smoked, one was on an antidepressant, the adolescent male had traces of steroids, and the adolescent female was a smoker and pregnant. The five Chinese samples were all adults. Five were smokers, one had traces of opium, one was on statins, and one had cancer. Of the six Afghans, two were malnourished, three had parasites, and four were smokers, two of them contaminated with opium.

The taste tests were punishing. The liver, kidneys, heart, and flesh of the statin users were described as foul. The lungs, kidneys, and flesh of the smokers were rated the same. Use of the flesh and organs of the ones on mind-altering drugs, antidepressants, and opium were forbidden by law.

The only samples that would have been economically viable would be one adult, an obese Texan female, and the adolescent female, as the smoking hadn't tainted her flesh yet. But, of course, the lungs couldn't be used. Even then, the adolescent would not normally be harvested as a single unit due to pregnancy. And finally, two of the Afghans were acceptable, but even they were too lean to be marketable. If things continued in this manner, the project would be an abject failure.

Synster was in trouble and he knew it. Almost all were

deficient in most of the necessary trace minerals, and their vitamin levels appeared to be near the bare minimum for health. All of them had elevated system-wide inflammation from an over-active, innate immune system. The Algorithm did not project anything like this. Synster knew a more extensive review of recent human history would be necessary to determine why these results were so extreme. He had personally reduced the deleterious effects of wheat to prevent this very situation. They would have to take many more samples. What had promised to be such a profitable venture was transforming into a debacle.

The Gradient Contact Protocol was being initiated. The Provenger had no desire to conquer a world. Theirs was a management program, an initiative to promote a species determined to be a valuable resource for their flesh and organs. It was much more cost-effective to manage a free and self-sustaining population than it was to conquer, consolidate, manage, feed, and slaughter the entire population of Earth. Everyone knew this. For this reason their project was highly regulated.

The next stage required secrecy in their interaction with humans. A human population alert to their presence would mean economic chaos and disruptions that would make Natural Proliferation impossible. It would force them to initiate Managed Collectivization.

The Gradient Contact Protocol allowed Synster one primary operative on Earth. It dictated a professionally and socially mid-level individual so that, if necessary, this person could be eliminated without too many noticing or caring. If the surrogates were at too high a level, they would have too much influence and be damaging, should they decide to reveal the Provenger presence. A mid-level operative could easily be made to look as if he'd lost his mind. Therefore, Synster's contact would have to fit the requirements as well as be positioned to influence by having higher level contacts within governmental organizations: one human that he could personally rely on to promote their interests. He had to choose strategically who this would be. This human needed to serve many purposes. He would need intelligence, contacts, and resourcefulness. And Synster would need to turn him from his own kind.

The others on his team also would have their contacts with humans on Earth, each one carefully handled, providing a broad spectrum of expertise. Each human that was contacted would need to be tightly controlled until such time as the individual had been tested. Each one had to have the proper motivation and ultimately see the logic and wisdom of cooperation.

The Provenger had always conscripted successfully, with few problems. When provided the proper motivation, their recruits would choose power, personal gain, and the relative security of their people over their own annihilation along with the extermination of their society's way of life. It seemed a simple choice.

Chapter 10

Thursday night Monitor

Rick sat at his dinner table thinking about Tony Carrian and what he might do about him. The thing that was most troublesome was that he didn't even know the guy. He understood how people could hate him, in the sense that he knows people might hate him for his NSA work, or any of the other things he'd done in his life. But since he didn't know Carrian, this meant someone else had put Carrian on to him. Someone must either be paying Carrian or he is a self-employed spy.

Dinner was on the grill and Rick heard Carson get out of the shower. He needed to check the food and moved toward the door. Barnes and Nobelle were whining and wanted to go out. They pranced to the door with him in excited agitation.

They must hear something out there, Rick speculated. He stopped at the door and they sat. Rick opened it and walked out. He said, "Go ahead", and the dogs bolted for the far side of the property. They ran to the edge of the lawn and started barking through the fence. Must be a deer or coyote, Rick thought. He checked the meat, zucchini and onions. They were done, so he piled them on a platter and brought them in, sprinkled on a little sea salt, turmeric, and pepper.

Carson walked down the hallway. "Is dinner ready? Smells good."

"Yep, just about."

"Are you going hunting this weekend?"

"Yes," Rick said, looking up, hoping he would ask to come along.

"Cause I have to run some errands, and I was wondering if I

could use the truck Saturday."

Running errands could be code for Christmas shopping, but Rick knew Carson also had some friends he wanted to hang out with.

"Where are you going?"

"Durango, downtown and maybe the mall."

"Alright, just drive careful. And watch out for elk." Rick was always concerned about his new driver. This time of year elk were moving to the lower country and might be crossing the road on the pass to Durango. Carson tended to be vigilant for other cars, but until you encounter an elk crossing the road, you really don't know what to expect. And when a driver hits an animal that big the results are fairly predictable. The car takes the animal's legs out and the body stops in the driver's lap, with the roof and windshield in between. "And don't eat any junk," Rick added as he put the platter on the table. "Actually, I think I'll hunt tomorrow afternoon."

Rick and Carson talked while they ate, and Synster stood motionless in the far corner of the room, fully cloaked, undetectable to the eye. He listened to their whole conversation with great interest. They spoke of Rick's work, a little about what he monitored from satellites. They talked about Carson's friends and what he might do over next summer now that he could drive. Then Carson asked if his mother would want him to visit over the summer. They talked about the government taking over health care and Rick's health internet site, Primal Estate, and how he'd like to expand it to a book. Carson talked about some other kids at school that were causing trouble, and hinted at his desire to get another hunting rifle. And Rick hinted that they couldn't afford it.

Synster already knew who Rick was professionally. He'd accessed all existing electronic records and had recorded all of Rick's activities in the last four days with his order of the level four surveillance. Synster even knew his blood type and that he had a pin in his right leg from being shot twenty-five years before. Most importantly, he knew that Rick's brother was the United States Deputy Secretary of the Department of Health and Human Services. Before Synster made contact he wanted to view Rick in person. He seemed to be the ideal target due to his position, abilities and contacts. Synster wanted to make sure. His future and that of his family could depend on this one selection.

Rick rose from the table and walked toward the back door. He opened it and whistled for the dogs, who immediately came running for the house. Synster decided it was time to leave. He also decided that tomorrow, while Rick was hunting, contact would be made. Synster touched his gauntlet and he was back aboard his ship, a billion miles beyond the sun, orbiting the planet Saturn.

After dinner Rick sat down at his computer and logged onto his web site. He checked his email and comments from the last few articles, and crafted a few responses. He'd been posting to his site for a few years now. It was one of many on the internet advocating the benefits of a whole foods diet, avoidance of wheat, legumes, and other mass produced agricultural products. The most important thing, Rick felt, was spreading the word about autoimmune disease, and how it could be healed by natural means. And that it cannot be healed otherwise, but only managed, and badly. It had been years since the discovery of zonulin and its regulation of the permeability of epithelial tissue, and doctors still didn't communicate to patients about the havoc overly permeable tissue creates. Most still didn't even know what it was. Why should the pharmaceutical companies want them informed? They were making their money from people being sick. Here it was the very gatekeeper, a regulator of the path to autoimmunity, and still no one seemed to know about it.

Years ago, while travelling in Africa, Rick had come down with a fever. After recovering from the acute symptoms, he had chronic health problems that no doctors could diagnose. He gradually got worse and saw no end in sight. Every so often Rick thought about how bad it might get. Would he become completely disabled? Would he be confined to bed? Would he deteriorate to the point where he was completely physically and mentally disabled? Killing himself at that point wouldn't be an option. It would hurt Carson too much. His stubbornness made Rick forge ahead. Eventually, after a few years, and acquiring symptoms that some thought might be multiple sclerosis, he figured out how to heal himself.

It happened slowly. Despite his health issues and weakness, his refusal to give up led him to continue his outdoor activities, though at a much slower pace. One afternoon he'd been scouting an area of the San Juan Mountain range, a place called Lone Cone. He'd stopped to rest, exhausted from a simple walk up a gentle slope

Sitting on a log at the top, suffering in silence, he looked up to watch an eagle working the updraft on a ridge. He was thinking how this bird was at the top of the food chain and so was he. Only predators, with perhaps the exception of extremely large herbivores, maintained this status, he thought.

All of the top predators on Earth were fewer in number than their prey, except humans. The success of all the top predators on Earth was an indication of the overall health of the environment in which they lived, except for humans, who seemed to survive in even poor environments.

All the top predator populations on Earth were either healthy due to a healthy habitat or their numbers in their environments were declining by either natural or unnatural means, except for humans. Humans were unhealthy and yet they continued to survive and multiply even in poor habitats.

What made humans so different in all these situations? Rick was suffering from autoimmune symptoms. His own immune system was taking him apart. How could that be even remotely natural? And this same thing was happening to hundreds of millions if not billions of people. How could this be? As if looking in a mirror for the first time in his whole life, and seeing his reflection, he could finally understand himself fully. The answer to the question why humans were many and their prey few, why their number was not an indication of their environment's health, why they were not only sick but increasing in number, had always been there right in front of him, and made perfect sense. Agriculture had kept them artificially prolific. Perhaps it had also contributed to health problems.

Man, with the same intelligence that had made him a superior predator through the invention of weapons, created foods for himself that were not foods for him. The foods that he'd always eaten in the wild, he now grew for himself, and enjoyed. The plants he knew would poison him immediately, he naturally did not grow. But what about the foods in between, the ones that were rarely used, that might serve a small purpose occasionally, but ultimately, over the long-term, were poison to him? What if he could just barely tolerate them, but in a way that he was poisoned slowly without immediately identifying it? And if he started farming such a crop and always ate it because he had a surplus, wouldn't he suffer? Humans eat so many different things; would he even notice?

Everything works this way, in a matter of degrees, Rick thought. There were poisons that acted slowly, and there were poisons that acted fast. What if there were poisons that tasted good, but acted so slowly that their effects could not be recognized. Rick stood and started home. He'd found what he'd been scouting for that day.

When he got to his computer he searched, "Common food allergies" figuring that if the human body doesn't do well with something, it would probably try to make it known with negative reactions, at least for some people more than others. He learned that there were eight very common allergies: milk, eggs, peanuts, tree nuts, soy, wheat, fish and shellfish.

Rick then asked himself, which of those are made possible through intensive agricultural practices? Certainly milk, but definitely eggs, peanuts, soy and wheat were the most affected by modern agricultural practices. Then he asked himself, which ones are the biggest part of our diet? And his answer, at least personally, was simple: wheat and soy. His doctors had already tested him for these things with negative results. He would conduct his own tests, the only real test, not contrived in a laboratory, but a test involving his own body

Rick was very motivated because he knew that at the rate his mind and body were deteriorating he would eventually lose his job, and become an invalid. His limbs were wracked with pain. His muscles were weakening, squirming under his skin and twitching all over his body. His headaches were getting worse, and he was often dizzy to the point of falling down. His hands and feet were always numb and vibrating. He would wake in the middle of the night covered in sweat, the sheets soaked through with what seemed like a puddle of slime. He could take his own pulse by simply sitting still, and feel it throbbing in his body. Shooting pains randomly cut across his flesh and aches seemed to erupt from the marrow of his bones. He was often angered quickly and easily over very little, and didn't know if it was from his pain induced sleep deprivation, or a fundamental change in his hormones or brain. He couldn't concentrate, learn, or remember anything. He was making increasingly bad decisions at work that could potentially have life or death results. Even typing a few words or sitting still in a chair for ten minutes was torture. He would never be able to endure writing the novel he'd always wanted to. He'd begun to lose control of his bowels, at times, waking in the morning lying in his own feces.

Rick devised a plan. First he ate nothing for a few days. This was easy for him to do because at that stage, not eating simply meant he wouldn't wake up in his own shit. Always a good thing, he thought.

After three days, Rick felt better. This convinced him that food might be the problem. Then he decided to cut wheat and soy out of his diet. Almost immediately he had no bowel issues, after a week his headaches were gone. After two weeks the tingling in his arms and legs had lessened, and the numbness was gone. After a month, his energy was back. After six months his muscles twitched less and on and on with most of his symptoms. In the meantime, he'd educated himself about all the ailments that people suffer, searching information that included the term wheat, soy, and their constituent parts that people suspected gave them problems. And a coherent model began to develop. The mass of modern humanity generally made predominant in their diet foods that were not intended for the species. They were not designed to eat these foods. They were as horses eating meat, or lions eating grass.

Rick began to see these diseases for what they were. Obesity wasn't a condition caused by gluttony, or the old and discredited "calories in, calories out" theory. It was a poisoning of continual starch induced insulin spikes and the resulting inflammation. All the autoimmune diseases weren't caused by genetics and ethereal environmental toxins, they were the result of unsuitable food substances creating an environment in the gut that results in a dysfunctional digestive system, allowing into the bloodstream foreign material, and activating the immune system. The intestines were at once too permeable, letting in undigested proteins, and yet unable to absorb vital, necessary nutrients. It was all so simple;

the correct foods for a species. Consume the foods the species was designed for, and health is the result. Consume what was not originally meant for a species and the animal will become unfit, slowly, almost imperceptibly, and painfully, until the body's systems are overwhelmed.

When he searched with the correct terms, all the information was there, the existing scientific literature explained it all, and yet it seemed few paid attention to it, even most doctors. All they'd wanted to do was give him drugs. Rick was both incredulous and angry.

He then changed his diet even further from what everyone else usually ate to what he thought would be a natural diet, what man could collect or kill, mostly animal proteins, meat and organs, with a variety of edible plants. But they had to be plant genera to which no one, or at least very few, had allergic reactions. Rick lost some of the allergies he had, and realized through experiment and research that proteins in wheat were allowing the permeability that led to his allergies of other foods.

This diet served him well, resulting in an almost complete elimination of his symptoms over a period of a few years. The way of eating was simple, it had only a handful of rules that were easy to remember because they were rules that had previously been imposed by the natural environment due to availability. Eat when hungry, if you can't, hunger is not bad. Eat only nutrient dense foods, avoiding starchy plants with negligible nutrition like potatoes and grains. Eat whole vegetable and animal based foods as naturally created as possible. Put nothing in the mouth that requires an ingredients list. Seek out variety. Consume, in quantity, natural fats, even saturated. Rick realized that this manner of eating had been his heritage for the last half million years, at least.

Then, as if it couldn't get any better, it did. Rick realized that occasionally, probably more than occasionally, over the course of his evolution, man would have tolerated periods without food. This would happen on a regular basis, he reasoned, probably between hunting forays. Those humans' bodies that found a use for this period of not eating would have an advantage over those that merely lost energy and grew weak. So nature found a use for the period of not eating. Nature hates a void. It always seems to find a use for everything. It could even find a use for scarcity.

When Rick fasted for a day his body's attention withdrew from digestion and his immune system calmed, focusing instead on fine tuning other structures. His body moved into repair mode. Efficiency and quality became his body's way. Profound changes took place.

Rick found himself eating half the food he had normally consumed, and he enjoyed it more. He never seemed to get thirsty and figured his body used water more efficiently. He figured he had fewer wastes to process. Rick only did his quick morning sprint along with his few other exercises and yet managed to stay fit and lean. He didn't need to spend hours at the gym.

When a meal was especially good, he gorged and amazed people by the large quantities he'd eat. Then other days he would eat nothing at all. He never suffered from hunger, even on fast days. He grew healthy, and never got sick, not even the flu or the common cold. This was mankind's right, his intended inheritance, to have his sustenance be his ally, not his foe. Agriculture, making both appropriate and inappropriate foods interminably available, had robbed humanity of this birthright.

Why hadn't the doctors told him of this, he wondered? He searched, and discovered the answer to that too. Doctors don't study nutrition. Even gastroenterologists, students of the digestive system, seemed to believe that food had little to do with the health of that system. The patient's problem was instead, some kind of disease. Rick was incredulous.

From that point on, Rick lost faith in doctors. They had offered him only drugs that would have confused his body's systems, allowed his underlying problems to continue, and destined him to a life of misery. Instead, Rick had used his own mind, his own logic to save himself, when the accumulated medical knowledge of the last couple hundred years had utterly failed him. How many millions had they also failed, and how long would this continue? How could this be?

Chapter 11

FrIday afternoon, fIrst contact

Rick pulled into his parking spot on the mesa above Ruin Canyon. He'd decided to take leave from work so he could get there by the afternoon. The weather was still mild and he wanted to hunt during sunset in that canyon. He knew he probably wouldn't see the lion again, but he still wanted to get it out of his system. It was something he had to do.

As usual there was no one around, as the area was only infrequently used by hunters and cowboys. Rick went through his routine, and before long he was at the bottom of the canyon cliff. As was his custom, he took a different route to the same general location where he encountered the lion before, but not the exact same spot. He set up his position and began to call. Far in the distance, he saw movement. Curious as he was, he broke with protocol and lifted his binoculars to get a better look. Sometimes a simple action changes more than it should. His life would never be the same.

Near the edge of the canyon wall, to the east, from the side he had come, Rick saw a man. He appeared to be wearing a kind of collar that covered his shoulders and a skirt or kilt, which appeared to be gold, and sandals on his feet. As soon as Rick got a good fix on him with his binos, the man looked directly at him and pointed. Rick couldn't imagine that he was pointing at him and wondered what was behind him. There was no one in between them. The whole situation was so bizarre that Rick thought maybe there were some people from California out there filming something weird.

Suddenly the man started running at a speed that Rick thought strange. His first impression was that people don't run like that. Rick followed him with his binos and led him forward in the direction of his sprint. In a moment that horrified him, Rick saw the target of a pursuit; it was a cougar running away!

Rick had the feeling someone was playing a joke on him. He blinked hard with his eyes still at the binoculars. Yes, the man was running after the lion. Leaping across boulders, around bushes, and through trees; the man closed with the lion.

The first contact was a smack to the rear of the cat with a powerful sweep of his hand. The cougar sensed this coming and turned its head as it ran, to snarl at the assailant. The hit to its hind quarters set it slightly off balance and gave the man an advantage in speed for closing the contact. The cougar sensed this and lifted its paw in mid leap to swipe back.

Rick could sense the cat's terror. Rick felt terror. Western mountain lions ran from men, yes, but were never chased by them, let alone seen by them. It was as if some ancient nightmare that the lion's genetic memory harbored, reacting on impulse, had come true and the man was again the superior predator. The lion was frantic. Rick could feel it as he watched in horror. This thing did not happen.

The man caught the lion's front paw swat with a sweeping slap to that forearm. This sent her spinning in a midair turn to engage a killer that could not be outrun. The man followed this hit with a grab to the lion's chest with one hand, and while reaching across with his other hand, he swiped across the throat of the cat in one swift motion. The two tumbled together in a pile of limbs, fur, and dust. Out of the red cloud he rolled to his feet, a man of considerable stature. He looked down on a crumpled mass of fur, reached up over his shoulder, and pulled a prickly pear out of his back. The lion was pawing at the ground in fits. She twisted onto her back and lashed with claws at the air, kicked her rear legs as if to keep running, and was then still.

Rick was having problems with what he was seeing. It should have been the opposite. He felt confused. He wanted to look away and look back to see something different, but he couldn't make himself. This was a man. He killed a cougar. He ran her down. This does not happen.

The man looked up, directly at Rick. He looked at me again! I'm hundreds of yards away. How could he look at me? Rick felt as if this situation had been staged. I should run now! This was impossible. He'd catch me. How could this be happening?

As the man stood over the cougar, Rick wondered what to do. He felt panic rising in him and the fear of succumbing to it. He considered going back to his Jeep. He just might run the whole way. He was instinctively scared of this person who had the capability of running down a wild cougar and killing it. The only person who would do such a thing so efficiently must have done it, or something like it, before and have the confidence and ability that he could do it again. Such a man was extremely dangerous. On top of all this, he seemed to be staging it for Rick to see, unless there was a film crew somewhere and this was some kind of elaborate reality show stunt. Rick's mind was racing for options. He was trying to fit an unnatural occurrence into the realm of reality. He couldn't do it.

Rick's rational mind took over. He decided that this must be what it was. A man unknown to him had actually run down a wild mountain lion. What would he do with such a man? Rick knew. In a moment of resignation that enabled Rick to bury his fear, he stepped out of the bush where he'd been hiding. He would have to speak to him. This man was not pointing to someone behind him. Rick knew there was no one there. He was pointing to Rick. This man was there for him. He was demonstrating for an audience. And Rick was the only one around.

A sudden sensation overwhelmed him in flashes of comprehension. Rick realized that from this point on, his life would never be the same. The quiet retirement that he had looked forward to was gone. He had resigned himself to a boring existence into oblivion, but he could now see that this was threatened.

He would confront this man because it was his duty. It was the responsibility he had been subject to his whole life but had rarely called on him. He now had to answer that call, and he felt old, simple, and dumb. Why had something like this come so late in his life? Those first steps in the direction of the dead cougar were the most tormented he'd ever taken.

As he walked, Rick tried to get control of himself. He realized he had an M4 with at least twenty-four rounds in it. He had his revolver. He was well armed, and the lion killer didn't appear to have any weapons. No matter how fast he could run, he couldn't outrun a bullet. That thought just made Rick feel worse. This stranger had just killed a lion with nothing. The man was alternately examining his kill and looking at Rick as the distance closed.

At fifty meters, Rick realized he didn't know what he was going to say. Was this man poaching? That was stupid. Give him an award, not a citation. Rick held his M4 close to his chest, relieving his shoulder of the weight of the sling. At forty meters, Rick clicked the selector to fire. The small sound seemed to echo through the canyon and the stranger looked up. Rick would keep his distance, not pose a threat, and get as much information as possible. He'd wish him good day. Then he'd get the hell out if the man would let him. Rick had a sinking feeling it wouldn't go down that way.

At twenty-five meters, sound came from Rick's mouth and he regretted it before he could stop. "You from around here, stranger?" What a fucking idiot I am. Who am I, John Wayne? Is this Silverado? Of course he's not from around here, you idiot! Men from Cortez don't hunt in gold skirts and sandals. People from around here don't run down lions on foot! His question hung in the air until the stench of its absurdity made Rick feel like a schoolboy. The man did not answer, which made it even worse, but only stood, as though he was savoring his kill.

Until now, Rick realized his main concern had been about his own safety. Would he be attacked? Would he get away? Why was he approaching this obviously dangerous person? Rick hadn't been assessing this threat. He focused. The best he could tell was this man stood about six foot three, two hundred thirty pounds, evidently thickly muscled under just a gold and blue fabric collar around his neck and shoulders. It seemed almost glued on. The skin around his right shoulder revealed heavy scarring from what must have been a devastating wound. Parallel line scars elsewhere on his body hinted it was from a previous hunt and seemed to indicate that not every lion he'd killed had been as easy as this one. He was bald and clean shaven, his features were strong and thick. Rick seemed to be looking at a cross between Mr. Clean and a giant, hairless Neanderthal. A kilt-like skirt covered him from the waist to just above the knee and he wore what looked like sandals designed for combat, with covered toes and sides. He had a kind of gauntlet on each of his forearms.

Rick stopped at twenty meters. He figured that even if this man rushed him, he could level his rifle and…Rick realized he was too close to this unknown threat. He'd been using standards for a normal human adversary. But this man had inhuman speed. Shit.

Rick stood still and waited. Alright, Mr. Clean, he thought. You want to be the silent type? I've got all afternoon. Rick thought about home and Carson, and getting back safely. Rick waited.

After what seemed like an eternity, Mr. Clean took a deep breath. Rick tensed and noticed, as Clean moved slightly, there were, projecting from the gauntlet down the back of each hand, two long, gently-curved blades with large wavy serrations down one edge, extending about eight inches beyond his hands, bloodied and starting to dry. So he did have a weapon. He was like a tall, hairless Wolverine in a dress!

As he moved, Rick raised his rifle to cover him. The giant looked at him and smiled as he reached down and began to un-crumple the cougar. "Would you like to help me skin her?" He asked in perfect American English.

Rick was surprised and wasn't sure why. "No thanks," he responded immediately, revealing his controlled fear. Rick wished he'd waited longer to reply, as if he'd had the courage to consider the invitation.

The stranger stooped over the cat, his back to Rick, and with his long curved knives extending from his gauntlet, began expertly dressing the animal. He tied it by its front paws from the large scrub cedar next to him. First he skinned it, placing the hide below it, flesh side up. There was very little blood as he'd killed it with a slash to the throat. He gutted it and put all the organs on the hide, carefully protecting them from the dirt. He picked up the liver from this pile and took a large bite from it. Rick had leaned against a boulder to rest while he waited patiently, forgetting momentarily the unnatural speed he'd witnessed.

Rick then remembered the speed and realized he might be falling for a scheme by this thing to make him less alert. There were perhaps three hours until sunset, but Rick didn't want to look down at his watch. Eyes on and rifle up. He could feel his arms tiring.

The butchering was done. Mr. Clean carefully took the hide from the ground with its contents of internal organs, and used the four legs of the skin as handles. He tied them together to make a kind of carrying case and hung it in a tree. He stroked the fur with his hand, sweeping the dust from it. Rick was determined not to speak first.

At last the stranger turned to him and spoke. "You are patient." He lifted his arm to point at him. "That's good." A bluish squiggling fog erupted from the blades on the gauntlet and hit Rick's midsection before he could begin to move his trigger finger. His M4 vibrated violently and crumbled in an instant, falling to the ground as dust. Rick immediately moved for his revolver under his jacket, knowing what he'd feel. As his hand hit the pistol grip, he felt it shudder and crumble, sending the same shock through his hand that took the rifle from him. Dread flooded him as he was becoming disarmed, helpless. "You don't need those," the monster said.

Rick felt like a child standing before a god. He would have reached for his knife if not for the feeling he imagined a fawn must have in the jaws of a bear. What's the use? It was probably gone, too. A second ago, he thought he had some sort of power over the situation. Now, he had nothing except for the knowledge that he was indeed witnessing something very unusual, and if he came to die, at least it would be due to powers beyond his control. His mind raced, and all his knowledge and training, in an instant, became irrelevant.

Just when Rick thought he might be getting control of himself, the god threw something to him. "Take this." His impulse was to catch it, and he immediately knew this was wrong. Half catching and half squirming to avoid it, he felt like an out of control child again. As the object hit his contorted arm in the midst of its aborted catch, it seemed to crawl to his wrist in an instant. He heard and felt a click, and the object, a sort of bracelet, was now affixed. Again, with the despair he thought must belong to a desperate animal succumbing to a predator, he knew all was lost. He was now trapped beyond recovery. Every caution, every concern, all his weapons and training had led to nothing but this one moment of being an easy victim to this thing that appeared human, that looked real, and that spoke to him but left him helpless. Rick's vision quickly dimmed to black.

Chapter 12

Rick oNboard

Rick had the sensation of cold stone on his fingertips. He moved them to confirm the slick texture. A bright light above him forced his eyes open, then immediately made them want to close. He blinked and tried to move, but couldn't. He struggled to get his elbows beneath him to get up, but they wouldn't go. He tried to lift his head, but the muscles in his neck immediately cramped. He realized his legs were being held down by something. His clothes were gone. The dread that he'd felt before came to him again. He'd rather be dead than feel this way.

Rick was strapped on a table – head, arms, and legs all secured. He was in a large white room lined with glass on the upper wall. There was a robotic arm above him with a large needle. He heard a voice command, "Be still", and a searing pain, like a red-hot skillet pressed to his neurons was raked across his brain. He could not move and wanted only for the pain to stop. When it did, he wanted only to die. And when he thought about moving again, the pain came back a little, reminding him of its torture and threatening more. He screamed as if to try to disgorge both his physical and mental agony. When he once thought to rip and tear at his bindings with all his might, all at once, the pain consumed his being. He thought this must be the fire of hell. After that, he remained motionless, simply wanting to die.

The needle moved slowly down to his face, entering his nostril and piercing his head somewhere deep in his sinus cavity. This pain almost felt good compared to what he'd just suffered. The needle came out and moved to his abdomen, where it inserted again just below his ribcage. This continued over multiple locations around his body. All the while he prayed for death.

Rick awoke not even knowing he'd become unconscious. He was on a bed and could feel a blanket on his face. My God, what a horrible dream! He thought he'd been poisoned and he …opened his eyes to see the nightmare was not over. It was reality.

Looking down on him was Mr. Clean, the large bald man who'd trapped him. Though Rick felt weak, he also felt remarkably good and otherwise well rested. He was wearing a robe that felt of silk and was extremely comfortable. His hair was slightly damp, and he smelled fresh, as though he'd been bathed.

"Come with me," the bald one commanded.

Remembering the pain, Rick complied, simply glad to be off the slab. His circumstances had improved. Could there be hope? Sitting up on the edge of the bed, he found simple sandals on the floor. He put them on. He looked at the evil bracelet still on his wrist. Rick stood and followed Clean to another room where they sat with a table between them. Rick thought, correctly, here it comes.

"Rick Thompson, I am Synster the Provenger. A long time ago, we introduced agriculture to your primitive species to encourage population growth so that we could return one day to harvest your kind from a sustainable population. Your species is our cattle, our livestock. I have chosen you to be my operative on Earth. You will consider resisting this proposal. To assist you in this decision, I must inform you of the circumstances.

"Your entire civilization exists because of our intervention approximately 12,893 years ago. If it had not been for our arrival, humans would still be scurrying around in the dust fighting with other animals for food, just as they had for the last half million years. You owe everything in your current, somewhat advanced society, to us. We are here now to complete our project on schedule. We are technologically advanced beyond any of your capabilities, and your resistance to us would result in complete failure.

"We have two possible plans for the future of the human race. The first is called 'Natural Proliferation'. This management method is similar to the method you use on your fifty acres of land. You set up the conditions for wild game to be successful and then harvest it as you need it."

Rick sat bewildered, understanding everything he was hearing but not wanting to believe it. He was afraid to speak from the pain he'd previously felt. Synster seemed to sense this.

"You may speak freely."

Rick had so many things he wanted to say. Curses, threats, questions, more curses and threats. He felt like a wild animal inside, yet knew that all his words were impotent. He couldn't think of anything. He just shook his head.

Synster continued, "This is how we plan to harvest from your population. You live out your lives mostly unaware of our existence. We harvest per our quotas – quotas, I might add, that we designed your current population to sustain many millennia ago.

"As a reward for helping us where we need, you get the following. You get to assist in assuring the continuance of, for a large number of people on your planet, their current way of life. You will be allowed to exempt from harvest anyone you want, as long as they touch your life in some immediate way, such as family members, your mailman, your senator, your lawyer, everyone in your town…you get the idea."

Senator and lawyer on a no-kill list? Rick wondered. Synster obviously didn't have a complete concept of human culture.

"You would also be empowered with the ability to include certain people or groups in the harvest, any who you feel might be a threat to you and your work. You will also be granted any Earth-derived material goods or pleasures that suit you. We believe these incentives are sufficient for you to freely decide to work with us on this endeavor. What I've described will be yours. If I haven't yet been clear enough, we are offering you the power over life and death, along with all the material possessions on Earth that you desire."

Rick had to agree this Synster had a lot to offer. He didn't consider himself a religious man, but this reminded him somewhat of a deal with the devil. Everything seemed too good to be true. Rick looked around the stark room for probes, thinking maybe he was being tested for what might be incentives for humans. Anything could be going on. Rick decided he'd have to ask a lot of good questions to assess this situation.

"And what if I refuse?" Rick realized he sounded like a movie again as he lowered his head in disbelief.

"We've put considerable effort into our preparations so far, and your refusal would cause me personal and professional inconveniences. I will promise you that if you refuse, I will personally use all of my authority to keep you alive as long as possible while on the highest pain setting that will allow your sustained existence. I will also abduct all of your family members, your friends, everyone that I can imagine has held any significance to you, including your dogs, Barnes and Nobelle, and see that they all get the same pain treatment. And when they appear to be at the end of their lives, you will watch as they are dissected while they still live, for the edification of our school children."

Synster was glad there were no recording devices in this room. He'd chosen it for that exact reason. While he was allowed to conduct vivisection on samples taken from Earth and use pain control to recruit his surrogate for the sake of the Project, the punishments he just promised could not be implemented with any kind of official endorsement. It would be the same kind of depravity that is forbidden during the Contact Protocols. But threatening was not doing. The only time the Provenger were allowed to commit such destruction on humans other than testing samples was during their ritualistic banquets. Synster knew he had to convince Rick how committed and serious he was, and how brutal the Provenger could be.

"Observe." Synster commanded.

On the white wall in front of Rick appeared a room containing six people, three women and three men. They were all mounted on individual racks that seemed to be floating without gravity. The image was so clear that Rick couldn't tell if it was some kind of projection or if it was an actual room on the other side of the wall.

From what he'd observed so far, Synster had no hair, not on his head or his arms. The people on the racks were obviously human because they had hair on their heads and looked scared. Approximately two dozen male and female Provenger entered the room. They wore only the gauntlets on their arms with shorter blades than what Rick had seen on Synster. They approached the racks and, as if on signal, took turns jumping into them. When near the racks, they would also float. It appeared that in the area of the rack there was no gravity. They used their gauntlet knives to hold and slice at their victims, cutting them repeatedly, gripping onto them with their curved blades. Blood shot directly out, but when it reached a certain distance, it seemed to touch gravity and fall with a gush and a splat to the floor. The Provenger clung to their meals and so became covered with blood. If they let go and drifted to the edge, they also fell to the ground in the puddle of blood.

In a very short time, every inch of their bodies was covered in the blood of their bound, screaming victims. As the Provenger clung to them and cut, they bit into them, drinking their blood as ravenously as they could. To Rick they appeared as hideous blood-soaked vampires. He waited with dread for the smell of blood to reach him, but it did not. He couldn't take any more. He closed his eyes and turned away.

"If this is happening now, please make it stop."

"This has happened." Synster turned it off. "It was some years ago, a banquet. We are a reasonable race. But we take what we want, what we need. When we first arrived on Earth, we were treated as gods. We can't have that now. But we still need the product from the resources we've invested in your species." Synster stood and continued. "It's simple, Rick. Your gods have returned, and we're hungry." He opened a door on a wall where Rick saw none, and gestured that they proceed. "Tour of the ship?"

Synster's plan was simple: extend unlimited benefits to the human, while promising unlimited horror if he did not comply. Show him they were capable of the horror in the form of terrible bloodshed, and follow that with a tour demonstrating their awesome capabilities. This human really had no choice. If Provenger had any compassion, Synster would have felt sorry for him.

Chapter 13

Friday eveninG on the ship

"So, what do you think?" asked Synster.

Rick didn't quite know what to think. He sat across the desk from Synster in a sparsely furnished office. There was no light fixture in the room, and yet there was light everywhere. Okay, technology, he thought. There are probably a dozen other things going on in this office that I don't understand. There was a white desk in the middle of the white room, the white chairs on either side that they sat in, and a strange bench built into the wall on the left and right sides of the room. Much of it was designed for sitting, but probably half was designed with curves and ledges, various protrusions to support various body parts in different positions from reclining through standing. They seemed to invite any visitor to assume the position that suited them.

The image of Saturn lay beyond the large picture window behind Synster, and Rick wondered if it was real. He didn't doubt it. He'd been given a half hour tour of the ship and was satisfied it couldn't be faked. Yet he still had a hard time imagining he was the first human to make it to Saturn. He doubted he was.

While in the Grand Corridor, a vast open tube that ran the circumference of the ship and provided the Provenger with access to most areas, he'd followed the flight of a shuttle as it cruised silently by. His eyes then fixed on a surprising token. He saw a long-haired person from a distance. He was at first surprised he'd spotted her from so far away and then realized how much she stuck out among the hundreds of bald heads around her. Rick had always been amazed at how people could identify gender from a distance, assuming it must be some kind of a survival mechanism, enabling them to identify a potential threat or opportunity as early as possible. When he saw her for that brief moment, he could not possibly have predicted the nature or the extent of the opportunity he had just afforded himself. That one chance glimpse would change the course of his life and the future of humanity.

Rick had already come to grips with the idea that he was a dead man. Any way he looked at this situation, he was a goner. No cooperation, dead. Try for revenge, dead. Run and hide, dead. The only thing he hadn't yet considered was cooperating, and when he tried, he still instinctively figured, dead. Strangely, the only thing that gave him comfort was that he knew he wasn't alone. The whole human race was in a similar fix. But, so far as he was aware, he was the only one who knew. This either put him in an enviable position or simply an informed one. Either way, he'd rather be in the know. Either way, he had the company of all mankind as the comfort to his misery.

He'd had some time to calm down and get a grip on himself. It's not every day a man learns that his entire civilization has been engineered by an alien race for the purposes of a food resource development project.

And now he was learning that even the original wheat wasn't natural and that it was possibly the first GMO, an alien creation designed to manipulate man. I'll have to completely reassess my crusade against Monsanto, Rick quipped to himself.

Rick sat in the office of a being whose natural diet apparently included him. This very Provenger was the being who created the food that screwed with his health for about five years of his life. Rick thought, actually my whole life; I just didn't feel it until that last five.

"Why me?" Rick asked Synster, much more in control of himself now, though with full awareness of the instrument of pain still on his wrist.

"We are required, as part of our contact protocol, to have a surrogate on Earth. It reduces the danger of Provenger being injured, killed, or discovered. It also serves a number of other purposes. We choose people with contacts and skills we can use.

Your previous employment with the military and NSA, and your brother being the Deputy Director of the Department of Health and Human Services was a factor. Those associations put you in a position we can use. On a personal level, you have shown great tenacity throughout your life. As a former Marine and hunter, you understand the natural order of the food chain. We have examined your medical records. As someone who has healed yourself from the effect of our engineered grain, you have discovered something of your natural history. This reveals the ability to reconfigure paradigms to new realities. It demonstrates your adaptability to new ideas, your ability to innovate. We are certainly something new to which any collaborator must adapt. Even the large jar of broken pottery on the mantle in your house indicates a healthy disregard for your government's laws when you personally feel they've been misapplied."

Rick raised an eyebrow in surprise. They had been thorough. How often had they been in his house, he wondered?

"Your internet presence through your website also gives you some influence among your people. We have measured your following. You have more that you think."

As perverse as all this sounded, Rick had to agree. But his feeling of vindication was quickly squelched by his caution against being groomed, lulled into complacency by his enemy with pretty words. Synster was trying to appeal to his pride. And it was working. Foreboding followed, as he imagined he'd be tasked with approaching his brother for something, perhaps many things. He realized how his world would start to crumble. As for his internet site under his false name, Rick had always harbored concern that this might somehow conflict with his NSA career. But he never imagined it would be a conflict of interest by serving an alien conspiracy. Rick pondered, he's already got you thinking how you're going to fit into your new position. Resist and think, you idiot!

Rick suspected that Synster considered this a question and answer period where Rick could satisfy his curiosity. Maybe Synster thought this might allow Rick the time to make the decision to join this scheme. He may never have a better chance to get his questions answered. He must seem random in his interests. He must get an understanding of their technology while not appearing to have questions that are too specific.

It seemed as though Synster read his mind. "Your interest in our technology will only be satisfied to a limited degree, but suffice it to say, we are advanced far beyond your species. You have nothing that can compete with us, and any attempt to use force against us will be anticipated and crushed."

Rick stared at him. In an inept move to throw him off, Rick asked, "Do you have a last name?"

Without hesitating, Synster replied, "Our last names are the accent and inflection with which our single names are spoken."

Rick thought about that for a moment. Shit, these things have language sophistication way beyond anything I can comprehend. "So you're pretty good at language. That answers my next question."

"Yes, as a rule we learn the languages of almost all the beings we interact with. It is an excellent intellectual exercise and a process we enjoy."

Rick didn't know how much time he had to ask questions. If they didn't like him, they might kill him. He needed to be the operative Synster wanted, but the least he could do was try to get something he could use. Rick tried to concentrate on the information he thought he'd need. He was not likely to be able to use this session to pull any interrogation tricks. He knew he was outmatched.

"How did you get here?" Rick tried his best to sound stupid. In his assessment, he was doing quite well.

"We use gravitational waves powered by a binary neutron star contained at the center of this ship. It gives us the power necessary to create something like what you might call a wormhole. This ship, due to certain technology that I will not share with you, is protected from the effects of the gravity waves we create. These waves are focused at the space surrounding the ship, and it is that space, with this ship in it, somewhat like a protective cocoon, that relocates in the galaxy. By manipulating the focus of the gravity waves, we are able to create and collapse the wormhole where we choose. This provides our direction. The ship remains stationary in the space, while that section of space is what moves, or possibly the entire universe moves around us. It can be thought of as one or both. That part is still up for debate, as our calculations indicate. This avoids the detrimental effects on mass that your Einstein theorized would occur to matter traveling light speed."

Rick had thoroughly read about Special Relativity and almost understood it. He knew there was a time passage issue in this whole thing and was struggling to recall the lingo. "Do the issues of time travel still effect the ship?"

"The effect of gravitational time dilation is significant. Ten years have passed for us since we were here last, almost twelve thousand nine hundred years for you on Earth. Enough of time travel." There were certain topics related to this subject that Synster didn't want to discuss. Best to impress him with the basics, but no need to give him the whole picture, he thought. "What else?"

Rick made a mental note of Synster's avoidance of the time travel issue. "Okay, why eat humans? Why not cattle?"

"With our introduction of agriculture, humans can produce their own food. Cattle are not smart enough to do this. Cattle don't explore, colonize new lands, or kill other animals that compete with them or prey on them. Humans do all these things for us while we are away. There are many exceptions, of course, but for the most part you manage yourselves, increasing your populations so that we don't have to. For us, this is a commercial venture, and we take our nutrition very seriously. Both efficiency and quality product are very important. Human flesh, if properly raised, is both very nutritious and flavorful. For Provenger, it is considered a delicacy."

Rick had never thought he'd be described as a product and even a delicacy. He inadvertently shifted in his seat as the notion of being a better food than a cow massaged an untapped portion of his ego. The image of a barcode tattooed on his arm then flashed through his head. "Don't you feel bad about eating another species that so closely resembles your own, that are self-aware, and you can talk to?"

"No." Strange question, Synster thought, coming from a species which has at one time or another eaten every other edible species on his planet, including many he can communicate with, to include his own kind. "You must see the hypocrisy of your question. We only consider cannibalism abhorrent. I might also add, since you seem concerned about the morality of what we eat, that if we had not intervened in the natural evolution of your species, you would have hunted to extinction all animals capable of domestication, as happened on the Australian continent and many islands around the planet. Where would you be without them? We stopped that. Without the animals you domesticated – the dog, the cow, the horse, and others – your development toward what you are now would have been permanently halted.

"You see, you developed hunting techniques as a race on the continent of Africa with coevolving beasts for prey. Since they evolved with you, they developed defenses against you. When you emerged from Africa with those hunting skills, even the wildest animals of the other continents could not defend against them. They had little chance. As your weapons developed further, they had even less."

Rick had always wondered why there wasn't the kind of large and dangerous animal diversity elsewhere in the world that there was in Africa.

"That is how humanity spread so quickly once it emerged from Africa. Humanity hunted its way across continents. When we arrived, your race was at its zenith. All was good and there was plenty of game. But within a very short time, with a population explosion and most continents exploited and with the recent development of the bow and other hunting methods, you were on your way to exterminating them all. We let the mammoth become extinct as it would have been disruptive to agriculture. I had mammoth for lunch yesterday, by the way. Excellent texture. We could create living mammoth from the tissue we have if we needed. We have a few planets we're looking at.

"So you see, Rick, as a race, you would have been much less without us. If we hadn't come, you would have hunted the relatively gentle cow and horse into extinction. Ever notice that there are only zebra left in Africa and no wild horses? What would have pulled your plows, carried your goods? You would be hunter gatherers reduced to chasing rats and eating grubs. We examined the outcome with our Algorithm. If not for our intervention, your population would be ninety-nine percent fewer. We made you what you are today. We can unmake you."

Rick understood his message. Mankind had regularly eaten

all kinds of animals, hunting the easiest first. Rick realized he was still digressing and needed to get back on track. "Since we do look so similar, are we related in any way?"

"We may be, as closely as you are related to a chimpanzee. We suffered horribly from a war not long ago. Much of our history was contained in electronic media that were destroyed in the conflict."

Rick inadvertently expressed doubt.

Synster sighed and continued. "Imagine if your entire civilization's academic community were destroyed in a horrible war along with all their records, computer files, and books. And all you had left to reconstruct your society was the military establishment that had managed to defend itself. That is what we endured. Those surviving Provenger reconstructed as much of our history as they could, but were not experts regarding all the details of all fields. Some large portions of our history were a complete loss. We have, of course, our ability to isolate our DNA and have found we do potentially have a common origin, if that's the answer you're looking for. But we are a very different species. We cannot interbreed."

Now that was a little more information than Rick was looking for, and he found it interesting that Synster added it, although Rick had already considered the topic himself during his brief tour of the ship. Despite the hatred and disgust he'd developed for the Provenger in the couple short hours in which his concept of the world had been crushed by them, he had to admit, they were very attractive, if you could get past the lack of eyebrows.

During his tour, he'd seen many men and women, and they were all, without exception, tall, of strong stature, with well-developed musculature. So much so, he found himself questioning under his breath, "What are these people on?" At first, they all looked somewhat similar, but when he looked more carefully, he could see a diversity. Some were stockier, some were slim, and others had very delicate features while some were hard and thick. He saw none that looked even remotely fat, weak, or diseased. They all had straight teeth, solid posture, and clear skin. They had the appearance of super beings.

After overcoming his shock and resigning himself to his situation, he was amused by their sense of style. The men went mostly bare chested, except for a circular collar draped from the base of their neck encircling it, with slight coverage in front, on the shoulders, and back. It was highly decorative and seemed so thin and supple that it was always in contact with their skin. A few wore a tunic, open at the front. Most had some kind of forearm coverings, somewhat like gauntlets, except without the knives that Synster had worn when he killed the cougar. They all had, hanging from their waists in the front and back, knee-length, highly decorative cloth panels that almost had the look of a kilt. Overall, their clothing looked very ancient in design. Rick felt like he was among warriors of ancient Sumer or Egypt. Most wore sandals on their feet, but many went barefoot.

The females were the most interesting. Aside from being completely bald and their unnerving appearance with no eyebrows, Rick thought he might be able to get used to them. The young females wore a dress that reminded Rick of pictures he'd seen of the Minoan people. The entire front of their dress exposed their chest and stomach down to below the navel, with their breasts slightly crowded to the center by the raised collar of their plunging "neckline". Their hemline was long to the ankle on one side and, vaulting up, it usually exposed the leg completely on the other. The dress was tight around the buttocks, possibly made of this same material that hugged the skin. It seemed obvious to Rick that this clothing was designed specifically to showcase their feminine attributes, and the effect was spectacular. "This is how our unmarried women dress in public," Synster told him when he saw Rick's surprise. If Rick hadn't been distracted by the end of civilization as he knew it, he would have thoroughly enjoyed himself.

"So you come to Earth thousands of years ago, introduce us to agriculture so we fill the planet, and return now to harvest us for food," Rick paused. "You get a full ship, then you go home, wherever that is, to sell your product?"

"That is a gross simplification. For us, it was less than ten years. But, yes, that is what we do."

"So," Rick continued, "how do you make sure, if your form of travel involves forward time travel, or time dilation, that you arrive back to a time where you have others of your people... um sorry, your kind, there to trade with?"

Synster was impressed with Rick. This was finally a good question. "We are all on the same travel schedule. We know when we must travel, and for how long, to rendezvous at the same place in time. It is all worked out before we depart."

"How many bodies do you need?"

"I will decline to answer that question."

That answer means the number they need is so great it would disturb me. A tenth, half the population of the Earth, Rick wondered. "So how long will you be with us?" Rick considered this information vital.

"I won't tell you that exactly. I will only say that we will benefit from your company for approximately two to twenty years," Synster said with a smile. "As for you, consider it a long-term relationship. Your future, Rick, lies with us."

Well, that narrows it down, Rick thought. "What other people will you be contacting? Will I be part of some kind of a team?"

"You will not know that unless we tell you or they are allowed to tell you. There is no team."

At that moment, someone entered the room behind Rick, and Synster sprang to his feet as his face became at once either surprised or irritated; Rick couldn't tell.

"I apologize. The threshold cloak was flickering and didn't indicate there was anyone in here," she said. It was a voice so feminine and soothing that Rick was shocked

"The cloak doesn't work properly when there is a tag in the area," Synster snapped while gesturing to the device on Rick's arm. "You should know that."

"Oh yes, I do," she replied while walking around to Synster's side of the desk as he sat down. "But how was I to know that before I came in?" She sat down on top of his desk and folded her right leg over the left, exposing them both from under the long side of the gown. She had a plate of covered food in her hands. She put it down in front of Synster. This should irritate father, Nwella thought as she put her left hand on the table, leaned on it, and planted a broad smile on Rick.

Rick could tell the good-smelling food was some kind of roasted meat along with something else he couldn't identify. Human flesh, he thought?

She was the most exotic female Rick had ever seen. For a

moment, he thought that if Synster offered him this beauty, he would consider delivering the body and soul of every human being on Earth, both living and dead. An instant later, he wondered if this could be part of his recruitment. Her left arm crushed into her side as she leaned on it, demonstrating lean yet sizable muscles. She was unmarried, as indicated by her bare, round breasts protruding from her dress. Her naked legs, freed from coverage by the left side of her gown, and folded on the table, were tan and smooth. With her legs uncovered, her arms bare, and the entire front of her body exposed, there was so much glowing bronze skin in front of Rick it gave him the impression that she was completely nude. Rick couldn't believe it when Synster said, "This is my daughter, Nwella."

Rick almost expected, or wanted him to say something like, "This is your prize for helping us eat all of mankind."

I must be in hell, he thought. She appeared to him to be about as young as a female could be while still being fully developed. Rick didn't know where to look. All he was trying to do was gather information in a feeble attempt to save humanity, and here he had to deal with this goddess distracting him, displaying just about everything she had, and she was the daughter of his enemy. Then he was suddenly aware that all he was wearing was a thin robe.

"I wanted to bring you your dinner since you were working late. And who is this?" She looked at Rick, turning her shoulders square to him, her breasts staring at him like a second pair of eyes. And he stared back.

"You know who…" Synster paused and started again. "This is Rick Thompson, a human. Of course, you know that." Synster seemed flustered.

"Yes," she said, looking him deep in the eyes, "How old are you?" Nwella found him very interesting. His shaggy silver hair reminded her of the primitives she'd met years ago. She still had fond memories of them. And this one had silver hair on his chin. It somehow made him look wise.

"Fifty." Rick observed her surprise. He knew he tended to look older than he was, due to his premature graying. But when his hair was cut close and his face clean shaven, he looked twenty years younger. He caught himself wanting to be attractive to this thing. Why was that, he wondered? He should want to kill her.

She smiled again. "Poor thing," she said pursing her lips.

I need to get back on task. Should I keep asking questions in front of her? Would it be rude? Rick decided to wait and say nothing.

"Nwella dear, we need to get some things done," Synster said, with irritation in his voice even Rick could detect.

Synster was incensed with his daughter. As soon as she'd come in, she'd released her sex pheromone. He caught it on the air as she sat on his desk. Why does she play games like this? They would have a talk later.

Before she left, Nwella walked up next to him, bent down, and put her nose next to Rick's mouth. He thought she was going to kiss him and Rick almost puckered his lips. She drew a deep breath as she smelled from his chin, up his face, and across his hair.

Rick was glad he'd been washed. He thought about how he normally didn't wear cologne, but noticed that whatever they'd washed him with smelled pretty good. He was careful not to exhale so she wouldn't smell his breath.

As she smelled him, he turned his head toward her and his eyes worked down her neck, breasts, stomach, and finally to her navel. He couldn't help himself. He felt a shudder leap from the base of his spine up to the vicinity of his bladder, then dissipate everywhere from his thighs to his chest. He was afraid it had actually made him move. She stood up and ran her fingers through his hair. She smiled at him one last time. Rick smiled back like an idiot, and she walked toward the threshold.

"Good evening, Father."

"Nwella," Synster replied.

"Nwella," Rick said unconsciously under his breath, as if she'd said goodbye to him. He was still smiling.

It was everything Rick could do to keep from turning around to watch her leave. He felt like he'd just made love to her, right there in front of her father, a mortal enemy. His mortal enemy! It never even occurred to him to reach out, grab her throat, and destroy her as quickly as possible. No doubt the "tag", as Synster called it, would have stopped him. Rick took a deep breath and tried to focus.

"So you mentioned this pain device on my wrist is called a tit-aaaa-tag? What does it do?"

"That is merely a device designed to identify and control you. It takes your own impulses to initiate an activity that we have forbidden and turns them against you as pain. The more intense your desire to do the thing we have told you not to do, the more intense the pain. It has a variety of setting levels. We can also initiate the pain for punishment or training."

"Can you take it off me if I promise to be good?" Rick once again felt like a child but didn't care. He was already playing that role to look stupid and once again, he was doing it well.

"No, we don't trust you."

Rick wished he could jump up quickly at that moment and lunge toward Synster without the intent to touch him, just to test the device, to see if it would activate even when he didn't intend to do harm, but he didn't. He was too close to its last demonstration of pain, and it had him scared.

With this thought of pain, Rick began to feel tired and abandoned hope of trying to maintain some line of questioning that would provide him with a foundational knowledge of the Provenger. His impulses for self-preservation kicked in.

"So what do you want me to do?"

"Finally, Rick, a question that serves our interests. We as Provenger love adventure, but we carefully calculate those danger variables. Dealing with un-tagged humans can be unpredictable, so we are disinclined to make frequent contact ourselves. For this purpose, we have surrogates. I have chosen you. Because we are currently operating under the Natural Proliferation Program, we are required to maintain secrecy. If our presence were to become common knowledge, then we would be required to move to the Managed Collectivization Program. As part of your responsibilities, it is important that you understand the difference between these two."

Rick knew his history and if the Provenger were consistent in the accurate use of their English, he didn't like the sound of the second program.

"The Natural Proliferation Program started with our introduction of wheat and a few other agricultural products thousands of Earth years ago to obtain results distinctive to our goals. We wanted to dramatically increase the human population. Your development of agriculture would do that. With the surpluses it provided, you would then develop vocational specialization, which would lead to the development of technology. Without limiting this technological development, we had no way of controlling how far it could go, and we couldn't come back to a population that was a technological threat to our harvesting project.

"To stunt technological development, we needed to limit the abilities and the lifespan of those who, over the generations, would contribute. We found through our calculations that each decade of productive intellectual contributions beyond the reproductive years would exert considerable momentum toward such progress. We, therefore, needed to limit the cognitive ability and lifespan in these decades. For our scheduled return, we had a ten year window, but Earth necessitated at least twelve thousand five hundred years to reach the population levels we need. If technological development had continued unabated throughout this period, we could possibly have arrived to face a belligerent and equal foe. By introducing certain deleterious effects in wheat, we could retard the growth of your technology.

"We engineered wheat to have long-term negative effects on the digestive and immune systems. These would slowly deplete the body's ability to obtain the nutrition that powers everything else, from the immune system to the nervous system. With all the organs of the body, including the brain, being slowly deprived of nutrients or harassed by a confused immune system, a variety of dysfunctions would occur, all dependent on the individual human's unique genetic makeup. Since these appear as very different problems, they work to hide the source of the problem. Even today most of your people, and certainly most of your traditional medical community, have no idea what causes your autoimmune diseases.

"Even so, we calculated through our Algorithm that by the time we arrived, your people would have discovered these causes and would be living relatively healthy lives, using the grains more as animal feed to produce the fat and protein in your own livestock that was the foundation of your natural diet. Instead, you have made the mistake of avoiding fats in your diet because they have a higher caloric density, and you believe they make you fat when they do not.

"We know that you personally have adopted this traditional diet and saved yourself from a chronic autoimmune disorder you call by the names dysautonomia, Gulf War syndrome, post-traumatic stress disorder, fibromyalgia, chronic fatigue syndrome, and a few others. Have you not?"

"I thought it was multiple sclerosis," Rick replied, interested at how this had taken a personal turn."

"Yes, it could have become that if you had one slightly different genetic expression and hadn't changed your diet. Our scans have confirmed that. But back to my main point; humans have certainly populated Earth, per our plan. But, contrary to our expectations, your technological development has fallen far behind where we thought it would be. Perhaps we have only ourselves to blame. One of the effects of nutrient deficiency, of course, is reduced intellectual capacity. Right about the time when many conclusions were being reached regarding the whole fat versus carbohydrate issue in the 1950's through 70's, we intervened to change wheat again. At around that time, we enhanced both the yield, to reach more cultures, and the deleterious effects of wheat, to reach certain body mass index quotas. We value human fat."

"Norman Borlaug?" asked Rick, taking a chance, suspecting Provenger involvement.

"He may have been a miscalculation on our part. His work to enhance the yield of wheat crops certainly enhanced some of the deleterious effects we had already carefully calibrated. While this aided our goals to fatten your population prior to our arrival, there is now a problem.

"Various decisions your healthcare researchers made during the last fifty years contributed to the health mess you find yourselves in and, therefore, the mess we find ourselves in. You see, Natural Proliferation would work just fine if you humans weren't all poisoning yourselves with drugs. Since you are, it is looking more likely that Managed Collectivization might be necessary for us to harvest our required quota. We require an organic product."

Rick squirmed in his seat. He knew exactly what Synster was

talking about, and this just happened to be one of the main topics on his web site. One in every three adult Americans was on some kind of statin drug, one in nine were on antidepressants, and the statistics for blood pressure medications were even worse. Almost all Americans ingested artificial sweeteners in everything from chewing gum to diet sodas. There existed a virtual cornucopia of drugs that, when tallied together, amounted to a very small percentage of the population that was unaffected. Rick and, recently, Carson happened to be two of the unaffected.

"I've been arguing against these drugs for years, so have many doctors and researchers. What more could I possibly do?"

"All of the research already exists," Synster related with obvious annoyance, "that shows these drugs are unnecessary if only people would conduct themselves properly. The only improvement that can be made is for your government to change its policy on the use of these drugs through its control of your mandatory healthcare system."

Rick knew this meant the heavy involvement of his brother.

"I've reviewed the history of your species' health care initiatives. It is so unfortunate that it's taken the course it has. Up until the 1960's, you had it right. Improvements in nutrition were seen as the first line of defense against disease. Then the industrialization of agriculture, the hybridization of grain and legume crops, and creative food scientists in flavor labs all conspired, resulting in the massive consumption of carbohydrates by your species. Instead of realizing this as the cause and reversing it, your healers decided to medicate. The alchemists you call doctors believed they could use their single compounds to improve a complex system degenerating due to an inappropriate internal environment. Their successes resolving infectious disease with vaccines and medications, a completely different health issue, made them feel comfortable with applying single medication strategies to chronic physiologic malfunctions. Your people moved away from the gene therapy that good nutrition is, and instead pursued a path of medications. You abandoned the source of the problem and toyed with the symptoms."

Rick seemed to feel that Synster was on a rant. He seemed very disturbed by all this. Was he desperate?

"Now they are finally getting back to gene therapy again but trying to change the actual genes instead of allowing them the environment in which they've evolved to work. How a people with the prowess you have in physics can let this happen is beyond my understanding. If I seem frustrated, you are correct. What simpletons would think they can correctly mediate something as complex as inflammation and lipid metabolism with single or multiple drugs?"

Synster seemed more than professionally involved in this, Rick thought. The level of intensity seemed personal. Rick wondered if Synster had pressure on him from his own kind. Maybe Synster was on the ropes regarding this project.

"I'll need you and your contacts to exert certain influences to change things. With my guidance, the population of Earth will eliminate medications and become healthier. We need to harvest an organic product to maintain Natural Proliferation."

Looks like you're in this for the long term, Rick joked with himself. This yahoo doesn't know his humans very well. They need you for something. In the meantime, you'll figure out how to fight them.

"The alternate method of harvest produces for us unpleasant inconveniences. For you and your people, it would mean the end of everything as you know it. Under the Natural Proliferation Program, we would slowly harvest from various segments of the population based on our needs, leaving the rest to continue with their lives, continuing to produce food and offspring in what we call a Perpetuant Cycle.

"Since you collectively decided to poison yourselves, destroying our meat and organ harvest, our reluctant alternative may be to initiate the Managed Collectivization Program. This would necessitate an overt approach. We would have to take control of large portions of the population to manage their diets and recreational activities. To merely take control of part of your planet, or parts of various populations, would guarantee that the rest would make war on us. We would need significant earthbound resources to manage our human ranches to turn out a nutritionally sound, un-medicated, antibiotic-free, un-poisoned product. I'm sure you can imagine the implications to your way of life, not to mention the significantly increased resources we would need to employ in security and management. We would literally need to become ranchers of animals to feed to our collectives of humans. We find this prospect to be incredibly wasteful of our time and resources. You have some land, Rick?"

"Yes, I do." Rick was jolted out of his visualization of the world as a gulag.

"You plant grasses there to encourage the success of animals so that you may return to hunt them?"

"Yes, I do."

"We are no different. These deer and elk on your land are your food. Suppose someone was to feed them sugar cubes and lettuce all day long because they like it and, therefore, figured they were doing them some good. Then, when their health suffered, they were pumped full of drugs to "cure" all the problems. If you couldn't stop these people and allow the animals to eat the way they were meant to, wouldn't you fence them in or fence the people out?"

"Yes, I would," Rick replied. "Or I'd have to go the grocery and buy my meat there, supporting someone else's managed collectivization," he continued in complete agreement. They have every right to do what they're doing, Rick thought.

"We were really expecting you humans to take care of these issues on your own." Synster didn't add that Natural Proliferation was his project, and if it didn't work, he would lose everything and Ryvil would be promoted to Project Director. Just in case Rick was pettier than he thought, he didn't want him to get any crazy ideas about methods of revenge.

"So if we get our act together, it's Natural Proliferation and you get your organic harvest. If we don't, it's Managed Collectivization, and you put us all in collective meat factories to manage our health for us?" Rick felt like he was negotiating a deal on The Price Is Right, except the total destruction of humanity was behind the next curtain.

"Oversimplified again, but yes."

"May I have a glass of water?" Rick inquired, and with his wry sense of humor continued, "Or whatever it is you think I should be drinking." Rick felt like he might throw up.

Synster appreciated this last comment and took it to be Rick's submission of will. It was not. Synster touched a panel on his desk and ordered the water.

This will be impossible, Rick thought. People treat food like a religion. They won't change for their own good. They'll resist, they've already been resisting the science for decades.

"This, of course," Synster continued, "is all background information and only necessary in that you understand the motives for your actions. You need to know that your activities will truly be contributing to the salvation of man as a somewhat independent animal, rather than a factory raised product."

A Provenger entered, placed water on the table, and exited.

"What you need to do will be coordinated, over time, by me. You will use your influence through your internet site, and you will need to use your contacts; your brother. I may contact others, and you will represent me when I choose not to engage them. Any duties that I require must be executed precisely as I've ordered. You will answer only to me unless I appoint an agent to act for me. Although we appear to have complete knowledge about your culture and your history, we've only had time to assimilate what initially interests us, leaving the depth of our knowledge lacking. I will need you to fill in the gaps. We will also need you to use your position with the NSA to inform us if your government discovers any of our technology."

"So exactly what do I need to do on my website? I've already been trying to get people to eat real food and get off meds."

"I'm glad you asked. When your government proposes our policies, many will seem questionable. You will express support, as opposed to your regular disagreement with the government. For example, currently around seven hundred thousand people every year have their gallbladders removed due to damage from their current high carbohydrate diet. Its function is to aid in the digestion of fats. With your government's advocacy of high carbohydrate, low fat eating, this organ is simultaneously inflamed and atrophied. Its removal is the only option once it becomes clogged and inoperative. The government will require these to be preserved and submitted for testing.

"In addition, the government will begin advocating and encouraging through insurance policy benefits the proactive removal of gallbladders for people with certain health issues. Since gallbladders help people to digest fats and dietary fats are thought by your ill-informed doctors to increase cholesterol and make people fat, we believe it will be easy to get gallbladders removed from people who are obese. We value the gallbladder for elixirs and may still be able to use them.

"With sixty-five percent of the people in your country overweight and cholecystectomy being now a simple procedure, we will be able to immediately fill our quotas for this organ. This will do much to delay implementation of Managed Collectivization. You will publicly support these initiatives."

Synster read the look on Rick's face. "This will all be painful for you. It will require you to break the laws of your country. And this is only the beginning, compared to the assassinations we may plan. Rick, you will also be my assassin."

There was a long silence. Rick could get around supporting things he didn't believe in on his web site. He could lie, cheat, steal, and quite possibly a great deal more, but the thought of killing people who had not tried to kill him, who had families, loved ones, and lives to complete…then he realized… "Why can't you kill them? Just take them like you did me and harvest them or whatever the hell you call it. Why make me do it?"

"We may need you to do it to prove your trustworthiness, or to make it look like a political statement of your own kind. We are unsure at this point. But remember your benefits."

There was another long silence and Rick tried to think of benefits that would make him feel right about assassinating someone. A lobotomy maybe? He looked out the window at Saturn and realized he had his cell phone on him. He could take a picture. He felt strangely calm and yet nauseous and resigned to a fate of destruction.

"Excuse me," he began with a tone of apology, "but I was still adjusting to the idea of being food when you told me all the goodies. Could we go over that again?"

"Aside from assuring the continuance of your current way of life for as long as possible, you will be allowed to exempt anyone you want from harvest, as long as you are close to them in some way. You will also have the ability to include certain people or groups in the harvest for any reason. It doesn't matter. We are very liberal with this issue under the Program laws. You will also be given any material goods or pleasures you want, as long as they originate from the Earth. You can't request anything we have created, for obvious reasons, though you may be provided with certain tools of ours from time to time to complete your mission."

"Can I get that deal in writing?" Rick thought he was being funny. One of his coping mechanisms was humor. What he really wanted to do was throw up.

Synster didn't get it. "No. I will leave you here now. You have five minutes to decide if you will cooperate. If you choose to cooperate, your efforts will be assessed on a daily basis and you'll be notified if you're deficient. You have five minutes." Synster rose from his chair, walked through the cloaked door, and disappeared from Rick's view. Looking through the threshold, Rick could see only a vacant science deck on the other side. It flickered once and Rick caught a glimpse of Synster. He had turned and was looking back in while speaking to another Provenger.

Chapter 14

Home Troubles

Synster arrived home after a long day. The threshold cloak was still malfunctioning, allowing him to catch flashes of Nwella inside. She was sitting in the lounge and must have just gotten home as she was still in her public gown. In that moment, he decided not to discipline her until after his mind had settled a bit. Synster walked into the home. "Hello, Nwella dear."

"Hello, Father," Nwella replied as she turned off her personal monitor and left the room.

Synster sat where she had been and looked at the view of Saturn. He dreaded having this talk with Nwella. She was really far too old to discipline, but as long as she was still living at home, it was his responsibility. And her behavior had been atrocious.

From the quiet, it appeared that no one else was home, and he eventually decided that now would be a good time.

"Nwella dear, come here, please."

Nwella had been trying to avoid him and was not interested in being talked at. She could sense he was going to be critical.

"What, Father?"

"Come here, please. I need to talk to you." Synster waited a moment. "I'm not going to yell to the next room." Synster waited.

Nwella took her time. She walked in slowly and stood at a distance from her father, saying nothing, a fist on her hip.

"Sit, please."

"Father, this is unnecessary. I know what you're going to say already, so you don't have to say it." Nwella insisted as she walked up and sat down.

"Alright, you tell me what I'm going to say."

"You're going to tell me that I was rude to you and that you're disappointed in me that I would fluem for that human, that I embarrassed you, yada yada yada."

That was pretty close, but Synster tried to act like he was thinking something different. "No. What I was going to do was ask you what you were thinking. I want you to be successful in life and you exhibited such immaturity and lack of professionalism at a time when I was recruiting a vital link in our operations. I even suspect you arrived at that time on purpose just to take a look at…"

"I was bringing your dinner because I knew you were working hard!"

Synster glared at her with an expression of doubt.

"So I can never just do something nice for you?"

"I'm not saying that," Synster rebutted. "What I'm say is that your behavior was not consistent with who I know you to be."

"Oh, so who am I, Father? Who do you want me to be?" Nwella got up and started to walk away.

"Don't you walk away from me!" Synster yelled at her.

In mid-stride, Nwella turned to the viewer and began walking toward it. "I'm not. I just don't want to sit." She stood looking at the screen, with her back to Synster. She acted like she was admiring Saturn, but she just wanted to be away somewhere else. She wanted to be free.

"Nwella, I want you to be as successful as you can be. This nation is very competitive right now, and both you and I need to be at our peak in performance…" Synster continued talking about the stress he was under, the project he was coordinating, and the dire consequences of failure. He spoke of the chances of Ryvil taking over and the pressure he was under to secure a position in the new nation ship when it arrived.

His voice faded out of her consciousness as Nwella's mind drifted far away to ten years ago and her first visit to Earth. She was twenty-seven years old, and the implementation of the project had just begun. The teams were all in place and doing their job, and she and her father were free to pursue adventure.

They had both gone to a remote beach on the southern coast of the Anatolian peninsula. The great floods caused by the small moon's destruction had not yet come, and the water there was still a beautiful blue green. They had gone there to swim and hunt. With their clothes hanging in a tree near the water, they also hung their bladed gauntlets. There were electronic components in their garments that could become compromised from the minerals in the water. They swam in the gentle waves and scrubbed their bodies clean with the wet sand, and then reclined on the slope where the waves and the beach met.

Two lions appeared from behind some rocks down the beach. Nwella saw them first and showed her father. It gave her such a thrill to see them. Synster immediately wanted to hunt them and made toward the tree for his gauntlet. Reaching it quickly, he hurried to dry his arms, put them on, and rushed after his prey.

Nwella begged him not to, as she wanted to watch them, but he wouldn't listen. Off he went, down the beach, with only his gauntlets on his arms. Nwella didn't care to watch and laid her body back in the sand, enjoying the sun in the massage of salt and sand that crawled back and forth in the light surf. She was irritated that he would interrupt their day together to go off on his own.

She should have known better, but there she remained, lying on the brown beach in the ocean wash, looking very small and very vulnerable to the additional lion crouched on the grassy dune immediately beyond the tree where her gauntlets and clothing were hanging.

With legs slightly bent, she felt the sand between her toes and swept her hands in the sand above her head. Without a care, she thought of the years ahead and the wonderful experiences she'd have when all their plans would come to fruition. Completely unaware of the wild territory she was in, and completely stripped of all defenses, she drifted in and out of consciousness.

At twenty-seven, she was fast and strong, and with her gauntlets had a chance to defend herself against any lion. But naked on the beach, with her eyes closed and unaware, she was dangerously close to being flayed by this wily cat.

The lions apparently had a scheme. The Provenger had never experienced animals so cunning before. They were primitive and yet seemed capable of intricate planning and complex communication that even the Provenger underestimated. The two cats up the beach were a diversion to separate the large prey from the small, as is the perpetual goal of the predator. The successful ones are those who can get a meal, any meal, with the least possible effort and threat of harm. For if harm comes to the body of the predator, the animal has no recourse but death. They live in a small margin where physical performance means success. Anything less brings ultimate failure.

This lion was the best hunter of the three, and she took a quick look down the beach and didn't see the large prey. He had disappeared behind the rocks. She could smell him, though, on the warm constant breeze that flowed down the beach. He smelled distant as his scent cone was thinned by many parts of air. Now was the time. Kill and carry away. While still crouched, the lion emerged from the grass. It was leaving cover and therefore moved at a moderate pace silently down the sand slope to the waterline, closing the time-distance gap. Complete focus on the flesh waiting for her, all systems shut down except for her senses, brain focused on the nose, eyes, total focus, make no sound, no breathing, closer, ready to lunge, closer, ready...

A shrill screaming from the other end of the beach made Nwella bolt upright, bounding from a prone position on her back to standing in an instant. She was so startled that she let out a small yell of her own. Then she saw the huge cat almost upon her and, from both fear and ferocity, the yell turned into a hissing scream.

The lion was startled from the sudden movement of her small prey off the sand into then a much taller animal, the screaming down the beach, and the shriek of this surprisingly large quarry. She hesitated. The clamor continued as Nwella backed slowly into the surf. This was the kind of drama predatory instincts reviled against. Bad surprises lead to injury. She wasn't that hungry, they'd just killed yesterday and had half a carcass to return to. Sudden change from the small prey to large, loud prey, two sources of human noises, outnumbered two to one, a possible fight in the water... The cat decided to run, and with a quick dash and a few leaps was back up the slope and over the dune.

Sprinting toward Nwella but no longer yelling was a man holding a long spear. His naked body was painted completely in swirls of black and white, and his chest was heaving from his sprint. He dropped his spear to show that he meant no harm. Holding his palms out in front of him, he blurted out a language she could not understand. From his tone and sign language she quickly deciphered his meaning. He had been a distance down the beach, seen the cat stalking her, and ran as fast as he could. Then he yelled to scare it away when he saw it begin its final rush.

He now stood before her, the panicked look calming and his large chest heaving. He was imposing for a human, young and healthy. His arms were strong and muscular, as were his legs. He had large eyes that were green with the bushiest lashes she'd seen on a human. He had long straight black hair pulled tight, close to his scalp and tied back, falling down the back of his head. This last feature, with his hair out of the way along with his large stature, made him look almost like a Provenger. Nwella's eyes danced across his body. What a great idea, she thought. The painted circles all over him excited her. His square features were a little different from the other primitives they'd encounter far away during the Contact Protocol, but this one was obviously not one of them. He was wild. He was beautiful, Nwella thought.

He was soaked with sweat and still rambling away. Nwella quickly recognized he was saying the same thing over and over, and since she had already figured out what it was, she wanted quiet. She gently put her hand on his mouth. He immediately jumped back and stared, startled from her act.

He began to slowly circle her, amazed. He'd never seen a woman like her before. She had no hair on her head, no hair anywhere, not even eyebrows or between her legs. Her body was completely void of any blemish and so clean. Her skin was a light bronze color and she had no weapons. He thought she must be some kind of witch or nymph from out of the sea, going about in such a dangerous place alone with no defenses. He felt a twinge of fear and thought perhaps he shouldn't look her in the eyes, or perhaps he should run. Or maybe he should fall to his knees. If she was a witch, he hoped that by saving her, some favor might come to his tribe. He looked down and got even more nervous. Her body was perfect. She looked strong, toned, and lean. Her breasts were full and her hips were wide. He instinctively wanted to have children with her.

Nwella looked over his shoulder, down the beach to where her father would be and didn't see him. Nwella knew she was on adventure, and that gave her a little leeway when it came to her actions. She wasn't sure if what she was about to do was outside of protocol for adventure, but she was tired of trying to keep track. Under these circumstances, if this man had been a Provenger, it would now be her prerogative to offer herself to him. Wasn't the wild and outrageous the standard for adventure? Wasn't there a very loose and forgiving attitude when it came to transgressions during adventure? Hadn't Father just left her to pursue his? He might be gone for some time. Shouldn't she have hers?

Nwella reached out, pushed his chin up with her fingertips and locked her eyes on his. Even in the blazing light of midday, her intent made her pupils large. He saw this as he instinctively stared back into them, and the completely unexpected became real. He imagined that a spell was being cast on him and his head began to swim.

Nwella slowly dropped to her knees as she drew in a deep breath, smelling her way down his still heaving, breathing body, dripping with sweat. His scent was of earth and of sunlight on skin, and the tip of her nose became wet from a droplet as it rubbed down his skin. Once on her knees she grabbed him with her hands and pressed her left cheek to the skin below his navel, turned her head slowly, and pressed her right cheek to the same spot. Nwella began to sweat and her heart beat faster. She could tell he was getting the right idea. Maybe these humans weren't so different, she thought.

She stroked him with her hands as she rose to her feet. He touched her body as their gaze met. While looking at him again, straight in the eyes without blinking, she let go with her right hand and drew it back. She smacked him as hard as she could with an open hand on his backside and jumped away from him, smiling.

His eyes bloomed wide, and a confused stupor gave way to a warm smile. He crouched slightly, raised his hands in front of him as if ready to attack. His muscles bulged, and he was rigid and looked huge. The deep gasping from his run turned into the rhythmic breathing of excitement, and he slowly stepped toward her.

She matched his steps forward with equal steps backward as

the two developed their own dance, a leap apart. He understood the dance, she thought. They already felt a union. After four such steps, Nwella shrieked with excitement, turned, and ran down the shoreline, in the direction away from where her father was. She ran as fast as she could, and he followed.

He was amazed at her speed and for a moment thought that she was really trying to escape from him until she glanced back at him, flashing a smile. Her body was trim and muscular, and the white sandy soles of her feet taunted him as he followed her with eyes and body, putting full effort into both. She must be a witch.

She felt free and wild with the wind billowing across every inch of her bare skin as she fluemed, filling the air in his path with her sweet, fleshy scent. He would catch her and take her.

As he pursued at a full sprint, his desire to catch her suddenly began to rage within, and a madness of lust compelled him. Just when he thought his heart would burst, she left the hard, wet sand, veered for the water, and dove into the waves. He followed, dove, grabbed her feet, and pulling her toward him, took her waist in his grip. She grabbed him, wrapping herself tightly and engulfing him around the waist with her legs. He held her thighs and stood as she released her arms, her hands clearing her face of water, continuing to the back of her bald head where they stayed as she gripped tighter with her legs and leaned back, flexing the hard muscles of her stomach. Her nipples poised on her round breasts turned rigid from the cool water and warm wind as he walked them both out to the sand. His legs quivering from the chase and their combined weight, he dropped to his knees, lowering her to the hard, wet sand, the salty foam flowing around them. Their breath was heaving in unison from the dead sprint, and their blood was pounding.

Nwella closed her eyes. His strong arms held at the base of her spine as she arched her back and bridged her head into the sand; his body curled over hers. She then gripped him and dug her nails into the back of his arms. Nwella felt like she was in the waves as the motion between them created its rhythm. She indulged herself in what she wished had been an eternity. The surf washed around them, pushing, then pulling their locked bodies against the firm beach. The warm breeze slid between the few gaps of their intertwined forms. Nwella felt a heavy thud that vibrated through her torso, and she lifted her head.

Opening her eyes, she was blinded by hot liquid shooting in her face. She turned away, tried to see again, and everything was red through her burning eyes. She smelled blood and screamed. She pushed away, and the man's severed head was lying next to her, eyes wide and staring. The stump of his neck was pumping blood on her chest and face, and her father was standing over them. Synster was dripping with blood, and one shoulder was laid open, flesh hanging off. He was white as lime, his chest heaving as though he was drowning, and he collapsed on top of them both. Nwella was pinned and squirmed out from under the two blood-soaked men...

"Nwella! Nwella! Have you been listening to a single thing I've said? You've got to stop with your childish action..."

"Stop!" Nwella screamed as loud as she could. "I've had enough of this." Her memories of that day had finally become completely clear. Her resentment surfaced, and she lost control. "The Project is failing, and you know it!" she shrieked. "We'll end up in The Bowels, and everyone who's watched me act superior during the protocols will jeer at me and treat me with contempt. I will be a joke in their talk!" Nwella screamed at him, losing control with the eruption of a building rage.

"Nwella, you little deviant, you don't have th..."

"No! You don't have control over anything!" Nwella was feeling vicious and wanted to hurt him for what he'd done on the beach. "Even your wife goes to that human at the sparring ring!"

Synster first looked at her in surprise and disgust. Then he lashed out with a lightning-fast strike to her face. The impact sent her crashing into the viewer and onto the floor. Spittle erupted from his mouth, "You should never talk...!" Synster stopped. He realized what he'd done. He could lose everything from the consequences. He looked around nervously as if to check if anyone had seen. He realized the threshold shield wasn't working properly and someone might have been able to see in.

It happened so fast that Nwella knew she'd been struck only after she'd hit the floor. Her sprawled figure lay still for a moment. Then she slowly rose to her feet. She knew what this meant. They were done. All her anger seemed gone. As only a

Provenger can, she rejected all emotions in the process of dissociating herself from the dominion of her parents.

Nwella stood erect, stared Synster in the chest, and tried to control her quivering voice. "I am declaring Disinterest in this family. I will be moving myself to the Lofts when there is an available cell. I am older and none will see it as unreasonable."

She'd said it. Synster couldn't believe it. His wife with the sparring human, his daughter leaving him. His world was quickly crumbling.

Chapter 15

Back on EartH

The musty smell of the desert was the first sensation Rick had. Then a thin rain fought for the attention of his senses as he roused from the trauma of a strange day. The sun had just set in Ruin Canyon with just a dim glow in the west, and he woke with the feeling that he'd suffered a horrible nightmare. But he paid little attention to his desire for it to be a bad dream.

As he grew more aware, the light rain slowed to a stop and Rick sat upright. He looked at the tag on his wrist and he knew he was not crazy. Now, the tag looked like a wristwatch but Rick could tell what it was. They must have changed it. It felt the same on his flesh and he couldn't find a way to take it off. Rick leaned back on a rock and wished again he'd just had a bad knock on the head. He hadn't. He thought about the things he needed to do since agreeing to Synster's deal. The issues flooded his mind, the assassinations, the threat to humanity, the danger to his world. Rick vomited a mixture of stomach bile and Provenger water down his chest.

This made him feel a little better in the stomach but left him even more depressed, feeling pitiful, covered in his own mess. He was surprised to find his pack on the ground to his right and pulled it to his lap. He unzipped it and removed a water bottle. He took a swig, swished it around in his mouth, and spat it out. He then pulled out a sweatshirt. Feeling as if he were drunk, he took off the jacket with the vomit and threw it to his left. He put on the sweatshirt and thought about shooting himself in the head. Then he remembered his gun had been destroyed by Synster. He felt remorse over his two favorite guns being destroyed. These would be the first things he'd ask for under their agreement. He'd ask for replacements and more.

Rick knew he wasn't thinking clearly. He was angry and wanted his life back, the normal, boring life where he would work, then retire, then grow old while supporting his son, and eventually die an obscure detail in history. He didn't want to be involved in anything but fading away. This beast Synster the Provenger has got to come back in my lifetime to harvest his meat, he thought. What are the chances?

Rick hadn't realized he'd fallen asleep, waking to the sound of a man yelling at him. Some guy was leaning over him, had him by the shoulders, shaking him, and it was annoying.

"You okay? You okay? I was just across the wash and I couldn't find you. I was zigzagging back and forth in the dark and eventually I found you from over there." The man pointed somewhere into the dark. "I saw you when you were taken and waited all afternoon. I was about to leave when I saw a small light in about the same place where I saw you disappear. I came down as quick as I could. You okay?"

Rick looked at this man and after his eyes cleared, he realized it was Tony with the flat tire, the guy who was following him. Rick rubbed his eyes slowly and held the sides of his head. "What time is it?

"About nine, nine thirty," responded Tony. "I saw the guy take you."

"What day is it? Is it still Friday?"

"Yeah, it's still Friday. Where the hell were you?"

Rick tried to stand but felt stiff and decided to sit for a while longer.

"Would you believe I was on a spaceship orbiting Saturn?"

"I don't know what to believe, but after what I saw that guy do, and you still went over to him; you've got some kind of balls! What happened?"

Rick continued to rub the sides of his head with both hands, still wanting to believe he'd had a bad dream. Slowly Rick took his phone from his pocket, activated the camera app and looked at his recent pictures. His smiling face stared back at him from the screen, a "selfie" he had taken while holding his camera with his outstretched arm, alone in Synster's office. The picture wasn't bad. He was standing in front of a window, the planet Saturn in the background outside. "Yep." He casually showed it to Tony and immediately remembered the tag on his wrist. Shit, he thought, I don't really know what this thing does. It could be monitoring everything we say. If it knows the words that I'm thinking, well, I'm just screwed. The least I can do is try to prevent it from hearing us.

With this thought Rick quickly dug a shallow hole in the loose sand, stuck his wrist in, covered it, and then pulled a medium size rock over it. And there he lay on his side.

Rick was tired and had expected to die numerous times during the last eight hours. He thought about concocting some story for Tony but was just too exhausted. He knew he couldn't pull it off. He needed to tell someone, to show the picture, to confirm for him that he was not insane, to believe him. Tony had already seen his abduction and was already talking about what happened. Rick caved to his weakness.

Rick put his finger to his lips. "Shhh. You're going to think I'm insane. He took me to a ship," pointing up to the sky, "orbiting Saturn, of course," Rick said in a low-toned whisper, but slowly and clearly, "...told me all mankind is a feedlot to be harvested for them to eat, and he wants my help to do it."

Tony looked at the picture. "I don't know if you're fuckin' with me or not, but I know what I saw. That guy took down a mountain lion with his bare hands."

"Knives actually."

"Then he destroyed your guns and both of you disappeared in a circle of light. I've never seen anything like it. I didn't know what to do. I couldn't run off and tell anyone. No one would believe me. So I waited all afternoon 'til now to try to find out what the hell was going on."

Being with a fellow human again made Rick drop all pretenses. "Hey, why the fuck are you following me, anyway?"

"Where did you go? What's going on?" Tony ignored Rick's

question.

"I already told you. They want to eat us."

"Who wants to eat us?"

"The aliens who came here twelve thousand years ago. They started agriculture for us. Gave us grains so we'd be freed from hunting, so we could settle down, specialize and populate Earth, so they could have enough of us to eat!"

"Why don't they just eat cows?"

Rick rolled his eyes and poked him hard in the chest with his free hand. "I asked the same thing! Apparently cows don't explore and settle new places like we do." Rick flopped his head back and sighed. "No ships...something about not being able to grasp a hammer with a hoof."

Tony smiled. "Well, that makes sense." There was a brief silence. Tony stared off into the desert. "I'm going to have to totally rethink my crusade against the NSA."

"Yeah. That's what I said," Rick replied, poking Tony in the chest again. "Kind of."

Rick started to feel a little vulnerable with his wrist buried in the sand and a rock over it, in an indefensible posture. He assumed Tony was a run-of-the-mill militia sort, but then realized he may have been there to do him harm. Or maybe he worked for Synster. Rick just wanted to be alone. If he couldn't have that, then he just wanted another human he could trust. The need overwhelmed him. Tony already knew what was going on because he saw Synster take him, so Rick wasn't telling him anything new. Rick figured that help from Tony was a possibility. Who else would he, alone, be able to convince of the whole alien story? No one. Besides, he was desperate, he was tired, and he wasn't thinking clearly.

"Okay, I get it." Rick started, wanting to define their new relationship before Tony made any confessions of a more sinister nature. "You're an antigovernment type. And you're following me because you figure I work for the government, and you want to know what I'm up to. Well, I'm not up to shit, other than wanting to retire sometime soon. So you can just forget about there being some evil government conspiracy against Joe Citizen. It just isn't there. The government couldn't find its thumb if it was up its own ass. We've got a real problem here, and I could use your help."

Tony gave him a blank stare during his rant and without changing expression said, "Go on."

"If you've got time to follow me all day long, you either don't care about working a real job, or you've already got some resources socked away. Judging from the look of the truck you drive, the rifle on your back, your dandy outdoor gear and nice boots, I'd say money is not a particular problem. Would that be accurate?"

Tony nodded and said, "Well, we all tend to live up to our means."

"So you're well-funded and following me. I don't know what you're planning, but as you can see, we've got bigger fish to fry. Are you on statins by any chance?" Rick asked.

"What?

"Are you on statins?" Rick asked again.

Tony just stared.

"Well, you might want to start," Rick said sarcastically. "I'm gonna forget your stance against me 'cause I understand; I can't stand the government either. Except for my day job, we're probably on the same side."

Tony's blank stare continued.

"What's your deal? What are you up to?" asked Rick. He held his gaze on Tony and waited for his answer.

Tony cracked easier than Rick would have thought. "I have a website under a different name."

How amusing, Rick thought.

"I want you to know I support the Constitution and will fight to support it."

"Me, too. Why were you following me?" Rick asked again.

"I advocate the disruption of government attempts to control our lives...communications, surveillance, healthcare. I have quite a following."

"How do you make a living? Donations?"

"No, family money. But I served in the Army," Tony replied, trying to legitimize himself.

"You live in Mancos, right?" Rick had already checked him out...knew his address, vehicles, and what his house cost.

"Yeah."

"What kind of a network do you have? People, I mean. Can you contact some Army buddies and put together a squad of armed killers?"

"Maybe. What do you have in mind?" Tony was intrigued.

"I'm going to work to earn these assholes' trust; meanwhile, you put your group together. If I can figure out how to get access to their ship and we have a group of committed people, we might be able to figure out a way to stop them. I know it sounds crazy. We'll communicate through dead drops. It'll help keep us from exposing each other. Do you know what that is?"

"Kind of, it's when…"

"Shhh, find a book on tradecraft and read about it. It'll even help you with your antigovernment work." Rick gave him a quick smile and lowered his volume to be as quiet as he could and still make a sound. "The signal location will be the U.S. mailbox outside the Cortez Walmart, a piece of chewing gum on the south side. The drop area will be…"

Rick fished a pen out of his pocket and wrote the drop location on Tony's hand. "Do you know where that is?"

Tony nodded.

"Under it," Rick said. "Check Tuesday, Thursday, and Saturday at 6pm. Follow the instructions you find. Good?"

"Yeah. How many of them are there?" Tony asked.

"Not sure." Rick rolled over to his back and sprawled as if to rest, his tagged arm still in the sand under the rock. "The most I saw at any one time were hundreds; I think this guy said they were millions. But numbers aren't the problem. It's technology; they're way ahead of us." Rick took a long pause and let his mind wander. "But get this. Their women walk around with bare chests."

Tony's eyebrows went up. "Are you sure we really want to kill them?"

They both smiled and Rick replied, "Yeah, I'm sure."

"What did you mean about taking statins? You mean the cholesterol drug?"

"Yeah. Apparently it makes our flesh bad. They don't like the flavors or something. Synster, that's the guy's name, said that we've poisoned ourselves with medication and destroyed their product. Now this is the important part," Rick realized, "they have to succeed, for a while, at least."

"What?"

"Yeah, they have to succeed until we can plan something. If they don't get their quotas covertly, then they will take over to make certain no one takes drugs so they can get our flesh clear. You know, we all live in gulags, concentration camps of the organic."

"Why do they have to be covert at all? Why don't they just take us?"

"This is a business for them. They don't want the expense and problems of the war it would start...civil disruption, people killing each other...or the costs of guarding, feeding, and housing a confined and belligerent mass of condemned humanity. Do you have any idea how badly that kind of stress taints the meat?" Rick said in a grim tone.

"So how do we stop them?"

"I have no idea, but when I figure something out, I'll let you know. Until then, I'll work my end, and you work yours. Get as many men together as possible. Quality is better than quantity. We aren't going to accomplish this by numbers." Rick paused. "You can't tell anyone. First off, no one would believe you, and you have no proof. Second, I think these guys can probably get access to anything on the internet, maybe even over the phone, so use the mail or talk in person." Rick paused again. "No wait...tell them you're training them for a variety of survival scenarios, something you could justify. Train for that and use whatever communication you normally would. But these guys have to be the type that when you get them together for the real thing, they won't back down. Can you find those types?"

"I think so." In the back of Tony's mind the fact that Rick was a fed kept coming up. Normally he'd be very suspicious. But then immediately he remembered what he'd seen. The feds could stage a circle of light, they could stage destroying weapons, alien guy's funky clothing. But how could they stage someone running down and killing a mountain lion. It was all too real. Before he had found Rick, Tony had come across the blood and hair that was left from the lion. He'd seen Synster throw the skinned carcass over his shoulder and carry the guts in the hide like a bag. When they had both disappeared, he had seen the white sphere and then the same thing again when Rick returned. He'd witnessed everything through his spotting scope from the top of the canyon. It had been as though he was standing right there with them. He'd even been sure to closely examine his scope for tampering as he waited all afternoon for Rick to return. Tony knew that what he'd seen was the real thing.

Rick wasn't sure what to do next. Were the plans to be in contact with Tony enough? Could he trust him? Would Tony start talking, and make a fool of himself? There was no way he could know. "Tony, I'll change the dead drop during our first communication," Rick whispered and couldn't think of anything more. His pulse was rapid, but he was exhausted. He just wanted to get home. "Okay, when I take my arm out from under this rock, we can only talk like I was lost and you just found me. You'll help me back up to my Jeep, and we'll talk like we're getting to know each other. You give me your history and I'll give you mine. That way we'll know who we're dealing with and what our skills are. Make sense?"

"Yeah, it does."

"If we definitely need to say anything regarding a plan, we'll have to call a stop to rest and write it down. No talking. Okay?

Tony nodded.

"Here we go." Rick pushed the rock away, removed his arm from the sand, and thanked Tony for letting him rest. He added that they'd better get going and excused himself to call his son. Then Rick remembered he was in the middle of nowhere and there was no cell coverage.

The two talked as if getting to know each other. By the time they climbed the long slope, picked their way up the cliff, and arrived at Rick's Jeep on the mesa top, they did know each other.

Rick only then thought to ask Tony where he was parked. "The other side of the canyon. I've been a lot more careful since the flat tire." If Rick hadn't been so tired, he would have felt sorry for Tony. He had miles of rough walking in the dark, back down into the canyon, across the bottom, and back up the other side before he could roll instead of walk. Rick knew the area pretty well but didn't even know there was a road over there.

"Oh, I almost forgot. Who put you on to me?" Rick inquired.

Tony smiled and stared back at Rick, not sure if he should tell him. "Let's wait a little on that. I don't like to put out too much on a first date."

Rick understood and didn't mind not knowing for now, but he would have to know soon. He'd get it out of him. "Be careful getting back to your truck, Tony." Rick smiled at him, gave him a thumbs up, and wondered if he'd ever see him again.

On his drive down the pine-crowded trail, Rick caught one last look at Tony, through the trees, trying to locate the best spot to descend. He kind of liked him. He wasn't a bad guy, maybe a little misguided.

Sleep again assaulted Rick's mind as he started drowsing behind the wheel. After the third nod, he realized this wouldn't do, and decided to pull over. The adrenalin crash from the abduction was hitting him hard. For hours, it had been pumping, and now all his mind wanted to do was sleep. Wouldn't he feel silly, he thought, having survived an alien abduction, trip to Saturn, the needle probe harassment package, the pain bracelet, and the trip back right into the hands of an antigovernment militiaman, all so he could fall asleep at the wheel to be killed in a rollover. He'd already made it to the land he owned. He pulled to the side of the road, shut the Jeep down, and turned off the lights. He tried Carson on his cell and, to his surprise, he got through.

"Carson, buddy, it's me."

"Dad! You must have had a great hunt being out so late. I was worried sick," replied Carson. "It's past midnight."

"I know. I'm sorry, yeah, I got a big one, as big as they come."

"What, you got a lion?!"

"No, I'm just kidding. I'm coming home empty handed."

"Are you okay? You sound tired. You haven't been drinking have you?"

Rick chuckled. "I wish. No, just a long hunt. I'm okay. But I am tired. I just pulled over at the Primal Estate. I'm gonna take a quick nap in the Jeep. Then I'll be on my way."

"You want me to come out, Dad?"

"No. Thanks, though. But if you don't hear from me in an hour...I'll call when I'm done napping...send out the posse, okay? I've just got to take the edge off."

"All right. I'm gonna go to bed, but I'll have the phone

nearby, so when you call…"

"Thanks, Carson. Bye."

"Bye, Dad."

Rick put down the phone and looked out at his land. His eyes were adjusting, and he had a little help from faint moonlight. He had too much to think about and was too tired to do it. He wouldn't tell Carson, at least not yet. It might be too much for him, and he didn't need the stress. He'd keep it from him for as long as he could.

Rick also decided not share it with any authorities. As he saw it, Synster wouldn't have recruited him if he'd thought Rick's alerting the NSA or any other authority couldn't be managed. If Rick did convince anyone that wasn't part of their plan, they'd probably just kill them and make it look like he'd gone nuts. That's why they pick a mid-level guy, he thought. Rick knew he'd have to do this alone.

Then there was the question of Tony. A nice enough guy; he might tell somebody, he might not, but that wasn't something Rick could have controlled. If Synster had been surveiling them, he'd do something about it. If not, Rick would have to figure out how to manage him. Otherwise, he'd possibly have a group together in case an opportunity presented itself. But Rick doubted it would.

The longer he thought about it, the more Rick doubted he'd be able to do anything with the people Tony put together. The concept was goofy, he thought. Rick recognized his whole encounter with Tony and the way he'd conducted himself had been under the influence of the trauma he'd just experienced. He'd been tortured and stressed in a very foreign place, and even though it hadn't been for that long, only a few hours, it had stressed him enough to influence his judgment.

The question remained. How could he get rid of the Provenger? How could he stop Synster, a superior being, who had superior technology, had been planning this whole thing with supercomputers and advanced biology, and had abilities of surveillance and weaponry beyond anything Rick could ever imagine? Rick rolled down his window and looked out into the trees on the edge of his field that he'd seeded days before.

A magpie landed in a tree right next to the truck and called out. The moon was just coming up, and Rick could discern the distinctive black and white coloring of the feathers. He'd never seen them out at night before. Strange. This bird always plagued Rick, announcing his presence to the world whenever he was hunting. It would sometimes fly in and perch somewhere over his head and scream to all the animals in the area that he was there. This night the bird sat and looked at him, tilting its head to get a better view.

The magpie made him think about the animals of the desert and how they interacted. Sometimes they were enemies, sometimes allies. The magpie made him feel very much more like a member of Earth's animals, rather than a human separated from the others. Rick thought about the cougar that had stalked him. If only I could be so cunning. Then he thought about the one that Synster killed. He hoped it wasn't her, but he suspected otherwise.

Rick looked out over his land. In the distance he could barely see movement along a tree line. First, he thought he saw a tail, then a face, then the whole cat. He believed he saw a mountain lion working the edge of his field not two hundred yards away. It stopped and looked directly at him, and Rick thought of Synster's hunt. Was his mind playing tricks on him? Rick refocused his eyes and looked again. He thought he saw the cat walking into the cover of the trees as sleep overtook him.

Images were suddenly crystal clear, smells formed landscapes filled with life, and sounds revealed the motives of plants and animals alike. Gliding through a forest making no sound, the structure of presence had its own existence. The hunt was not forced and fatigue was blind. Rick was stealth and patience, and silence was the spoor of the ghost. He felt his place. His dream was of existence, not as a man but as an animal of Earth.

"Dad, Dad!" Rick woke to Carson yanking on his sweatshirt. For the second time that night, he'd been ripped away from his peaceful unconsciousness. His heart did a little dance in his chest, and before he could think, he said, "God dammit, boy! You scared the shit out of me!" But Rick had something on his mind that he knew was important. He had to write it down.

"Dad, you okay? I never got a call from you, and I couldn't get through, so I came out."

Rick needed to focus on what he'd seen and couldn't talk. "Carson, go back to the car, I've got to write something down." Rick found the pen in his pocket, grabbed a scrap piece of paper out of the glove compartment, and wrote down four words. *I am the lion.*

Carson drove his father home, helped him into bed, and turned out the light.

Chapter 16

The dEbriEf

"I think that went well," Synster told Streyn as they sat in his office on the science deck. "Rick is a careful man and he won't do anything stupid. You saw how he took a photo of himself with the window in the background? Humans can fake that type of picture, so he didn't take it to prove anything to anyone else. He took it to prove to himself where he'd been, to eliminate the possibility that he'd imagined it, or been fooled in some way. He's smarter than he lets on." Synster had a lot of issues to deal with and was trying to console himself that things would go well. Inside, he was wound tight.

"I hope so," Streyn replied. "He'd better be because with conditions the way they are, we'll barely meet our quotas. I know the third world sample statistics are suitable, but they are still so close to our margins, we have no room for error."

"We'll reach our quotas through harvests from the less developed nations," Synster stated confidently. "And by the time we have reached the optimal sustainable harvest from those nations, we'll get the medical community and the developed nations' governments to correct the errors of the last seventy-five years." Synster, trying to think of ways they'd been lucky, asked, "Can you imagine if the subsequent run of the Algorithm hadn't been done? Can you imagine this Project without the Finishing Protocol? We'd be finished."

Streyn admitted, "What concerns me is that the Algorithm suggested a course of action to serve one purpose, but instead it served to benefit us in a completely different way."

"Continue." Synster was especially interested in Streyn's analysis of the issue, since he was the one who led the Finishing Protocol.

"Well, the Algorithm identified the goal of the Finishing Protocol as making wheat universally available for consumption soon before our harvest in our high population areas. It would allow two full generations' time for wheat to become dominant in these diets, and assure us the carcass fat content we desire. While this was certainly accomplished, one side effect was that the human turned to drugs for the illnesses that resulted, making them inorganic and therefore undesirable. The other side effect was to make wheat available to developing nations, something that wasn't our focus. It is what has saved this project. It was a huge digression. Very disturbing. We can't rely on luck to muddle our way through this Project."

Synster considered the implications of this. Streyn was right. It was a huge digression. The Algorithm had told them to conduct the Finishing Protocol to make wheat more productive to grow, as well as a little more addictive. This would fatten large population groups prior to harvest. It did. But it simultaneously made them sick and subsequently drugged by their doctors. The only large groups left for harvest were in developing countries not part of modern pharmaceutical distribution systems. It would be a longer and more troublesome harvest. This kind of error was very disturbing. Could there be a major flaw with the Algorithm?

Perhaps, Synster thought, there was something they'd missed in the Algorithm's motive. Their method of getting the proper breed of wheat to the humans had been complex and had many risks. They'd had to conduct their intervention covertly. They couldn't just deliver a bag of properly hybridized wheat seed with a sign on it that said "Use this really great stuff!" without raising some suspicion. And they could plant it somewhere and wait for it to be discovered; it couldn't reproduce independently. They had to spoon feed it to the humans so they would think it was their own.

"Streyn, I want to test my thinking of the Finishing Protocol. Give me a concise synopsis of your perspective of the development and execution of this Protocol."

"Certainly." Streyn cleared his throat, reflecting on his own involvement. "As we gradually phased out of gravitational dilation during our arrival, initial scans of the populations indicated that strong cultural influences, even in high population density areas, had prevented the full adoption of wheat products, to the extent that it would limit the optimal fat marbling in those populations during harvest. Since the completion of our phase travel would encompass many years on Earth, we ran the Algorithm with the new information and determined that in post industrialized societies, a reduction in the price of wheat flour would result in its almost universal use by food companies as well as adding to availability for animal feed.

"They would reformulate wheat flour into a large variety of foods tuned specifically to the flavors humans crave most, to which they are most likely to develop addictions. This phenomenon would be strong enough to break the cultural bonds with traditional food choices and render these new products a universally-used commodity among diverse cultures in high-population areas. The best way to reduce its price would be to increase its yield. So the Algorithm's intent was primarily to break culturally-guided food habits by decreasing price by increasing yield. It would serve as a pre-harvest fattening program.

"To that end, in August of 1950, Earth time, I took a team in to begin this project. Since we wanted Kylamity Base anyway as a safe haven for terrestrial Provenger operations, we took corvettes of the First Brigade – my cousin, Ryolf, is their commander – and established the base on the North American continent in the mountains of what is called the State of Idaho. Great hunting up there, by the way.

"From that location, I established Class II contact with scientists Orville Vogel in Pullman, Washington, and Norman Borlaug in Mexico City, Mexico, as selected by the Algorithm. Both were working on methods to advance the productivity of wheat agriculture and appeared to be on the correct path for our needs. Over the next fifteen years, we fed them information that guided development of the strains of wheat we needed to make it a universally, economically desirable product. Vogel contributed the dwarf wheat aspect while Borlaug hybridized Vogel's contribution with his work on the problems farmers were having growing wheat in tropical and sub-tropical environments. You know, drought and diseases."

"Stop!" Synster interrupted. "That's it. Tropical and sub-tropical environments! The location of most developing countries on Earth. If the Algorithm had suggested some scientist working in North America, then the strains we prompted them to develop would have been adapted only to temperate climactic environments, theoretically."

Streyn interjected, "Borlaug was working in North America when he was identified by the Algorithm. He moved to Mexico later, before we got to him. I don't know why the Algorithm didn't see that."

"The only answer would be that the Algorithm was hampered by its information collection during the phase cycle, so it was not as complete as it would have been otherwise. We were making choices and decisions on old information and acting on it at a much later date. Elements had changed between the data collection and your deployment. There were too many confounding variables. We should have run the Algorithm again immediately before we made contact with Borlaug and Vogel, for the best outcome.

"So with the development of highly-productive tropical and sub-tropical adapted wheat, we inadvertently saved the project. If I recall correctly," Synster continued, "so that Borlaug could increase the rate at which he could crossbreed, you suggested he get two crops per year by growing one in northern Mexico then another in the more tropical south. This led to a sub-tropical adapted wheat. Isn't it great how things always seem to work out right?" Synster mused.

"Yes. You know, he didn't initially want to try the double crop per year cycle. He thought that the wheat grain needed more time to rest before it could germinate. Remember how I convinced him?" Streyn asked.

"Yes, that was an amusing story."

"That was an exciting time." Streyn missed it.

"You told me just last week."

"Yes," Streyn realized, feeling a little silly. "For me the incident was years ago."

"We'll have to record our observations of the Algorithm's quirks and assure there are notifications for future runs." Synster paused. "So now we have massive populations in developing countries that would have otherwise yielded little. Now one out of every three at harvest age has the correct body mass index for our quotas. And, for the most part, they haven't been medicated yet. I've reviewed some of the information generated by Earth media. You know what they're attributing the weight gain to in third world regions?"

"With meat and fat being the most expensive foods available, please don't say meat and fat." Streyn winced.

"Meat and fat!" parroted Synster. "It's amazing. Borlaug made wheat cheap and easy for them to grow. They even called it the 'Green Revolution'. They lauded him for saving millions, if not billions, of lives. They gave him the Nobel Peace Prize for providing the world with grain. And when those millions of people augment their traditional diets with flour, what do they think is making them obese? The two major groups that don't cause obesity, meat and fat!" laughed Synster.

"You know," Streyn suggested. "I've had my concerns about these humans being too clever, but I don't think I have much to worry about."

"We shouldn't let those in the third world live too much longer, should we, Streyn?" Synster grinned at him. "Otherwise, all the profit will go to Earth's drug companies and not to us! We'll have to triple our efforts in these affected nations."

"Already working on it," Streyn assured.

Chapter 17

Tony's Purpose

Tony woke quickly from a deep sleep. He'd been up almost all night crossing the entire canyon after walking Rick back to his Jeep.

He was a very different man. Yesterday morning he'd been contemplating the evils of his government socializing medicine, conducting surveillance on its citizens, and possibly assassinating them. Now he was friends with a fed in the very organization he most vilified. Yesterday he'd been plotting against the forces that threatened his Constitution, and now he was plotting against the forces that threatened his planet. Tony didn't consider for a moment that it could all just be a bad dream. He'd spent too much time all yesterday afternoon waiting for something to happen after Rick disappeared. When Rick returned, it was clear confirmation of everything he'd been suspecting.

Tony slowly pulled himself to the side of his bed and sat up. Out the French doors of his bedroom, he could see across hundreds of acres of clearly lit desert scrub. He had three hundred acres along with the house that his father had left him when he died. He'd moved to Mancos two years ago, knowing he would never need to work again, as long as he managed his money well.

His long-time girlfriend from New Jersey refused to come with him, but he decided to leave anyway. His job in Jersey wasn't going anywhere, and he wanted to experience life in the West and enjoy his father's house. At thirty-six, he felt like he might be getting a little old and probably shouldn't be alone. But he was working on that, still trying to get his girlfriend, Rachel, to move out. He was even thinking of proposing.

Tony stood, stretched, and ambled to the kitchen where a cup of coffee was waiting in the machine. He only got one swallow down before the phone rang, and he answered before the second, "Yello."

"Mr. Carrian, I want to talk to you about our agreement. I don't like the way things are going. Did you get anything this week?"

"Aw shit, lady, what the hell are you doing calling me this early in the morning?" Tony asked.

"It's two in the afternoon!"

"Oh, I guess it is." Tony glanced at the clock for the first time since he awoke. "Still, I told you I'd call you if I had anything. And I don't have anything."

"I have an appointment with Government Health Services in a week, and I need something!"

"Well I don't have anything, and you know what?" Tony grew irritated and considered his new relationship with Rick. "I don't think this is going to work out."

"What do you mean, won't work out? We have a deal!" she screeched.

"Yeah, well, the deal isn't working," Tony countered.

"Well, you'd better make it work because the cops might be interested in your anti-government activities, not to mention the fact you've been spying on the NSA."

"Hey, hey, hey…Listen Sarah, you give me one tip about him being…you know what, with promises of more if I do my part, and you come up with nothing. The deal isn't working out. Besides, the way you've been dealing with me, I'm starting to think you're full of shit."

"Mr. Carrian," Sarah said in a suddenly calm voice, "when I get off the phone with you, my next call is going to be to the Montezuma County Sheriff's Office. I'm going to tell them that you told me you have automatic weapons, and that you've been conducting surveillance on one of their citizens without any authority to do so."

"Listen, lady, I didn't tell you anything about weapons, and don't threaten me!" Tony found himself getting angry very quickly. Calm down Tony, he thought. Just get rid of her. He took a deep breath. "Listen, I'll tell you what I have so far, and we end this thing, okay?

"No. I won't agree to that. You tell me what you have first, and then I'll decide whether or not we end it. You owe me. So far, I've got nothing."

"Well, I don't think there is anything to know. Rick lives a pretty clean life, he seems to care well for Carson, and he hasn't seen his girlfriend in months. Now I've got just one bit of detailed information on him, and I'm not going to give it to you unless you swear to leave me alone."

"Okay, I swear," Sarah lied, desperate for some dirt on Rick. "But if you screw with me, I'm going to screw back."

"Whatever." This lie needs to be good Tony thought… "Yesterday morning I went to my favorite breakfast place, and I'm sitting there at the counter. Rick walks in and sits right next to me. Next thing I know we're talking about the weather, some local issues, and he starts telling me about his son. So I see this as an opportunity to get some good intel for you. I lead the conversation a little, and he starts telling me about his cancer and how he's doing well. So I fake like I'm acting surprised and he agrees with me, you know, regarding the trouble getting appointments and rationing and all that, and tells me that although it's a pain in the ass, he's doing what the government is telling him to do. So I'm like, you mean waiting for appointments? And he says, no, he means doing all the treatment."

"Really?"

"Yes, really."

"So what was he having for breakfast?"

"What do you mean what was he having for breakfast? I don't remember what he was having for breakfast."

"So you sat there next to him, having breakfast, and you have no idea what he was having for breakfast."

"I don't know…pancakes. I think he was having pancakes."

"Are you sure?"

"Yeah, I'm sure. It was pancakes."

"Bullshit! Rick would never eat pancakes!"

Tony heard a couple smashing sounds on the other end of the line and then a dial tone. She'd hung up, and she sounded really pissed. Shit. She said her next call would be to the sheriff.

Tony started to panic and thought of the three fully automatic rifles he had in his house, the case of C4 explosive he'd lifted while in the Army, and his two grenades. He knew he'd never told Sarah about them, but that didn't matter. She didn't know he had them, but she was going to report him just to make trouble. He tried to think about what probable cause for a search warrant would be, and wondered how long it would take the sheriff to get one.

Rick had given him his phone number last night, to be used only in case of a dire emergency, and Tony decided this was one. He couldn't have his weapons or explosives taken. They might need them to fight the aliens. And he wasn't going to prison. He wouldn't say anything about the aliens while on the line; this didn't concern them. He justified making the call.

Rick hung up the phone from his call with Tony and couldn't understand why the world was conspiring against him. He'd just spent the last hour trying to calm Tony down while the man ran around the house trying to find a spot to hide his guns. Aliens were going to harvest the human population, his wife was conducting a covert op to undermine his custody of Carson, and his new domestic terrorist partner was panicking that the Sheriff was going to hit his house any minute. Life had taken a turn to the absurd.

Rick thought it very unlikely that Sarah would call anyone. She was always making threats she didn't keep. The stress from his new interplanetary duties, frustration with Carson's situation, and anger with his ex-wife were all brewing inside him. He needed relief. Rick drank and posted to his website for the rest of the day, which is never a good combination, and went to bed early. Maybe he'd wake the next morning to find it had all been a nightmare.

It took about five hours for Tony to calm down. Rick had tried to reason with him. Meanwhile, he'd found a pair of sunglasses, a set of keys, one sock, and two gift cards he'd lost. Simultaneously, he'd located some really great hiding places for his contraband, places he'd never even thought of before. He was amazed how fear had focused his creativity for locating remote crevasses of his home, and secreting weapons in their spaces.

Once calm, he considered the task ahead, putting his army

together. He immediately thought of three like-minded friends that he knew were reliable. Others, he would have more difficulty choosing. He went to his email and began filtering through contacts to get a feel for who might be right. He needed recruits to be unwitting soldiers for a cause no one knew existed. He scheduled training at their local range and even went for a drive to some public land, to check to see if it had potential for additional training. It took his mind off the horrors of what the future might hold.

Chapter 18

TRial by oRdeal

Rick stood before Synster and almost shit himself. He'd spent his Sunday morning in idle thought, waiting for something. He'd wanted to arrive at some profound conclusion about his place in life, discover something that might aid him in his survival. He didn't want to have to deal with work and hadn't taken leave for about eight months. He needed time to think. He'd just completed some major projects and had already spoken to his supervisor about taking some time off. Nothing new had been assigned to him so he phoned his boss in Denver at home, apologized for the Sunday call, and told him he'd like to "take the next two weeks off, if that is at all possible."

After checking schedules, his boss gave him a disgruntled "no problem" but "give me more notice next time." It was a good thing he'd made the call because Rick now had secondary employment.

Carson had left to meet his friends then go to a movie after. Rick had been home alone for about five minutes. He was about to sit down to watch a movie when his eyes went dark. He was back on the Provenger Ship.

Synster immediately noticed him shaking and thought it sufficient. "Did we frighten you?" It was good practice to make Rick think he could be snatched at any moment. It made this human think the Provenger were virtually all-powerful, and that was something that Synster needed.

"It's been a rough weekend, and I was about to sit down and relax." Rick's fear began to turn to annoyance and then to anger. "What the fuck do you think you're doing zapping me out of my own home?" Rick wanted to scream at Synster. But he didn't. Instead, he said, "I think we need to plan these visits better. My son could have seen me vanish."

"No, we saw him leave your house. But I will give you this." Synster tossed Rick a small object, and Rick immediately and deftly stepped to the side, allowing the object to sail right by him with a good two feet of clearance from his body. Synster laughed as it skipped across the floor.

After Rick got his heart out of what felt like his right lung, he also laughed, nervously. Then he stopped but forced a smile. He thought, Oh, isn't this nice. Earthling Rick and alien Synster share a little laugh together! Rick really wanted to kill him.

"Not this time Rick. That was a device that will enable you to signal me. It will only do two things. It will signal me to come to you. I may or may not, depending. And it will signal me that you want to come to the ship. Be aware that the intent of your subsequent actions are being monitored by your tag and will warn me if you have anything but our interests in mind." Synster bluffed. The tag didn't have that capability. "Do you understand?"

"Yes." Rick mustered all the courage he had, walked over to the thumb-drive sized device and picked it up off the floor. "Where does it go?"

"Put it near your tag, and it will find its way in," Synster replied.

While Rick really didn't want to do this, he definitely wanted to feel he might have some kind of control over when and where he'd get zapped across the solar system. He moved it toward the tag, and when it was about an inch away it leapt at the tag and imbedded itself. The tag still looked like a watch; it even kept time. "When do I get this thing off?" Rick asked. His sensation of hatred and fear of it were almost overwhelming.

"When I am reasonably assured you are invested in our relationship to work together to save your species from Managed Collectivization."

"I am committed to that. Can't you hook me up to a polygraph or something, to test me…that I'm committed?"

Synster was enjoying watching him squirm. He knew that the longer Rick felt this anxiety about getting the tag off, the more grateful he'd be when it was finally removed. By that time, he would already have been convinced. "Soon."

Rick was still breathing heavily from his surprise transport but was starting to calm. It had made a big impression on him. To think that he could be removed from anywhere at any moment, that they could see anyone come or go from his house, and that he had the power over immediate life or death, or worse yet, pain; this was terror.

He did have one angle so far. Rick had information from his first visit that the threshold cloak mechanism they used might not work reliably when a tag was around. He'd been clued into that when that gorgeous hunk of flesh called Synster's daughter had come into the office. If that was the case, as long as he had this tag around, he might be able to detect a cloaked Provenger inside his home.

Rick couldn't stop thinking about her.

"Now, we have some business to do. As you can see, we have the ability to bring you here at any moment we desire," bragged Synster. He then thought, If Rick only knew how much of my budget was blown by this little transport stunt, he'd know we could never do this again.

A regular transport wasn't that expensive, but not so with a surveillance assisted transport. It required a number of Provenger scanners diverted from other duties outside of the pre-established cloak mechanism, with improvised cloak modifications to prevent them from being detected, in just the right locations to obtain the necessary information. That all required a huge amount of energy, which necessitated a special request from the committee along with the accompanying fees. The resources and energy for the request needed to be diverted from the general fund, which took resources from each individual Provenger's recreation energy and transport allotments. Synster's first trip to abduct Rick consumed eight percent of his project's energy budget. Creating the standing wave gravitational cocoon and moving the space was what consumed the most energy during any transport. What weight or volume it involved, within reason, had little bearing. But good surveillance and counter surveillance was expensive.

"We need to know you are still committed to saving your world from Managed Collectivization. We have a twofold test to assess your loyalty. Keep in mind, I am currently monitoring your emotions. The amount of stress that you feel while providing us with our proofs will determine whether or not you are cooperative. Do you understand?"

"Yes." Rick's heart raced. A dread began to overwhelm him even as he began to realize now was the time he had to be his best. This bastard was going to ask him to do something, and he was going to have to say he'd do it and mean it. And perhaps, he would have to do it immediately. How committed am I? Then it happened.

Synster touched something on his desk and a panel popped up in front of him. "You need to give us something, and you need to ask something of us."

Rick's heart was racing.

"First, you will designate a family member that we will take, in harvest. You have thirty seconds. Demonstrate to us, Rick, your commitment." Synster stared at him, waiting for the answer.

Rick's head was pounding. He thought back to his Marine Corps days when some terrorists he'd captured told him they'd heard Marines had to kill a member of their family as part of their training. He'd had a rotten night sleep, nothing to eat yet today. And he felt like crap. His stress level was soaring, and he could feel his heartbeat in his extremities. Nothing could make him give up Carson. Maybe this is some kind of test. Maybe what he could ask from them was the promise that they wouldn't harvest the person he designated. No, that's stupid. That's Hollywood shit. They really want somebody, as a test. His parents? A cousin? All his cousins had kids. And they needed his brother.

"Fifteen seconds. Answer or we take your son."

Rick's mind swirled. His thinking would be clear right now if it weren't for Tony's call yesterday, and all the trouble caused by…

"Sarah," Rick said. "Take my wife, my son's mother, Sarah." Rick remembered that Synster didn't know that humans frequently don't like their lawyers. Maybe he didn't track on the whole divorce thing either. Rick took the chance and called her his wife instead of ex-wife. "She would be willing to sacrifice for this cause," Rick lied, "and I would be willing to give her to you, to save Earth from Managed Collectivization."

Synster studied his panel. He seemed to be checking a few

things. "She lives in Denver. Why?"

"She works there." It was an honest statement and Rick hoped he'd buy it. Hopefully any stress he measured would be interpreted consistently with what they'd expect. At any rate, he'd bought some time.

"Done. The order is being given now. She will be dead in ten minutes. You have made the decision." Synster touched a portion of his panel. "Now you must take something from us, and no, it cannot be a weapon of ours. Don't be stupid. It must be something of the Earth." Unknown to Rick, the Provenger considered the taking of an object or receiving of a favor as an overt demonstration of commitment between two parties. The Provenger had seen this process of bonding in their studies of human culture and erroneously thought it carried the same weight.

Rick thought. What an opportunity! Still trying to overcome the mixed feelings about the demise of Sarah, he realized she would no longer be a problem regarding custody over Carson. His mind still racing, Rick then concentrated on what he could do now, for his cause. Then a brilliant idea flashed into his mind.

"When you gave me a tour of the ship, I saw, from a distance, a woman with hair, long hair. She was obviously a human. I choose to take her." And in an attempt to be consistent with the low opinion Synster must have of his primitive species, Rick added, "I have given you my wife, and I will need a replacement."

Synster was shocked. He didn't expect such a request. First, he wasn't even aware that Rick knew of Shainan's existence. That's what happens when you give a tour, he thought. You try to show them things to impress, and they see them. Then Synster reflected on whether she would be available for him to give. After making this show of force and authority, he could not deny Rick's request. It would make him look weak. And even though she was "of the Earth" as Synster had formerly stipulated, she was in their custody and the responsibility of her keeper. He was undecided and was aware of Rick's stare. This human seemed to have quickly turned the tables on him.

"Turn away from me. Face the other direction," Synster commanded, as if speaking to a child.

Rick thought it strange, but he obeyed. He pondered, If he buys all this, it means he is dealing with me as he would deal with a Provenger. This is all very bizarre. He's treating me as if he knows that my customs are the same as his. But they aren't. This whole face away from me thing is weird, too. I think I've caught him off guard.

Synster knew he could deny this request based on some kind of reasoning that he could make sound legitimate, but he allowed himself a few more moments to think. He knew that Shainan's keeper was not being compensated for her and was responsible for her until she died. He'd already been paid for the sleep studies they'd wanted, and they'd been completed. He had no reason to want to keep her. She had been carefully managed and knew nothing of the ship or its operation.

Synster was also aware that Shainan and the fighter, Yootu, had been allowed to see each other. As the science director, he'd approved the visits himself. He knew that the visits were continuing and that they both enjoyed them. Synster began to hatch a plan. He could achieve a number of things simultaneously.

By giving Shainan to Rick, he could demonstrate his power to Rick and incur Rick's obligation. He could simultaneously incur the obligation of Shainan's keeper by alleviating him of her expenses. Why he would ever need this, he had no idea. But that was not his main objective. What Synster really wanted to do was get Yootu off the ship to eliminate Provenger females' access to him. Since Yootu and Shainan had been put together and they had behaved well and enjoyed their visits, they had been promised more. Synster saw his opportunity.

If Yootu was to hear of Shainan's release to Earth, never to see her again, chances are he would become unmanageable. This would put Bryock, Yootu's keeper, in a tough situation, being responsible both for Yootu's behavior and his upkeep. Later, Synster would go to Bryock and propose that Yootu be released to Earth. Synster would tell Rick to take him. Yootu was an idiot anyway, and had been isolated on the ship even more than Shainan. Both of them only spoke their own ancient language. If it was even possible for them, it would take years before they would be able to effectively communicate anything about the Provenger, and by then it would be too late.

If he could accomplish this, then the source of Synster's anger would be removed. Vwannan would never see Yootu again.

She would never again be able to embarrass them. Hopefully, this could be accomplished before any rumors began to circulate.

Without knowing for certain if he could get it done, Synster replied, "And so it is. She will be returning with you. You will be responsible for her. If she raises any suspicion on your planet, under the laws pertaining to this Project, she will be terminated. She speaks an ancient language and you will not be able to communicate with her. You will be expected to complete all your duties while caring for her. She will be briefed by us before she leaves. Do you understand?"

Rick was stunned. How could Synster be so stupid? Then Rick thought about it. Maybe she was an imbecile. Maybe she'd been given a lobotomy or a memory wipe of some kind. He started to regret this request. He was hoping he'd be able to learn something about the Provenger from her, but Synster gave her up so easily he began to doubt he could.

"Yes, I understand," Rick said in a defeated tone, half pretended and half real. "My wife won't be hurt, will she?" he asked with genuine concern.

"She will be dead before she even knows she is being taken. She will be as you were when you are transported, but never wake."

Synster reviewed a few rules with Rick regarding their relationship, what his responsibilities were and what was expected of his behavior. He would be allowed to inform certain people of the Provenger existence, but only to further his operational purposes, and he was to be responsible for their behavior afterward. They would be terminated if they caused problems, and his contract would be reviewed and he could be terminated.

Rick was then asked for his list of those he wanted to exempt from the harvest. He made it as extensive as he could. He included everyone in the town of Cortez, then expanded it to the entire county. Synster would not allow him to include anyone living beyond that. Rick included all of his immediate coworkers and friends who lived elsewhere, and all his immediate and distant family members that Synster would allow him to justify. Rick even surprised himself by naming his divorce lawyer in Denver, not because he liked him but because it would suit Synster's preconception. Rick was glad that he could save so many but felt evil for having named Sarah.

Rick was then put in a separate holding cell that was void of all objects, even a light fixture, and yet the room was still lit. He was tired from the day before and honestly didn't know what was to become of him. He always had to leave open the possibility that he'd said or done something that Synster didn't like, and would be terminated. When the solid door closed behind him, it both looked and felt like all the walls in the room. After pacing around the room for a few minutes, Rick realized he'd lost track of where the door was. He started to get anxious and realized this was not good use of his time. Rick sat, then stretched out on his back in the middle of the floor, and immediately fell asleep.

Something woke him, and he turned his head to the left, toward a sound. Still on the floor, on his back, Rick tried to recover quickly from his deep sleep. He had been exhausted. He opened his eyes as wide as possible as though this would make them work better. He slowly began to focus on a form in front of him. He thought at first he was dreaming. It was the form of a woman. He sat up, then quickly stood, feeling as though he'd been caught snoozing at the office.

This must be her, he realized. I'm still on the ship; this must be her. The door closed behind her, and she looked back for a moment, as if to acknowledge the end of an era. Her movement was slow and confident. Rick hadn't thought about this meeting because he didn't know if it would actually happen. These guys don't waste any time, he thought. He took a better look at her as his eyes fully focused, then said aloud, only half joking, "Good God, I've hit the jackpot."

"Googo-divitdejikbot," she said.

Shainan was beautiful, about five foot ten, standing eye to eye with Rick. The light brown eyes observed him with a cautious but curious confidence. She was not happy; that he could tell. For a moment, Rick thought it possible she might attack him. Her frame was imposing and her figure, covered by a tight white t-shirt and shorts, was near perfection, if there even was such a thing. She had long, thick, auburn hair that was loosely braided, hanging down her left side. It meandered to her waist. Her complexion was a healthy peach, looking like she may have recently been to the beach. Rick wondered where the tan lines might be. He mused, Rick, you're now the proud owner of a twelve-thousand-year-old Paleolithic, twenty-something, red hot super model. How am I going to manage this?

Then, recovering completely from his sleep, in a flash, he remembered Sarah. He saw her when she was a young woman, when he loved her and she loved him. He saw them all together when Carson was just born, playing with their baby in a field of wildflowers that grew near his parent's house. He wanted that time back. He wanted that time back and nothing else. Tears began to form in his eyes as he imagined she might already be dead and any small hope for reconciliation that he might have had was now gone forever. A tear broke from his lower lid and ran down his cheek.

Shainan knew his pain, whatever it was. She could sense his humanness and knew he must be feeling any one of the hundreds of losses she had felt over the last ten seasons. She walked to him, held him, and they grieved together.

Too rooms away from Shainan and Rick, on a slab, lay the body of Sarah, along with four hundred others, the gray matter of their brain scrambled by the action of a focused disruptive energy wave. They were ready for processing. It had only been one hour since Rick had uttered her name.

In that moment of compassion expressed by this person completely unknown to him, Rick's mind cleared. For the first time, he could really think. He knew who he would now have to be. Energy seemed to flow from her, and he felt more human, more of the Earth than he imagined possible. He would relinquish all thoughts of normal life or behaviors, he would be determined to adjust to this situation at all costs to himself or any living thing.

How could he fight them? They seemed all powerful. He recalled the magpie that landed in the tree next to his Jeep. He thought about his hunt and the lion. A predator who is less technologically advanced can overcome, but it has to be more cunning, more patient, and obtain and use as much advantage from its foe as possible. Like the lion, he must not see or be seen; he must be the ghost whose spoor is silence. He must infiltrate the Provenger as deeply as possible, figure out how to gain Synster's trust, and gain as much as possible. It will take time, patience, and deceit. He must consider himself dead from this moment on so he can move forward without fear or compassion for any living thing, like the lion, the ghost. His spoor must be silence. He must let his instinct and intellect guide him, but not his morality. He must be unpredictable. This would be the only way to ultimately save humanity. Be as Earth animalistic as possible, because this is what they are least likely to understand. He devised a plan, simple and adaptable. Their weaknesses must become his weapons.

Chapter 19

YOOtu's last date

Yootu sat calmly in his apartment cell waiting for his visit with Shainan. This time he'd decided he wanted them both to act as if they were home with their tribe. He had it all planned. He braided his hair into two strands on the side of his head and tied them back away from his face, with a strip of cloth he ripped from his clothes. He'd bathed for her and rubbed one of the lemons he'd ordered in his hair to make it smell like Earth, rather than using the colognes the Provenger provided.

He'd also ordered a large fish, and it was laying on the table next to his cooking surface. That would be their meal, but he also would act like he'd just returned with a kill. They would pretend to skin it together, and he would build the imaginary fire bigger to accumulate the ashes to cook in. She would prepare the meat and tell him of all the other foods she had found that day and how she was preparing them. They would talk about the children they would have and the things they would teach them.

Yootu had been thinking about this since her last visit and couldn't get his mind off of it. He'd gone over every detail. He could almost smell the fish cooking and feel her soft skin next to his. She was born before the great flood and remembered the time when the Provenger did not control their lives. Though Yootu had been born after their arrival, he had never cooperated nor followed Provenger ways. Yootu and Shainan were souls of the same spirit.

He'd not had red meat or taken prepared food from the Provenger almost the entire time aboard the Ship, since the time he realized they were eating people. He'd always insisted on meats that he could identify as a species that was non-human. And he always cooked it himself. For this reason, he ate mostly fish, a staple of his people for much of the season anyway.

The Provenger loved their meat in all forms, and accessing variety was not a problem for Yootu. He had even experimented with meats from other solar systems for a short time. He would cook it well, then eat a small portion of it, waiting a day or two. This was the way of his tribe with all new foods. After days of focus on how he felt, he would either continue if he felt well, or stop that food at the slightest sensation that something was off.

One day while experimenting with something new, he had a bad experience. He was cooking a small portion of meat from some unknown animal from some unknown planet. It had been frozen when he put it on the hot surface, and he had turned his back to choose some seasonings he was allowed. When he faced it again, the chunk was trying to crawl across the cooking surface, making a kind of sucking sound that made Yootu feel that it might be in pain. He suspected some of his handlers had provided him with this new kind of meat, knowing he would find it horrifying. He disposed of it quickly and never experimented again. From that point on, he always asked for his food whole, so that he could identify exactly what it was. And he always requested something from Earth. He determined that he was not made, body or mind, for anything foreign to his world.

When Shainan arrived, they would live a day at home as a family. He couldn't recall wanting anything more since he'd been captured, other than to be freed. The knowledge that she would soon arrive had him giddy, like a child, and he began to think that, perhaps, if he could spend it with Shainan, his life might take a turn and mean something. Perhaps the misery he'd endured would be infused with some joy.

Bryock approached one of his observation windows. The look on his face made Yootu snap out of his fairytale and realize where he was. A feeling of dread overcame him. Bryock told Yootu, in his ancient language, that Shainan would not be here to see him. She had been released back to Earth and was gone for the foreseeable future.

Yootu's first reaction was an overwhelming conflict of the rage at his confinement and not having control, combined with immediate joy that she was free. Then, in a moment, he became suspicious that none of it was true. He tried to question Bryock, but he would only repeat what he'd already said. Yootu begged to see her one last time but was repeatedly told by Bryock that she was already gone.

Slowly, waves of emotion, grief then anger then denial, all combined with the frustration of his captivity and hit him with tremendous inertia. A searing heat seemed to develop in the core of his body. In a rage, with his hands clenched before his face and his soul escaping through his screams, he looked at his arms through eyes stuffed with blood and fire. He thought he could see the sweat boiling from his skin. The barbarity in him grew, and he felt he couldn't bear to live. Yootu hurled himself across the room at the unbreakable door of his cell, trying to get to Bryock, hitting it head first with such force that it gave way under his impact. His legs giving out below him, he fell back stumbling and collapsing to his knees. He wanted only death or revenge. In a delirium, his thoughts were of a vow: he would kill the next Provenger he could get his hands on, or die trying.

Yootu looked at the door in front of him as his vision blurred. It was made of a material the Provenger had told him could not be broken. It was bent and bulged outward from his impact. In the center, there was a crack. He fell off his knees and to his back. The trauma to his head sent a searing pain down his spine. He struggled for breath as he stared vacantly at the ceiling. He thought only of his love, of Shainan, as his heart stopped and death took him.

Chapter 20

Shainan Visits Cortez

Rick found himself home again, but this time something was different. Held closely in his arms was Shainan. Back on the Provenger ship, before being shut in the room to wait, Rick had been guaranteed that Shainan would be vaccinated against all modern human diseases to which she would have no prior immunity. Synster had instructed Rick that to prevent the vaccines from adversely effecting her body, she should be kept on a strict diet of whole foods to include only meats and vegetables for at least the next month. Synthetic chemicals, refined carbohydrates, and especially the deleterious proteins found in all forms of wheat could, through various pathways, make the membranes of her body more permeable to the vaccines she'd been given and shock her immune system that was responding to them. A proper diet was critical to prevent potential autoimmune reactions.

Rick was told Shainan would be briefed regarding what was happening. She was to remain at Rick's home until he allowed her to leave. She was to obey him and learn what was appropriate for her behavior. She had already been informed that she was thousands of seasons in the future and that she would not see anyone she knew from her tribe, nor would she see the area in which she had lived. She was told they were all dead and it was all gone. Her life would be very different, and she would have to relearn everything.

What no one knew, human nor Provenger, was that Synster had promised her that Yootu would be following some time afterward, as long as she obeyed the rules she was given. She was ready, she thought, as long as she had a hope that Yootu would be joining her soon. She had no way to fight them; she had learned that. She had only one option, and that was to cooperate and believe.

Rick tried to feel embarrassed and stupid about his crying so that he could stop. He couldn't indulge himself in grief. He'd decided to dispense with all things that did not lead to the destruction of the Provenger. He must be single-minded.

Shainan let go of him, and her arms flopped to her sides. Barnes and Nobelle growled for a moment but then, seeing Rick's calm, walked cautiously over to them both. Shainan hadn't seen a dog in ten years. She'd had many that she'd called her own. She felt they were part of her family and had missed them as much.

On seeing them, she immediately knew she was no longer on the ship. The Provenger hated dogs, all pets, in fact. They didn't understand them; they weren't capable of loving them. Shainan ignored her immediate instinct to remain aloof from them, and she dropped to her knees and held her hands out to be sniffed, eager to greet them. The dogs were cautious at first, smelling the Provenger-made clothing she wore, but they sensed her genuine nature and in a moment moved in to lick her face as she scuffed their necks. She made a breathy panting sound with a heaving chest. She swayed her hips side to side as they moved about each other, playing with them as she had as a child. The dogs were immediately touched with love for her.

Rick wiped the last tear for Sarah from his cheek and stood there looking down on Shainan and his dogs with his mouth slightly open. This wasn't exactly what he'd imagined when he considered the return of the Paleolithic woman. But after witnessing the joy beneath him, it made perfect sense. They both spoke the same language. It was an innate semantic, a language shared by two different species of the planet Earth, two species with a long and ancient history of living and working together. Perhaps she could tell the dogs how to use the toilet, Rick thought, if she even knew herself.

This love-fest between Shainan and his dogs came to an abrupt ending on Shainan's terms. In a moment, she established her dominance over them as she decided their greeting was done. She stood and looked at Rick, directly in his eyes as if she wanted to remember his face forever. She then quickly looked around and spotted the sliding glass door and darted for it. It was evening now, and the subtle reflective glare showed her that the glass was in place. Rick thought she might run through it, but she put her hands out in front of her. They hit the glass as Rick followed up behind her. She began pleading, frantically. She obviously wanted to go outside. Rick could understand that. He reached down, unlatched, and slid the door away.

Shainan ran out into the yard, just past his patio of concrete pavers, and dropped to the ground. She ripped at the poorly kept sod with her hands and came up with fists of grass and soil which she put to her face while she drew in a deep breath. Rick followed her out, closed the door behind him so the dogs wouldn't get out, and watched in amazement from the patio. Then, on her knees in a fetal position, she splayed out her arms as if to try to embrace the earth. She stretched out and rolled over twice, coming to a stop on her face. She was crying and laughing at the same time, and Rick thought it was a good thing he didn't have any close neighbors. She remained that way for about five minutes as Rick let her have her reunion. It was about fifty degrees outside and dark now, and Rick began to grow concerned about her. Then all hell broke loose.

Shainan stopped her sobbing and jumped from the ground, whimpering and talking, obviously nothing of which Rick could understand. Then she began screaming and pulling at her clothes. She tore off her shirt, by pieces, directly from her body, not over her head, and tried to do the same with her shorts, but the fabric was too strong. She fell to the ground as she lowered them down and over her legs. No sooner did she have them in front of her, she began looking around for something, still ranting.

Shainan spotted the concrete pavers lining the patio and leapt for one. She picked it up with a single hand like she was grabbing a small stone, then turned on her clothing with murderous intentions. She knelt in front of her garments, apparently cursing in her language, epithets not spoken on Earth for perhaps ten millennium, and repeatedly plunged the heavy brick into the clothing until it turned into a shallow hole in the ground. Despite the cold, she worked up a sweat.

Rick continued to leave her to it. He realized she might have some issues to work out, but he was beginning to become alarmed. He had an absolutely beautiful naked woman in his back yard, pummeling her clothing into a hole with a large paver, uttering swears in a dead language with all the passion she could muster. Rick found himself glad to be on the sidelines during such an aggressive outburst.

For the second time, he found himself a little fearful of this ancient woman. He wasn't quite sure how the evening would be resolved, but he was pretty sure it wasn't going to be normal. And then there was Carson. What would he tell Carson?

Rick turned toward his house, and there was Carson, standing behind the sliding glass doors with his hands in the pockets of his blue jacket and his mouth hanging open. He was staring at a beautiful naked woman in his back yard using a patio paver to hammer a hole into the ground.

Carson had been out to the movies with his friends. Nothing special was going on afterwards, and despite numerous suggestions and invitations, he decided he'd just get home and go to bed. He wasn't feeling that well, and he was tired. As he walked to the front door, he heard something in the back yard and thought it might be the dogs. He went inside expecting to see his dad at the computer working on his blog while ignoring the dogs who wanted to get in. Carson walked through the kitchen, into the living room, turned left and up to the sliding glass doors to find the dogs on the inside looking out, whining with the occasional bark. He looked past his father to see what he was watching. It was quite a spectacle.

Sometimes his dad surprised him. It was typical of him to have innovative ideas, eccentric interests, and unconventional projects going on. But this time, Carson thought, he really had to hand it to him. He never doubted that his dad had things under control; he just couldn't imagine what the explanation would be. So he stood quietly watching, waiting for it. He thought for a second he might turn and walk away, give him time to straighten things up. But then he thought he'd stick around to see what happened. Besides, whoever this woman was, she was pretty hot.

Carson watched his dad put his head in his hands and slowly massage his temples. He walked slowly to the door and looked up at Carson who asked through the double paned glass, "Should I let the dogs out?"

Rick looked in and threw his hands in the air. "Why not?" Carson slid the door open and gave the command to go through; "Go ahead." They bolted out and surrounded Shainan. She collapsed in exhaustion and grief, lying on the grass. The shepherds huddled near her, plowing their shoulders to the ground and running themselves into her, their way of sharing her pain. Rick and Carson took one last look.

"This might be a stupid question, but is everything okay?" Carson asked. Then added, "Should we leave them out there?"

"Yeah, they'll be fine for a while," responded Rick as he walked in and closed the door. "It's only a two dog night."

Rick walked over to the kitchen, opened the door of the fridge, and took out a bottle of wine. He grabbed a juice glass from the drying rack next to the sink. He poured it to the top and beckoned Carson to have a seat. "Do you want something?"

"I'll have what you're having," Carson replied, joking with a smile.

"Okay, but let's not make a habit of it," Rick replied, much to Carson's surprise. "You're gonna need it."

Rick poured his sixteen-year-old a glass of wine, and they both sat down at the kitchen table. Rick didn't speak for a while. The only sounds were the humming of the refrigerator and the muffled crying female and whining dogs emanating from the back yard.

Rick was wondering how he should start, and he was trying out the order in his head. I'm a spy for aliens. Your mother is dead. We've adopted a cave woman. Humanity is a feed lot. Hmmmm. Maybe start with feed lot; that will put everything else in perspective. Or should I use 'good news, bad news'? What's the good news? It might be the cave woman part, but so far, it didn't appear to be panning out that way.

Rick and Carson talked for a little over an hour, a remarkably short period considering the subjects covered. When it was all over, and Rick had told Carson everything, almost, he couldn't even remember the order in which it came out.

He didn't tell Carson about his mother yet. He thought that would be too much for him. Carson was in disbelief throughout the chat. The two were so absorbed that half-way through their conversation, they finally became aware of a tapping on the sliding glass door and looked up to find a very naked and cold young woman and two dogs who wanted in. Rick brought her in and wrapped her in a bison hide he had over his couch.

Large, luxurious animal skins draped around the house were one of the benefits of being an avid hunter in Colorado. And it seemed especially appropriate for her. She seemed to appreciate it. He told the dogs to lie down in front of the wood stove and motioned for her to take the couch, giving her a few pillows. She seemed more than happy to comply, and she was asleep in minutes.

When the talk continued, so did Carson's skepticism. He suspected some sort of game. Rick's only two proofs were his tag and the woman. The tag looked to Carson like a watch. Rick challenged him to try to get it off his wrist. He couldn't. He had Shainan as proof, but, as Carson pointed out, you could get one of those most anywhere.

"Not one that has hair on her legs and under her arms," Rick replied.

"So she's European. You picked up a tourist at Mesa Verde today, and she's a nudist who loves dogs and hates lawns," Carson quipped. "It's not my birthday," Carson joked again, "so I don't think there is any kind of a themed surprise party." Whatever it was, his dad seemed sincere.

Carson would take him at his word for now but really believed deep down that this whole charade would morph into something realistic in a matter of time. In the end, he expected the whole thing to clear itself up, probably by morning. Carson was growing tired of considering the possibilities and told his dad that he didn't feel well. He wanted to go to bed.

After Carson had gone to his room for the night, Rick woke Shainan, who had fallen fast asleep in the large wooly hide. She was slightly panicked at first but quickly calmed and seemed very happy. Rick tried to take her to the guest bedroom, but she wouldn't leave him. He tried numerous times to explain to her that this would be her room, but she kept talking and appeared to be getting worried.

At some point in their interaction, Shainan smelled the wine on his breath. She saw the glasses on the table and insisted on having some. When Rick produced the bottle to pour a glass, she took it from him with a smile, and holding it in her fist began to drink. Rick stopped her.

"No, no, that's enough." He tried to take it from her, but she wouldn't let go. Rick figured she was just thirsty, but when he offered her water, she declined it, letting him know that she clearly preferred the wine. Rick then realized it was the alcohol that she wanted.

She continued to press him for something. He finally understood that she wanted to know where Carson was. Rick went to his room, woke him, and brought him in. To both their surprise, while holding the bottle in one hand, Shainan parted the enormous bison hide surrounding her and gave Carson a big frontal nudity, engulfing, embrace. Carson, initially annoyed at being woken, was groggy but now thrilled.

Through sign language and pantomime, she communicated that she felt they all needed to sleep together. After dealing with her for about fifteen minutes, Rick could see that Carson was tired, and he acquiesced. After Rick had gotten Shainan into some pajamas, all of them slept the night together in Rick's room. Bison hide wrapped Shainan, Rick, Carson, and Barnes and Nobelle all slept on Rick's king size bed. Best purchase he ever made. The entire night comprised a cacophony of snorting, scratching, and grumbling. The dogs made a little noise, too, but thankfully no sleepwalking.

Chapter 21

BrothEr DavE

At six a.m., the phone started ringing. Rick didn't get up. The answering machine picked up, but no one left a message. The calls continued. Rick was tired and wanted to sleep in. Between all three of them crowding the bed, he hadn't gotten much sleep. He knew Shainan would be adjusting and didn't want to be too hard on her the first night. He let her have her way. But from this point on, he would have to lead. He knew that.

At around six thirty, the dogs were up and had to go out. Rick was surprised but glad they'd slept so late. He dragged himself out of bed. He didn't feel well. Something about his whole life turning upside-down the last few days had unsettled the normalcy he'd wanted for the last ten years of his life. He had a headache.

Rick watched his dogs run around the back yard, and he started to calm. All this stress had made him remember he was a dead man any way things went. He had completely lost control over his destiny, and it seemed to free him. He could do just about anything right now, and it wouldn't matter. Planning for retirement, not an issue anymore. His own health issues, not an issue. Custody of Carson, not an issue. Carson. Actually his health was still an issue. Regardless of what happened to Rick, Carson must live on. He would have to. Rick wouldn't have it any other way.

While Rick was contemplating his vision of the future, Ryvil was planning it. On board the Provenger ship, he had reported to his station for the day and then slipped away. He had obtained temporary use of a Provenger battle gauntlet, a weapon not normally available to the average Provenger. His plan was to transport to Rick's house.

It had taken him days to access the file regarding the location and layout of the home. It was still early in the day on Earth, and he hoped to catch Rick by surprise. He would have to eliminate anyone who saw him. He couldn't risk discovery.

He was running late. Ryvil knew that Rick had been through a lot lately and would be tired. He guessed that he would still be in bed. Ryvil had to keep his presence in Rick's house at under two minutes; otherwise, the Provenger scans would notice, so he had to work fast. He would arrive cloaked, even though he knew Rick might have his tag on him and the cloak might not work. Ryvil knew he might be discovered, but he needed to act now. He was desperate and was running out of time.

Ryvil entered the coordinates, tuned his disruption wave to a needle thin beam, and initiated transport. Ryvil found himself standing in the corner of Rick's bedroom. He knew he needed to work fast.

They were both there, crumpled in numerous layers of pillows and blankets. Under an animal skin was the woman that had been given to Rick, sprawled with her legs sticking out. Next to her was Rick's form under a blanket with a pillow over his head. They were both fast asleep. They probably already had sex, Ryvil thought. That's not good. Go for the chest, he considered. You don't have much time. Ryvil aimed for Rick's torso, high in the chest, and gave the slightest pulse. I can't create too much damage, he thought. It would be too obvious.

After the shot, Ryvil saw movement. Good. A hit. As Ryvil initiated transport back to his ship and only twenty seconds had passed, he heard a bell ringing in the other room and was back on board the Provenger ship.

The phone started ringing again. Rick was standing next to it in the kitchen drinking his coffee. He picked it up. It was David, his brother, the successful one of the family. He was the one who'd always gotten good grades, had become a doctor, and was now with the Department of Health and Human Services, the lead policy advisor for the Department on all things medical. Rick and his brother had a falling out over the government healthcare takeover and hadn't spoken in years. Dave was panicked.

In a matter of about thirty seconds, he told Rick about what had happened to him the night before. It was either real or a dream, as he said, and at the end of it he was instructed to consult with his brother for confirmation. Apparently, the Provenger had anticipated that all humans, upon being released from their abduction experience, would question its veracity. The only way to confirm it would be to check with another person, someone they know and would trust. So now Rick was to be the collaborator.

"So what do you expect me to say, Dave?"

"I want you to tell me I'm losing my mind!" David pleaded.

"No, you aren't," Rick responded, wondering how many of these calls he was going to get now, realizing, almost hoping that his role would be only to act as a reference, advising people that the Provenger were not a figment of their imagination. "They're for real. So is the tag on your wrist." Dave hadn't yet mentioned it, but his silence on the matter confirmed that he had one.

There was continued silence on the other end of the line. Rick understood. He'd been there a few times himself, trying to assimilate this information into his personal form of reality. Everything gets upset; everything has to be reordered. Some beliefs need to be obliterated; some need only slight modification. It starts the moment you hear it and the implications percolate for days after.

Rick was patient. He waited. Then he felt like he was waiting too long.

"Are you still there?" Rick asked.

"Yeah."

"You need me to say it again?"

"Yeah."

"Okay. The Provenger are real. Obviously, I don't know exactly what they told you, but they are here, and more than likely you're going to have to do what they say. I've seen what they're capable of, and we have to cooperate." Rick added this last part, thinking as he spoke that he had no idea who might be listening to this call. He'd better sound on board, he thought. "Every indication is they monitor everything we say."

"They told me that I would have to conform health policy to their guidelines. I've got a list of pharmaceuticals here as long as my arm that they're telling me to recommend as dangerous. They want us to recommend that people stop eating wheat; start eating whole foods, avoid preservatives, artificial sweeteners, and wean themselves off their medications. This is insane! I thought aliens invade and destroy things, not issue dietary guidelines!"

"Yeah, those are Hollywood aliens. Real aliens are very health conscious. A straight-up fight would almost be preferable, if I thought we'd have a chance," Rick added.

"I can't recommend these things. I'll be the laughing stock of D.C. I'll be asked to resign. Then I'll be useless to them." Dave started sounding whiny.

After all Rick had been through, he wasn't in the mood. He had to deal with a patriot whack-job building a private army per his direction, a pain amplifier masquerading as a wristwatch attached to his arm, and a Paleolithic woman in his bed with his son and two dogs. Rick had never let the dogs on the bed! Five years of training down the tubes all because of a drunken Cro-Magnon with a nice smile and an incredible rack. Now, all his brother had to do was make some recommendations that would actually help people, and pass them off as the government's. That was his difficult task. "Yeah Dave, the government recommending things that make sense would immediately make people think aliens have taken over."

"This isn't a joke, Rick!"

"You're right for once. My advice would be to make the recommendations. Then, if your boss tells you to resign, do it. And be glad you have no more responsibility. Hopefully, they won't kill you as long as you keep your mouth shut. You'll be glad to know I put you on my no-kill list."

"You have a no-kill list? I didn't get a no-kill list."

"Believe me, Dave. They've contacted others, and those people are being told to do the same thing. The quicker you come out with the recommendations, the more you'll look like a leader, a maverick…if it's your career you're worried about."

"Dad!" Carson yelled from the other room. "Dad!"

"Carson, I'm on the phone with your uncle Dave. Hold on a

second."

"Dad!" Rick heard Shainan yell.

He threw the phone down, finally letting their tone register in his overburdened mind and knowing something must be wrong. In two strides, Rick was at a sprint and rounded the corner to his bedroom to find Carson on the floor in a fetal position. He was in Shainan's arms, throwing up blood. Shainan looked up. Rick jumped down to him and asked him if he could breathe.

He nodded and said, "Uh-huh."

Rick glanced quickly at Shainan and thanked her with his eyes. He grabbed the phone to call 911 and then stopped. They'd take forever to dispatch an ambulance. Then he'd wait forever for a doctor. Then they'd do something for him that probably wasn't good. He'd have to explain Shainan. What if, he thought, he went to the Provenger for help? Synster had promised him anything he wanted. They could get to the ship immediately. The Provenger medical technology had to be far superior. Before Rick thought much more or could even reflect on the implications, he'd activated the contact on his tag.

"Help is on the way, little man." He whispered in Carson's ear as he and Shainan cradled the boy.

Chapter 22

Red mooN waxiNg

During Bryock's initial panic, the minutes slipped by without account. His surprise with Yootu's charge at the door was only displaced with his amazement at the bulge in it and the crack that ran down its center. This was his facility, and he knew how it was made. The material in this door was supposed to be harder and thicker than anything in Yootu's body, not to mention a steel battering ram. He had obviously been conned by the supplier. He'd make his complaint. He was angry at the thought that all this time the only thing separating him from the possible vengeance of this angry beast was an inferior door not manufactured to specifications.

Then Bryock focused on Yootu. There was little doubt in his mind that he was dead. Such an impact could do little else, even if the door was below grade. Bryock initiated a physiologic scan of Yootu's cell and confirmed his suspicion. Dead.

Bryock had mixed feelings. On the one hand, he was now relieved from having to care for Yootu for the rest of his life, but on the other, he had grown to like and respect the human. Still, he didn't mind getting rid of the costs. The food, energy resources, and rent for the apartment cell were all adding up. And Yootu's sparring revenues had been sliding. Soon they would not have been covering his costs.

Bryock went to his office to cancel the class that was scheduled to view him this period. Thankfully, they hadn't been there to see the spectacle. That age group hadn't yet reached the level where they were allowed to see such a thing. Bryock then called for a disposal crew to make a report and remove the body. He would also make a call to Synster, he thought, and explain what had happened. Perhaps, since this was all a result of Synster's removal of Shainan due to operational needs, there would be funds available to compensate him for his loss. He wanted to get an estimate on the door before he confronted Synster regarding compensation. It was a longshot, but the more expenses he could justify, the more he was likely to get.

Bryock returned to the cell door to find a serial number. He looked through the cell's window to find Yootu standing at his sink washing his face. Bryock's first impulse was to open the door and tell Yootu how relieved he was that the scanner had been wrong, but then he quickly recalled the reason for this whole mess in the first place, and he began to fear Yootu. The skin on his bare scalp tingled. Best keep him isolated; he might still be angry. In fact, I'm certain of it, Bryock thought as he watched Yootu slowly turn his head and glare at him. A chill ran between his shoulder blades.

The class didn't come, and Bryock canceled the disposal crew. He kept Yootu in isolation. He would need to spend the next few days trying to think of a way to get rid of him. He was too unpredictable now. He was too dangerous to even consider sparring appointments and certainly too dangerous to make available to females. Since Synster had been the cause of all these problems, Bryock would press him for a solution. As to the display of violence and the broken door, Bryock would keep that quiet. Should he be allowed to sell Yootu, no one would want a killer.

Chapter 23

The emerGency Recombinant

In ten minutes Rick, Carson, and Shainan were on the Provenger Nation Ship in an examining room. Carson's bleeding had been stabilized, and he was resting comfortably. Shainan had gone berserk and could not be consoled. She had to be sedated by technicians before there was peace. It took four of them to do it. Rick suspected she knew something he didn't but then chalked it up to raw fear. She was secured in an adjacent room.

Rick watched Syrjon closely. He was an old Provenger and appeared to be responsible for the entire physiology unit as they called it. It looked much like an emergency room on Earth, except that is was much cleaner, smelled nice, and had quick service. Syrjon was a solid man of about six feet, and had wrinkles, which was strange, as most Provenger did not. He had rounded features with a nose and ears that looked a little too big for his head. His torso was thick, which seemed to be more from the shrinkage of age than from a weight issue. Rick hadn't seen any fat Provenger and didn't consider Syrjon to be in this club. He walked with a slight limp, which Rick took to be from the standard afflictions of age.

Rick and Carson had been directed to don robes similar to the one in which Rick had found himself during his first unfortunate visit. But this time he felt he was being treated as a patient, not an experiment. Then Syrjon did something that took Rick completely by surprise. He removed a device about the size of a cellphone from a drawer and waved it over Rick's tag. The evil thing released his arm and dropped into Syrjon's palm waiting below.

"You won't be needing this anymore," Syrjon stated.

With surprise apparent in his voice, Rick questioned, "Did Synster say you could take that off? I mean, I'm glad it's off." Rick paused for a moment, looking Syrjon in the eye. "You must know I'm glad it's off. I guess what I'm asking is if you trust me now." Rick felt awkward. *Why am I acting so stupid? I must be under a lot of stress. I certainly needed a good night sleep,* he thought.

"We are going to save your son's life. Would you like us to continue, or are you going to grab me and use me as a hostage for some impromptu and ill-defined plan for revenge? " Syrjon asked, with a smile.

"No, certainly," Rick responded. "I was just surprised."

"Don't worry. You'll get it back. It has your contact chip on it." Syrjon put it on a countertop and looked at Rick. "I am three-hundred and eighty years old, but I assure you that I'm quite capable of defending myself."

Rick looked at him in amazement.

"Have a seat, both of you." Syrjon motioned to a row of four black reclining chairs. "I'm going to need to hook both of you up to some sensors before the Recombinant can be calibrated to know you. This will not hurt. We need these waves to be able to flow from the source to the cap, through all the tissue in your body. We will make you both healthy and effectively young."

Syrjon recovered some wires that looked to be hanging from the back of the chairs and proceeded to attach them with small cushioned clamps to everything on the body that came to an end. After what Rick had been through with his first visit, this provoked considerable anxiety. Carson just appeared embarrassed. After placing the skull cap, the remaining attachments involved all of their fingers, toes, and their penis. Syrjon sensed Rick's apprehension.

"You don't want it to stay old do you?"

"No, sir, thank you," replied Rick.

When it was his turn, Carson had a worried look. He asked, "It won't get smaller, will it...you know, because I'll get younger?"

"I'm not sure," Syrjon responded, almost in anticipation of

the question. He then winked at the boy. He'd studied Earth humor as part of his research on human health. It was a big factor, apparently. "You're already young. The things we repair on older specimens that make them young do not reverse their growth, if that's your concern. The repairs simply eliminate the damage that time and toxicity have inflicted on DNA."

Rick, watching everything, had to remind himself that this being, and all Provenger, considered him food. When he discovered the Provenger would put Carson through a machine that he knew nothing about, he insisted on staying with him. After an initial analysis, Syrjon actually recommended they go through the process together. Syrjon told him it would help with the Recombinant's accuracy of the repairs necessary to eliminate Carson's cancer. Since they were human, having a blood relative present would give the Recombinant an additional frame of reference for the repair of Carson's DNA. He also mentioned to Synster that it would ensure the health and fitness of his chief operative on Earth. Synster had agreed.

Syrjon explained that this was a machine they would both have to walk through for a brief period, after which they would need to recuperate for days, possibly a week. Since Rick was fifty years old and Carson had cancer, as well as a laceration of the lung, their bodies would lose considerable cellular material. This would necessitate the temporary bypass of many of their organs, particularly their kidneys, so they wouldn't be overwhelmed by the waste products. They would be kept alive by Provenger technology that would act as their bodies' filters. Syrjon told Rick that if any of their organs were compromised, they would take what they needed from Shainan. Syrjon assured him this was very unlikely. Rick declined and argued, but was not given an alternative. This all fell under the provisions of the Project, and there was no negotiating.

Syrjon completed his preparations. The attachments were not painful, and Rick could feel what seemed like a small energy vibration through them, mostly where the attachment was fixed to the skin. The sensation seemed to fade as it progressed up the body. Rick was preoccupied with what might happen to poor Shainan. Carson was concerned he might get an erection.

Syrjon read the apprehension on both their faces. "The waves moving through you now are familiarizing our computer with your body, your metabolism, all of your common and unique parameters. When you walk the Recombinant, it will know you and be able to adapt to your body's reaction."

"Will it completely cure Carson's cancer?" Rick wanted to make certain they were getting their intended results.

"Absolutely," responded Syrjon. "Better than that, the second you emerge, both of you will be less likely to get cancer than anyone else on Earth. Now, relax."

Rick wanted to spend this time well. He needed to know things about the Provenger that would help him devise a strategy to defend himself, his family, and maybe Earth, if that was possible. This old guy might divulge something valuable. Rick knew he needed to get him talking, and people talk most about the things that interest them, so Rick knew what to do. He needed to ask the right questions. He also didn't know how much time they had. I'd better get started, he thought.

"Can we talk?" Rick almost begged, "Can I ask you some questions?"

Rick thought he'd start out with what would appear to be self-interest regarding this immediate situation and then work toward information about the Provenger. "How is it that Carson got his cancer?"

Syrjon looked at him for a moment. He had been authorized to answer questions they might have about human health. Syrjon had been briefed regarding some of the issues aggravating the harvest, and he knew that Synster wanted Rick to be educated regarding the true nature of their chronic disease problem. But he also knew he couldn't be too specific. He decided to speak in very general terms.

"Why have you not learned anything from noticing that your species originated in the tropics? You are a warm weather animal, as are we. You would be almost free of chronic disease if only you lived in an environment consistent with what that animal requires."

"Do you mean we need to live in the tropics?" Rick inquired, genuinely believing he should assume he knows nothing.

"You need to create, both inside and out, an environment that comes as close as possible to the one in which your species evolved. By doing this, you give all your processes their best chance at maintaining homeostasis, at living the culture they were born to live. You cannot expect to remain healthy otherwise."

"But some people just have genes that cause them to have a disease. What about genetic predisposition?" Rick inquired, repeating a commonly held belief to see what kind of response he'd get. A conversation about genetics could lead to information regarding flaws of both humans and the Provenger.

"Do you actually think that millions of years of evolution weren't able to identify errors or weaknesses in your genetic makeup? Quite the contrary. Millions of years were spent eliminating weakness to the environment in which you thrived as they popped up. That time was spent adapting you to a specific environmental set, from the surface of your skin to the DNA in your cells. The genetic trait that you think you see giving someone a chronic disease is actually a gene's reaction to an environment that has stretched its adaptability to the limit. The body enters survival mode; it gets desperate. There is always an exception to this, damaged genetic code, for instance, but this situation is the extreme exception."

"But humans have evolved to live in a huge variety of places. Isn't the ability to adapt one of our greatest...adaptations?" Rick asked. Maybe he could get Syrjon to start talking about where the Provenger originated.

"Most organisms have that ability. But if the environment changes too quickly, things will go wrong. The ability of the organism to leverage adaptability is limited. For instance, in your culture you were born and raised to attend backyard barbeques. Imagine how you would do if I invited you to a Provenger dinner party. Would you feel awkward? Would you express yourself, in an attempt to survive the situation, in a way you were meant to behave? Suppose we started tearing into a human corpse roasted on a spit. Would you sip your gin and tonic and make polite conversation?

"I doubt it. You would not behave well by your standards, or ours. In fact, you wouldn't even know what your standards are in that particular situation. You would be completely out of touch with what is normal. If we invited ten of your friends to that same situation, we would get a large variety of behaviors. Some people would get violent, some would act normal, and others would faint.

"In other words, some would appear normal, and others would express opposite extremes. But all those people would be under extreme stress. Your cells and their genes are no different when you put them in an extreme environment. In fact, Rick, you have no idea how similar people are to genes. You commonly hold both people and genes responsible for their decisions, when usually these decisions, in both cases, are made precisely due to the subtle input of the surrounding environment. With people, you call it free will. With genes, you call it epigenetics.

"We have introduced foods to your culture with the intent of purposely pushing these limits of behavior. We wanted you to populate your Earth at a specific rate without advancing your technology too rapidly. To achieve this rate, we needed you to become slightly less productive intellectually and creatively, and not live too long, thereby preventing you from more effectively building on the accomplishments of you predecessors. Wheat served this purpose exquisitely. It is a plant product that you didn't evolve with and is not a human food."

Syrjon checked some readings on his monitor.

"For example, humans were meant to live in a certain range of air temperature. They create that temperature wherever they go by using clothes. They take their environment with them. But if they were to live in the appropriate temperature water, they would certainly die. Your bodies are not designed to deal with the constant influence of water. Imagine the slow and chronic ailments that would follow; follow until death resulted. It would be truly horrific. Your skin would soak and blister, things nurtured from water would begin growing on it, in it. Infections and disorders of all kinds would result.

"This is what is happening inside humans. Your skin needs the environment of air for health. Your intestines also need the environment that your species has evolved with. But we have put wheat in your bellies. We have created a foreign environment. You have not recognized it, and you suffer grievously for it."

While Syrjon was talking, Rick shifted in his seat and slightly raised his hand like he might make a comment. He didn't know how much time he had, and this old-timer just wouldn't let him get a word in.

"You have more foreign cells in your intestine in the form of bacteria than you do in your entire body. If you feed them correctly, you are in symbiosis, and they help you. If you feed them incorrectly, you are fostering an adversarial environment. Kill them with insecticides or antibiotics and you've leveled the greatest city of your metabolic society."

"But when..." Rick tried.

"The body's cells are similar to people in how they survive. They are social. The lone person in your pre-history, living and hunting in isolation, was an anomaly predicated, no doubt, only by some catastrophe. The human cell works in the same manner. Alone it would perish. Working together with other cells, it can be a part of great accomplishments."

"…when the Provenger…"

"When confronted by some new environment that is foreign or less than optimal, the cells have to make decisions. Human DNA is incredibly adaptable in this respect. When confronted with a challenge, the genes will make decisions taking cues from that environment. These decisions lead to action. They make different tools, communicate new terms to the cells and organs around them. Then those cells and organs experience an environmental change and respond accordingly. It creates a cascade effect with multiple feedback loops. They act differently; their culture changes."

"Well, that sounds like adaptation, not disease," replied Rick.

"When pushed to the extreme, it is the process of chronic disease. Keep in mind that the environment we are talking about, your intestines, the digestive system, is the place where you absorb the nutrients that make everything work. Compromise that environment, and you compromise the source material and energy for all other systems. It is the single most important system of your body for ongoing health. Continually demand that your body perform within an adverse environment, and it will start making compromises, mistakes. It will initiate a triage to the detriment of certain organs. Anywhere in this process, a reoccurrence of the old, friendlier environment will return the organism and the cells to their natural, healthy, rational state. They will be allowed to return to what is familiar, where repair and healing becomes easy and crisis management is no longer an imperative. This is accomplished by returning to an original diet that doesn't include anything on the fringes of what is appropriate for the species. It's that simple."

Rick squirmed in his seat and put his finger in the air as if he was going to make an interesting point.

Syrjon gave no quarter. "In the case of your son," Syrjon motioned to Carson, who was hanging on Syrjon's every word, desperately trying to ignore the vibrating sensation of the wire clamped to the organ between his legs, "some cells' DNA became damaged from the antagonism or inflammation caused by this persistent change of environment. Their motivation morphed to self-interest. Now, all they want to do is keep themselves alive."

Syrjon knew they only had a few more minutes in the chairs, and this course of his monologue was now turning toward Rick's son. He'll be more interested now, Syrjon thought, and stop trying to drive the conversation into some subject he can use against the Provenger. "The other systems responsible for noticing this and terminating the self-interested cells are weakened by the same confused culture, as well as the stressful internal environment created by inappropriate foods, deficient nutrient absorption, and other environmental input. It just so happens that one of the main sources of inflammation and the source of preferred food for these cancerous cells is the same: glucose. That is what the starch from our wheat turns into."

I give up, Rick thought. He's on to me.

"Chronic disease is almost always the result of an inappropriate diet for a species. Being based in the digestive system, the immune system always suffers with it. Because the immune system is so unique, and due to the human's genetic individuality as well as a result of past exposures, the reactions across populations are usually different. This is also where the varied diet of humans comes into play. And the process starts out very slowly. This has complicated your ability to identify the problem."

"So how do the Provenger play into all this, and how can we get rid of you?" Rick figured it was time to simply ask his questions, suspecting that Syrjon was already wise to his attempts to gather information.

Syrjon smiled. "As for getting rid of us, Rick, forget about it.

That would be like any of your animals on Earth trying to rid themselves of humans. The trick will be to work with us." Syrjon contemplated the implications of what he'd just said and wondered if Rick really heard him.

Syrjon speculated. If only Rick knew the degree to which he was really working with us, from his first step through the Recombinant to the depths of his soul, he might be encouraged, or he might be horrified. We were lucky to get approval to put him through after Ryvil's botched mission. I must relate this conversation to him. He will be very interested.

Syrjon continued. "The tragedy is that you haven't noticed these effects of chronic disease sooner and managed them yourselves through your diet, the thing creating them."

"I noticed them," Rick insisted.

"Yes, but you were desperate and generally distrustful of people. You were almost forced to make your own decisions. Most do not. Your background as a warrior and an investigator compelled you to eventually rely on your own wits, to take responsibility for yourself and not defer to others when their reasoning or logic was unsound. Any doctor claiming to be able to treat a problem when they admit they don't know the cause of that problem cannot have logic on their side.

"We knew, due to our Algorithm, that the trend of agriculture would perpetuate and eventually dominate human societies. The cultures that adopted it were simply better able to compete, even if they were less healthy. They had ways to survive famine and feed their armies for the conquest of others. Large scale war is difficult to make without large food reserves. Agricultural stores made war possible. It created societies with excess wealth, something for an enemy to covet. Besides, since most of the bad effects of wheat come after the best age to fight and breed, agricultural societies maintained primacy. Your pacifist organizations should be boycotting whole grains, not red meat."

"I was hoping you'd give me something more," Rick confessed.

"Well, if you're referring to chronic illness, there isn't much more. But if you mean you want me to tell you how to dispose of us, I'm afraid that won't happen. I don't generally get to talk to anyone about this," said Syrjon. "It was quite pleasurable, even if you had a mind to pump me for information." Syrjon smiled. "Both of you are done, and we'll proceed to the Recombinant."

The two were unhooked, and Rick helped Carson to his feet. He was still weak from his blood loss not an hour ago. They walked to an adjacent room. It was the size of a small warehouse with a large, circular, tube-like tunnel in the middle, big enough for an elephant to walk through. It had ridges of color-coded tubes running down the sides, its full circumference. Rick thought it looked like a hybrid of a cyclotron and giant undersea tubeworm with an appreciation of the rainbow.

Syrjon approached a panel and started punching codes into a screen. Two beds emerged from the flat wall next to them, and the entrance to the Recombinant appeared in the side of the giant worm. Rick and Carson looked at each other, impressed.

"You will enter and move together counterclockwise. Keep moving, use all your muscles, breathe deeply, flex your abs, wiggle your ears, tighten your sphincter…you get the picture. The more you use it, the more it will be repaired. Don't concern yourselves with your internal organs; they are also working. The idea is to move through the space while the organ is being used. Do not stop. Carson, be gentle on yourself. You've recently stopped bleeding. When you hear a high-pitched tone, move to the door and exit. When you get out, you will feel tired. You will move directly to the beds and lie down. You will be sedated and, shortly afterward, put into a coma and monitored by our life support systems. You will be roused when you are done. Do you understand?"

Rick and Carson nodded eagerly at Syrjon. They were both unusually confident in him. He seemed experienced and discouraged any fears they might have. Rick caught himself feeling happy that Carson might actually be rid of his cancer, and Carson was excited to be healthy again. Just last night he'd felt very weak and was contemplating his death. Now, he was going to be healed by an alien race that, by all appearances, was motivated to help them. His adjustment to this new paradigm was faster and easier than his father's.

"Do you have any questions?"

They looked at each other again and shook their heads. Then Rick actually thought for a moment about work, glad he'd already taken two weeks off. "How long will it take to recover?"

"No more than a week," Syrjon replied.

With that, Rick and Carson moved through the hatch of the Recombinant. They started walking normally but then began to move their arms in all manner of positions. They then mixed in squat thrusts and then twisted their torsos in various positions as they circled counterclockwise through the giant tube. There was a dull, low-toned vibrating sound, but they otherwise didn't feel a thing.

Syrjon made adjustments to the control panel. They were small changes but nonetheless important. Syrjon smiled. He enjoyed his work with Ryvil. Together they would see that the Provenger fulfilled the destiny that was set for them long ago, a destiny much farther reaching than the current, short-sighted resource projects.

Looking at the monitor on his panel, Syrjon watched them, amused by the creativity of their motions, Rick encouraging his son to a great variety of contortions while simultaneously cautioning him against too much. Twisted facial expressions and weird dances engaged the two during their walk.

Syrjon rarely had the opportunity to put beings unfamiliar with the Recombinant through the treatment. But when possible, he always gave them the instructions about movement to see what they would innovate. Those who didn't understand the technology would believe anything, he thought. All they really had to do was walk through it. They could even shuffle if they wanted, as long as they moved. He was getting it all recorded. He and his associates would watch it later for a good laugh.

Streyn entered Synster's office armed with the results of the physiological analysis of Carson's wound.

Synster noted a concerned look on his face and figured their suspicion had been confirmed. Streyn placed the document on his desk and took a seat, knowing that Synster could read his expression.

"How much evidence do we have?" Synster asked.

"Only the nature of the injury. There is a signature of Provenger technology. The tissue laceration has no discernable etiology. So clean it must have been a disruption wave, very narrow. Nothing else that I can think of would have created such a clean effect. I couldn't find any evidence of Ryvil's absence from his schedule that day. If he transported under the recreational energy allotment, there would be no record of the transport if he'd wanted to hide it. There is the mandatory cloak travel mode for Earth right now, so we could identify a cloak during that timeframe, but we'd have to find the exact gauntlet he used. I could initiate a comprehensive search, but I think that might complicate issues regarding this Project. The Nation is already anxious about our progress. Such a search might make it seem like we've lost control. Should I begin?"

"No, not yet. I agree. A search would be bad. I think for now we should assume that Ryvil did this and proceed accordingly. We'll put protocols in place to monitor everything he does or as much of it as we can. Meanwhile, I think we might have another way to deal with this." Synster told him, with Rick in mind, "Let me handle it. Speak to no one about this."

The first time Rick awoke, he immediately looked for Carson and saw him lying on a bed a yard away. He could see he was breathing but asleep. He had no wires or tubes attached to him. He could tell from the folds in the sheet over him and the position he was in that he had moved for himself, as that was how he often slept. Rick then thought to look for Shainan, or for Syrjon to ask about her. He closed his eyes and the exhaustion that he still felt overcame him. He slept again.

Rick dreamed of a cool mountain slope with aspens all around him, swaying in a stiff breeze. He was cold then suddenly warm. The warmth was then soft, with the tenderness of human skin that seemed to melt around him. It was then dark, and he could smell a woman but couldn't recognize the smell. He felt pinned, as with weight on top of him. His uneasiness grew as the weight turned into Nwella, and immediate horror deflated to apprehension as his excitement inflamed to exhilaration. She was on him with her face buried in his neck, her arms and legs surrounding him, crushing any possibility of movement. She leaned back, and he felt her rise in front of him with her breasts bulging from her gown, begging him, her eyes boring through his soul.

"Dad, Dad," Carson shook Rick awake. He was excited and wouldn't leave his father alone.

Rick moved his head side-to-side, trying to make sense of something. As he gained consciousness, Carson rambled on about how good he felt and how he believed the process had worked. Rick was confused and wondered where he was.

"That's great, buddy." He forced a smile. Then he made an effort to conduct his own assessment. First, he felt incredibly well rested. His back didn't appear to hurt as it had for the last twenty years or so, and everything seemed so quiet. Then he realized it was because his ears weren't ringing. Rick raised his arms above his head and stretched, flexing every muscle in his body, turning his head to the extreme left and right, forcing the side of his face into the pillow. It was her. Her scent on the pillow. Rick realized he could smell Nwella on his pillow. He'd noticed the same smell the first time he'd met her. Either he was going crazy, or she had been there. He strained to remember but could not. Then, the dream.

Rick brought himself to a sitting position on his bed. He examined Carson. He looked good. They were still alive, and he felt well. Syrjon was behind a window in another room and looked up at Rick. Seeing him awake, Syrjon moved for the door and walked into the room to welcome back his two human subjects.

"It's nice to see you up. Things went very well," he said with a smile.

"How's Shainan? You didn't need to use her, did you?" Rick asked.

"No, she's fine. She doesn't like to be here, but she's fine."

Thank God, he thought. The family was almost together. "How many days has it been?" Rick asked, concerned about his dogs. He had an automatic waterer for them, but they hadn't eaten since he'd left. Rick knew they could survive perfectly fine for a week without food, as could he, but it wasn't pleasant. They might get loose by digging under the fence.

"It's only been five days. We took you off of life support after day three and let your organs take over. You've been perfectly fine and simply sleeping under mild sedation for the last twenty-four hours or so," Syrjon replied.

"Who were our visitors?" Rick asked.

"Synster stopped by a couple days after the procedure and then Nwella did about twelve hours ago. I believe you are familiar with both? I didn't realize you were conscious. Why do you ask?"

"No reason. Just curious," replied Rick.

Syrjon motioned for Carson and Rick to take a seat on Rick's bed. Syrjon sat on the other.

"Your bodies have been cleared of all advanced glycation end products, and repairs have been made to the telomeres on your DNA strands. Also, any cancer or pre-cancerous cells have been removed from all parts of your bodies. Any distortion from what your genetic composition originally intended has been eliminated. Carson, your cancer is gone, and you are in perfect health. Rick, repairs to the damage of your DNA have been made, and you are now the equivalent of between thirty and thirty-five years old, as best as I can tell. You haven't taken a look at yourself yet, but you'll appear considerably younger over the next few weeks. You'll experience some sloughing of old skin from your body for the next few days, part of a similar process you have been experiencing internally. You will need to do something about your hair. You will no longer be gray; it will grow out its original color now. Obviously that would look strange and draw attention. You might want to shave it off and keep it that way."

Rick stroked his silver beard in disbelief. Though he had gone prematurely gray in his early forties, he'd grown attached to his look. He felt comfortable with it. He knew he looked younger without the facial hair and people never failed to tell him so when he occasionally shaved it off. His hair, he wondered, how would it look when it began to grow? He'd have to either dye it gray or dye it some other color so it wouldn't look like fake gray, but like fake something else. Problem was, he thought, everyone who knows me would never believe that I would dye my hair.

Syrjon completed his brief, advising them that they might have some strange symptoms – headaches, digestive issues – but nothing major.

"Any strange dreams?" Rick asked.

"Not that I know of. But you raise an interesting point. We've experimented with the Recombinant on a variety of species.

Without exception, all have benefitted with no problems, even for the long-term. All have been rendered functionally younger and have lived vastly longer lives than control groups. But we have only rarely used the Recombinant on humans.

"We kept Shainan with us for many years as we recognized some strange occurrences with her because she walked in her sleep. We studied her for years, finding her dreaming very interesting. Provenger do not have dreams the way humans do. We then took a look at some other Earth animals that we had taken as specimens – canine, equine, bovine, corvine, cetacean, cervine, off the surface of my memory – and all did dream. We have not found this trait with any animals we've encountered on other planets.

"We eventually drew a correlation between dream activity and what we call our spectral scan results. They are a broad array of frequencies that emanate only from Earth creatures. I would consider this a major difference and something you ought to be aware of. So if anything strange does happen regarding dreams, let me know." Syrjon knew Rick wouldn't really understand his meaning, but he wanted to plant the seed in Rick's mind that dreams were interesting to him. And he knew Rick wouldn't mention Nwella's visit.

With this final statement by Syrjon, Rick knew that Nwella not only visited him but had sex with him while he slept. While he didn't mind, he felt like he should be upset. Why would she do that? Then the realization came. If they could be food, why couldn't they also be sex toys? Fuck'em then eat'em. Entertainment and a meal. Rick hoped she'd never get to the eating part. One twisted little bitch, he thought.

Chapter 24

ThE mEEting with Tony

Rick had been home with Carson and Shainan for about an hour. It was late afternoon. He had fed the dogs, who had faithfully stuck around for five days. He had just started working on his web site, adding some of the perspectives Syrjon had provided, when he realized he'd missed the first two scheduled signals for Tony. Rick wondered what progress he'd made and knew he had to contact him as soon as possible. It was Friday night, and the next signal could be given Saturday at 6 pm. He could contact him tomorrow.

Rick looked around his living room. Carson was curled up on the couch wrapped in his favorite bison rug, alternately watching three of his favorite shows on TV. Shainan was on the floor playing with the dogs, just glad to be back on Earth again. They were all decompressing.

Rick kept doubting the Recombinant and wanted to see results, still concerned about Carson. Rick walked into his bathroom and examined himself in the mirror. His head and face still had their gray hair, but the skin on his face was tight and had the imperceptibly small pores of a younger man. Not a wrinkle to be seen, almost. He'd had a lot of skin flaking off his face and scrubbed it vigorously when he first got home.

Rick put on a baseball cap, went to the mirror again, and covered his beard with his hands. He looked too young. He felt he might even get carded the next time he went to buy liquor. Fifty years old. He certainly hadn't imagined this kind of benefit that first time he'd been abducted and strapped to the slab on the Provenger ship. At this point, if he could just see them all through this thing and stay alive, he'd be happy.

That evening, the three of them sat down to dinner. Shainan thoroughly enjoyed some salmon from McPhee Reservoir, asparagus, and onions sautéed in a garlic butter sauce. They all ate ravenously, replacing tissue and energy spent from the days with the Provenger. While there, Shainan had refused to eat, either as a kind of protest about being on board or actual inability because she was so upset. Rick was unsure.

Again she insisted on having wine and that they all sleep together. Rick's new, younger body was arousing some stronger feelings. After one look at her getting into bed, Rick wondered how he would manage to steer clear of involvement with her. Then again, maybe he wouldn't. People who don't know better think that stressful circumstances curtail sexual desire. Rick knew otherwise. Stress demands stress relief.

He wanted to suggest the possibilities to her and held her close, spooning her from behind. He reached around her front with one hand and held her high on the ribcage with his forearm. He intertwined his legs with hers. He imagined her accepting his advances, both of them getting out of bed, going to the other room, and making love all night long.

Shainan gently took hold of his hand and moved it off of her. She turned her head toward him. Her lips touched his earlobe and she whispered, sinking her voice and her breath so deep in his ear it made him tremble. "Nen shanista ek net valka Utu shun sheh." She turned away from Rick and grabbed Carson, who was in front of her, pulled him over her, and plunked him in between herself and Rick.

Rick deflated and thought about what he'd heard. The best he could figure, she said, "Maybe later. I have a headache," or "Not if you were the last man on Earth." Or maybe something in between.

Carson, at the moment she was flipping him over her, thought he might get lucky. These prehistoric women were very unpredictable; he'd learned. Then he realized he was being positioned as a speed bump.

The next morning Rick rolled out of bed early, leaving the pile of two dogs, Shainan, and Carson on his bed. This would have to stop soon, perhaps when things got back to normal. When would things ever go back to normal, he wondered? He briefly looked back at them thinking it was just about the best thing he'd ever seen.

He went to the kitchen, started the coffee, and turned on the small TV screen over the desk. He flipped on the news. Had this still been a normal life like the one he'd had weeks ago, he would have been curious about the victims of the hurricanes, earthquakes, floods, and other disasters, such as ships and planes gone missing, that he heard about on the news. But because he didn't have a normal life any more, he saw things differently. What he noticed was that most of the victims of these catastrophes were missing, their bodies having been swept away, consumed by fire, dropped into a crevasse, or just plain gone with no explanations. And he was in the unfortunate position of knowing exactly why. The Provenger.

Most of the catastrophes happened in third world countries. These people were less likely to be on drugs, he thought, whether they were prescription or from the street. Their bodies were those of people who led lives largely untainted by the introduction of chemicals contrived to make them feel better. They either lived healthy lives in their somewhat traditional environment, or they were living under circumstances that prevented them from being subject to the marketing machine, the drug culture, the commercial engine that pumped pharmaceutical products into the near perfection that the human body could be. They didn't have convenience stores that peddled doughnuts and chips and crackers.

How soon would others recognize that people were disappearing? How long would it take before there were whispers, rumors, that something was going on. As long as these harvests happened in the third world, people hearing the news would expect emergency services to be inferior. They would expect people to be missing.

As Rick sipped his coffee and looked out at the morning with the sound of this news in the background, he heard his dogs leaving their new best friend, Shainan. They approached him, tails wagging, and bothered him to go out. He slid the door open and gave them the command. They ran out not knowing if they should play first or poo first, following whatever instinct guided them.

Rick thought of all the humans that might have been contacted by the Provenger and tried to imagine them keeping their secret. Could they tell only those people they needed to and convince them not to tell anyone? How the hell would that work, he wondered? It wouldn't. It wouldn't at all. Some would tell and many would not believe. Some would believe, and they would tell others who would believe. Be they wackos, or people who could be logically convinced, there would be many who would know. How could this all be kept secret? Things would fall apart quickly.

Rick realized that it could not remain a secret for long. It would eventually come out. It would be revealed. Everyone would know. Panic would grow. And then it would start. If the Provenger were as smart as Rick thought they were, they would know all this. They must know what would happen. Rick looked out at his dogs playing in the back yard. He noticed their subtle communication with every movement and gesture, acting and reacting to each other, instantaneously.

If this were the case, then the Provenger must know that they have a window of opportunity, a period where they can collect or "harvest" people and do it without detection. This period would offer them the optimal efficiency they always seemed to be looking for. They could collect without opposition, without resistance. It would cost them less. Once everyone knew or suspected, wouldn't they tighten security? Wouldn't it be tougher to get to them? Rick feared it would. How would the world grow accustomed to people disappearing all around them? They wouldn't. They would panic and fight.

In one of those flashes of realization that should have been there all along, the worst case scenario came alive in Rick's mind. What if the project they were managing was not a single process of creating expansive civilization through agriculture, but instead, was numerous cycles of creating agriculture, then population, then harvesting the vast majority of that population, then destroying that world, then doing it all over again starting from the beginning. A key point would be the number of people they intend to take, Rick thought. They couldn't possibly leave us with our technology and come back in another twelve thousand years. Imagine the progress that we'd make. We'd be a threat to them.

Would they destroy this world when they were done with their harvest? How many times had they already done this? The thought left Rick with only one last big question with many parts. How would he and the ones he cared about survive this cycle? Should his goal be that they, and only they, survive? Should he try to save the world, or should he try to save his world?

Rick got up and walked to the bathroom. In the mirror he saw, once again, a very different man. It was a man not ready to retire, but one with another life in front of him, perhaps a new family and a second chance. Rick reached under the cabinet and removed the set of electric clippers he used to cut Carson's hair. The plastic attachment that cut a half inch length was on the clipper. Rick took it off and threw it back in the bag. He moved the lever forward to allow the closest cut, and he started to shave his scalp. He needed to get the gray off so the new brown growing in wouldn't show a line, just as Syrjon had suggested.

He first shaved his head to the skin with the clippers. Next, he shaved his beard. Rick stepped in the shower and shaved his head and his face clean with a razor. After he had rinsed himself off, stepped out of the stall, and dried himself with a towel, Rick looked up at the mirror. The effect was profound. Not only did he look even younger, but to his horror, being completely bald, he looked like a Provenger. I'd better put on a cap, Rick thought. I don't want to scare the shit out of Shainan.

Rick needed to decide what message he would leave for Tony. If he had followed his original instructions, he'd spent a week identifying and recruiting as many high-quality, reliable individuals as he could, the core of a force that would be able, or at least willing, to fight the Provenger, if that was ever possible. To this prospect, Rick wondered if he'd been insane. He realized that when he first spoke to Tony, he had just been back from his abduction and that he'd been tired and stressed. But now he really began to question his judgment. What had he been thinking?

He was almost afraid of what he might find. He had a small army forming for him, supposedly, and didn't have any idea what form it would take or what he could do with it. The only one of them that even knew the real target was Tony, and all the rest were probably antigovernment, conspiracy-theory wackos. Hell, Rick speculated, when they find out I'm NSA, they might want to kill me. How will they react when they find out who the real target is and what we are really up against? They'll think we're crazy.

Even Tony was suspect. Rick didn't really know him. He seemed like a solid guy, but all he knew was what Tony had told him on their walk out of the canyon. He'd served in combat as an Army Ranger. He'd then completed a degree in political science and wanted to go on to business or law school. At some point, he'd decided to apply to the New Jersey State Police. He'd gone through the extensive application process and cleared their background checks. He was accepted shortly after. He'd started with a class at the academy and after just three weeks had been caught screwing one of his classmates in her room. She happened to be the daughter of one of the officials at the academy. He was sent packing the next day.

That had been the peak of Tony's legitimate career history. From that point on, he'd taken some business classes, started his website exploring the federal government's trashing of the Constitution, then come into some money and moved out west.

It had been Rick's job to figure out how to get through the Provenger technology, or steal it, and use it for some kind of half-baked bum rush suicide mission at their ship. What the fuck was I thinking? Rick shook his head, realizing his stupidity. They couldn't get at the Provenger that way.

Rick left the signal at the designated spot. Tony was right on time and checked it in a surprisingly professional manner. Rick only saw slight surprise on his face as he watched the reflection in the side mirror of his car. He was using a monocular concealed in his fist and held to one eye. He was parked in a busy lot about seventy-five yards to one side. Tony walked to his SUV and drove off in the direction of the drop. Rick watched for other cars leaving at the same time and saw none that looked suspicious. Rick's main concern was not the Provenger; it was anyone that Tony might have recruited or any law enforcement that might be investigating Tony for any missteps he might have made.

At the drop location, Tony would find a note telling him to return immediately to the Walmart to meet in the fabrics section in the store. Rick figured that was one spot where they might be able to notice anyone lingering if they were being followed or surveiled. They needed to talk in person.

Rick waited for Tony to return, again observing nothing suspicious during his arrival back at the parking lot. He watched Tony get out of his SUV and walk directly into the Walmart. He appeared to be alone, and it seemed no one was following him.

Rick got out of the Charger and went inside. He had some food shopping to do before approaching Tony. Let's see, how do I shop for a cave woman who hasn't been to Earth for the last ten years and wants to party, Rick wondered? He already had all the elk, venison, and fish he needed at home. So he was really just there to replace the vegetables that had gone bad in his fridge over the last week and pick up some onions, garlic, tubers, cabbage, and maybe a few tropical fruits as a treat and surprise for her.

As Rick pushed his cart down the aisle, he saw an acquaintance from his gun club up ahead and was going to make polite conversation. But just as they neared the distance that dictates a greeting among friends, the guy looked away and went about his business. Rick wasn't even recognized. He was clean shaven and wore a baseball cap and sunglasses. Even with the cap on, people could tell he was bald underneath. Okay, that's understandable, Rick thought, a little nervous. I must look like a completely different person. Chances are Tony won't recognize me either.

Rick completed his shopping with a stop at the spices section. Most of these will be a real treat for her, Rick thought. After all the food selections were complete, Rick caught himself imagining Shainan's first trip to the grocery store. Except for being outside on his property, she hadn't really been out yet to see this new world. Shainan was about his height and could wear his clothes, but he made an effort to buy her a few women's things, being careful to conceal them in the cart, a little paranoid about people discovering his new live-in.

He rolled through sporting goods to the ammunition section to check prices and then went to find Tony. He was there, a bolt of fabric in his arms, examining a few yards of red velvet. Rick did a casual three-sixty around the isle Tony was in, scanning for anything unusual as well as trying to smell anything that might be a cloaked Provenger. Rick didn't know if he should bring the tag. It could be a listening device. He hated the thing and had left it at home, choosing instead to rely on his senses. He then approached Tony and took off his glasses. "Long time no see," Rick said.

"Where the fuck have you been?" Tony asked in an excited but low tone, recognizing Rick's voice more than anything.

"It's a long story."

"What's with the hairless look?" Tony asked, brazenly reaching up and grabbing the bill of Rick's cap and pulling the hat off. Rick immediately grabbed it from him and casually put it back. "Damn you look young without all that gray shit all over your face."

Taking a cap off is sometimes used as a signal in law enforcement and elsewhere to initiate a team action, and Rick wondered if Tony had done it to see what might happen, if anything, before they started talking. "Yeah, I know. A lot has gone on since the canyon. My son Carson had some serious health issues and a few other developments."

"Is he okay?"

"Yeah, he's fine now, better than ever, actually." Rick changed the subject abruptly. "I need to know your progress. Things are even more complicated now than you might think."

"Well, I've got a half dozen that I've been working on, may get a dozen with more time. I'm not going to give you names for their protection. I've done a lot of thinking about this. I think we need to send these things a message."

"What do you mean a message?" Rick snapped.

"A message that they can't just come down here and do whatever they want."

Rick had a bad feeling about this, what he'd been dreading all along. "Tony, we've got to be very smart about everything we do. You have no idea what their capabilities are. So think carefully. What are you talking about?"

Tony gave a heavy sigh and began, "You know when Lewis and Clark did their expedition in the Louisiana Territory? Well, if the Indians had just killed them, they would have been fine for a long time, the Indians that is. When the next expedition was sent, they should have killed them. And so on and so on. They could have delayed the onslaught of settlers for decades or longer if they'd just had that resolve. Same way with the pilgrims."

"Tony, this is not the same situation. We never know exactly when or where they'll be."

"That's your job. You're supposed to figure out how to make that happen," Tony retorted.

"Yes, I suppose I could, maybe, eventually." Rick saw Tony looking down at his arms.

"Where's that thing you had on you wrist?"

"They took it off. I still have it, but I don't have to wear it. They said if I put it on, I'd be able to take it off on my own, but there's no way I'm putting it on, so I loop it on my belt. I left it at home in case it can hear or record us. These guys can cloak themselves, too, so we have to worry about that."

"You mean like invisible cloak?

"Yeah, invisible."

"Why do you still have the wrist thing? What does it do?" Tony asked about the tag.

"It allows me to call them. Then they either come to me, or I go to them." Rick was regretting the words as he spoke them.

"Well, there you go right there. That's how we can trap them."

"But it's not a matter of killing just a few..." Rick shut his mouth abruptly as a woman rounded the corner, looking at fabrics.

"You know what?" Rick suggested, "We should get out of here. I've got to pay for this stuff," nodding at his cart, "and I'll meet you outside. We can walk and talk."

Tony nodded, and they went separate ways.

After Rick had made it through the checkout line and out to the car, he saw Tony standing by the propane refill cage. Rick packed the groceries in the car and walked over to Tony to continue their conversation. Tony's mood had grown sour. He accused Rick of being soft. Rick accused Tony of being impatient.

Rick realized the relationship could crumble quickly if they stayed on this tack, so he changed the tone. He knew he needed to be useful to Tony, give him something that would seem to help. So he told Tony about the abductions, the natural disasters in the news lately, and told him to get anybody he really cared about,

211

family members and members of the team, on statins as soon as possible. Rick explained that the drug would probably do the least immediate damage to their health, but the effect on the entire body could possibly prevent the Provenger from being able to use any part. It might be enough to prevent them from being harvested.

Tony was grateful for the advice. And he immediately worried about his mother, who had recently stopped taking statins due to some book she'd read. He wondered how he could get her back on them when they made her feel bad.

Rick's conversation with Tony had gone from unproductive to lousy. They parted with that inconclusive and always barren notion of agreeing to disagree. Rick would continue to look for ways to infiltrate, and Tony would continue to build a group of true believers radically dedicated to saving something.

Rick drove home with the weight of too many issues crushing his mood. He still had the issue of Carson's mother to reconcile. He needed to tell him what he'd done, what he'd been forced to do. She hadn't made her usual weekly calls to Carson, and he hadn't said anything about it yet. But Rick knew Carson would probably suggest they call soon. He must have figured she was just neglecting him but would want to call soon, just to see that she was alright. When she was reported missing, an investigation would begin. There was no avoiding that. Rick wondered if he'd better approach the situation first.

As Rick pulled up his driveway, he thought again. He imagined himself as the investigator driving up to the house, knowing that in any missing person's case, with absolutely no leads, the ex-husband would be the prime suspect. Since the Provenger took her, there would be no body. With no body, there would be no time of death. Rick and Carson had been gone on the Provenger ship for almost a week after Rick had given up Sarah as the required family sacrifice. The police would suspect him. There would be interviews. He'd taken leave from work during the period that she'd disappeared. He'd called his boss at the last minute and asked for two weeks! He couldn't show that he wasn't in Denver because he couldn't show that he was anywhere on Earth. No one around town would have seen him for an entire week. This could put him on the top of the suspects list, and he had no alibi. On top of all that, he had a smoking hot Cro-Magnon living with him that had no identification. This quick assessment made Rick realize he couldn't tell Carson.

If his son knew the Provenger had taken his mother, it would be very difficult for him to carry off a series of believable answers to an investigator's questions. Any cop who knew his job would get suspicious. Carson's reactions to his mother missing needed to be genuine. Suspicion of murder was the last thing Rick needed.

He lingered on that thought. Rick had murdered her as much as if he'd pulled the trigger himself. He began to wonder if even he would be able to squirm out of an interrogation. No, they could not draw any suspicion. Instead, he and Carson needed to get their story straight; in Carson's case, for the benefit of school officials or friends inquiring as to his whereabouts. He would brief Carson to say that he had been sick, which he had, that he'd stayed home for the week, and that his Dad had the flu and forgot to call the school. His father had been with him the whole time. The lie, in this fashion, would be easier. They should probably hide Shainan in the basement. The only problem was, they didn't have one. The horror.

Chapter 25

Nwella and Rick

After two weeks, Rick had finally gotten Shainan into her own bedroom, along with the dogs. Not so coincidentally this was also the first night he'd been able to keep her from drinking. He'd hidden the four bottles of wine he had left in the garage and was able to convince her there weren't any more. He felt bad for her. She seemed to know exactly what she was doing when she started drinking. Rick figured they had some kind of alcohol in her time because she'd immediately recognized the smell of it on his breath. From that point on, she'd wanted it.

Rick feared it might become a problem. Whenever she started drinking, she didn't seem to stop until it was gone. She seemed to have no control. With the first sip, any resistance to drinking more was gone. He hoped it was merely an adjustment. Although she was very happy to be back on Earth, she seemed very sad or lonely, or both. She was friendly but somehow distant, tough to assess with the language barrier between them.

Rick wondered what the term for "high maintenance" was in Shainan's ancient language. That night she had insisted they build a large wood fire outside. She found an almost flat rock, put it in the fire, and covered it with coals. Then she took one of Rick's elk steaks, laid it on top of the coals, and then put more coals and ash on top. After about ten minutes, she fished it out with a fork, brushed off the chunks, cut it into portions, and served it to Rick and Carson. Out of curiosity, he tasted it first without any seasoning. To Rick's surprise, it was good, perfectly cooked, but it did need salt. It wasn't burnt anywhere. When Rick tried to brush some small bits of black charcoal off, Shainan stopped him and motioned for him to eat it. Hesitant at first, he popped a chunk of meat in his mouth. The charcoal had no flavor, was crunchy, and quickly dissolved. It wasn't at all unpleasant, completely not worth the effort to brush off the small pieces. When Rick added salt, the flavors of the steak exploded. It was one of the best he'd ever had. The ash added a flavor he'd never experienced.

He realized that a people with limited tools or continually on the move must have cooked this way, probably for hundreds of thousands of years. It beat holding the meat over the fire with a stick, and a grill wasn't necessary. Rick wondered why he hadn't been cooking that way all along. You needed nothing but the meat and the coals and hot ash.

After dinner, Rick got on the internet and searched the nutrient content of wood ash. Most of the sites he found were related to putting ash on gardens, not on food, with the exception of some high end restaurants. But the nutrients in ash made perfect sense. Wood ash was loaded with calcium, and many of the trace minerals needed for cellular metabolism were there: potassium, magnesium, phosphorus, zinc, iron, copper, cobalt, all probably in a form that would be readily absorbed by the human body. According to what he read, ash also enhanced the body's ability to digest and absorb protein. Sulfur, important for proper cholesterol transport, was possibly infused into the meat while cooking, and the small particles of charcoal appear to have the effect of absorbing chemicals that are poisonous to the body.

Flaming, which creates harmful hydrocarbons in grilled meat, didn't occur because the meat was in the ash, making the meat healthier. The only questionable issue was that some warned of heavy metals in the ash. But at most, there seemed to be only the slightest trace amounts, not enough, most sources said, to worry about.

For the next few days, the three of them settled into a routine. One evening, Rick thought it was time and suggested Carson call his mother. Of course, he got no answer. A few days later, they were visited by the Cortez Police as a courtesy, to let them know that Sarah was missing and to ask a few questions. Then the next day, they were contacted by the Denver police and questioned over the phone.

Carson had a rough time with it. He loved his mother, as any son would. After what they'd been through, he feared the worst. He regretted some of the harsh words they had traded and the missed opportunities. When answering questions, Rick and Carson were helpful and stuck to their story. They offered to assist in any way they could and waited for further developments. Rick told Carson that when investigators came to question them in person, they wouldn't make an appointment; they would just show up. If there were two of them instead of one, that meant they considered him a suspect in the disappearance. Rick still didn't tell Carson of his involvement.

Meanwhile, Rick was working on getting Shainan some kind of identity. Because she wouldn't be applying for a driver's license any time soon, that wasn't a priority, but he did need something in case the police arrived to question them. His plan was to introduce her as his second cousin visiting from Armenia. He and Carson had talked it over extensively. "It's a small country but still European to match her looks," Rick explained to Carson. "She's much less likely to run into someone from Armenia." It was a legitimate concern since, even though they lived in a remote area, they had a healthy flow of foreign tourists due to all the national parks in the area and Mesa Verde National Park right there in Cortez. As a final strategy, if they ran into someone from Armenia, they would claim she was deaf.

Rick was halfway through an elaborate plan to have her assume the identity of a dead girl when he realized he should delegate this to the Provenger. Within eight hours, she had a full identity as an Armenian immigrant with a green card and bank account with twelve thousand dollars in it, delivered to him by a messenger from Synster. Through sources at work, he checked the identification. It was all legitimate. The twelve thousand was an interesting number, Rick thought, small enough to not draw too much attention but large enough to be an immigrant's life savings.

Rick was a cosigner on the account. I've just gotten my first cash payment as a collaborator, Rick thought. Now it's official. Then he started thinking about what else he could get and found himself browsing the net for guns, tractor accessories, and the antique muscle car he always wanted.

A little over two weeks had gone by since Rick had left the Provenger Nation Ship and Nwella had raped him while he'd been sedated. She'd been pleased with herself. She'd done something she shouldn't have, just like last time with the wild man on the beach, except a head hadn't rolled this time. She felt like she had finally completed something of which her father had deprived her. She had to admit to herself; she had done it out of spite. But there was another reason.

When she'd met Rick Thompson that first time, something about him had intrigued her. Something about his smell meant freedom. Something of his look was exotic. When she'd gone to check on the progress of Carson and Rick, sent by her father to keep her busy, she'd had no idea what she was about to do. She had merely been going to ascertain their progress and report back. But she'd acted on impulse.

She'd seen through the wild white hair to a face that was strong and young. It seemed to promise her something. Whatever it was, she could not resist. He had been helpless, sedated. Syrjon had left for a distant section of the ship and she knew they were alone, except for the unconscious Carson. She had secured the cloak to that cell so no one would see or walk in. This was a Provenger recovery room, so there were no monitors. Only the viewing room was a danger, and she'd made it secure. She could have her way; she could dominate him and take from him something sacred. The thought excited her.

She was now sitting on a lounge in Observation Deck Beta when she received a message through her com-monitor that she was to report immediately to the science deck. She had been thinking about her triumph over the human and now had this summons. A panic ran through her as she realized how unusual this was. She had never been called to the science deck before in this manner. Her job was now to be the available unwed daughter who had recently declared her separation from the family of the Science Director, Synster the Provenger. She didn't get officially summoned there. She had brought him his meals occasionally of her own accord, when she was still considered his full daughter, but she was not an employee.

Did he know? Her paranoia approached slowly, as if from a distance. When it caught her, she became overwhelmed. If he knew, he would accuse her of being a deviant, and she would become even less than his outcast daughter running occasional errands at his request. And that was the best that could happen. She had already declared her separation from the family. She no longer had the protection that her former status offered.

As the shuttle hurried her toward the Science Section, her angst grew. She was certain as she walked to the threshold of her father's office that her time, even as an outcast of the family, was over. Things would now get worse. She entered the office prepared to accept her fate.

Synster looked at Nwella with disappointment. She had so much promise. Her sexual deviance on Earth ten years ago had been excusable, barely. And he'd forgiven her after her prompt action to save him from bleeding to death. Even though it had been her scream that day that distracted him during the hunt, he blamed himself for the injury. He had glanced away from the lion for only a moment. That was enough to give her the advantage to inflict a grievous wound. He should not have allowed the distraction.

And even if he'd known the encounter with the wild man was by her provocation in pursuit of adventure, he would have killed the nasty devil anyway. That day was so unfortunate. Synster felt he still owed her something.

"I've called you here to request that you act as agent for me in regards to contact with my primary human operatives. I'm heavily involved in the Harvest and ensuring that the Algorithm is regularly aligned with events unfolding on Earth. This will give you something to do, keep you involved with our progress. It may lead to employment in a field superior to where you're headed now."

Nwella bristled at his last comment. They both knew she was headed nowhere. She was angered by this expression of disappointment and his power to dispense favor on the unworthy. She now felt even more isolated. But her anger was tempered by her relief that she was not there to be disciplined. He must not know that she had slept with the human; otherwise, he would not have given her a role involving more interaction with Rick. How interesting. How relieving, she thought.

"What would you have me do, Father?" Nwella asked innocently. "Are you sure I'm qualified?"

"Nwella, I've been talking with you about this Project since it started. You know exactly what we need to do and how to get it done. Despite your little stunt in this office with Rick Thompson, I know you were just trying to irritate me, and you succeeded. So we're done with that now." He paused as if to let the words sink in. "I know you are done with that," Synster added.

The problem was that Nwella was not done. She had only started. "Alright, Father. I will do it."

"I need you to handle the following people." Synster handed her a list. She looked at it and immediately saw Rick's name at the top. She didn't look any further. How sweet, she thought. In her mind, all kinds of twisted thoughts mingled with weak notions of her official duties.

"Linked to each name is a summary of their specific missions and overall goals. I will, of course, be keeping track of their progress, but I want you to handle their intermittent contact. Do you think you can do that?"

Nwella looked at him. She didn't know if she had acquired some kind of exotic virus, had some strange genetic mutation, or was just plain twisted. What prevented him from understanding her state of mind? She had divorced herself of all concern for his project. She was essentially an outcast among her own people. Had he lost his mind asking her to handle these humans for him? Was he still clinging to some ill-conceived hope that he had not completely severed their relationship with his assault on her? One of them had gone mad, and she wasn't sure which one it was.

"I think I will be able to handle it very well," Nwella replied confidently with her sweetest daughter voice. "You have my guarantee."

"Excellent. This will free me of much of the concern I've had with these individuals. I believe they are all convinced to cooperate and remain fully committed."

"This will require regular transport to Earth," Nwella clarified, trying to sound responsible. "Am I to assume the funds for this are available through the Project account?"

"Yes, they are. That is not a problem."

"Very well. I shall return to my quarters and begin studying their histories. Am I dismissed?"

"Yes," Synster replied. "Report to me at the standard interval. And Nwella, thank you."

She nodded at him and exited. She felt the smallest twinge of remorse because of the way he said "thank you." But she knew he said it because he was glad to get rid of the duties, not because he appreciated her. If he only knew what she would do with her new assigned duties, he'd probably kill her in a rage.

The evening was cool but not cold, and Rick was sitting by the fire pit designed into the pavers of his patio. He'd put everyone to bed and come outside for a little fresh air. He needed to think and to listen to the sounds of the night before turning in. Nwella arrived, cloaked, around the side of the house, and moved slowly and silently to the back of Rick's patio. She didn't expect any interactions with humans, so she was still wearing her public gown, rather than the standard, ugly gray operational clothing. She looked around quickly for the dogs and, not seeing them, moved closer, studying as an anthropologist might observe a primitive tribe.

He looked so much younger now without the hair, though he'd lost some of the wild look that she admired. If he would take that silly looking hat off, he would almost look like a Provenger, except for his smaller stature. Both times she'd seen him he hadn't been standing. The first time he'd been sitting. The second time, of course, he'd been on his back. She wanted to see him stand. She walked around him curiously, hoping he'd do something, but he just kept staring off into space. For a moment, he raised his head, as though he'd thought of something and might get up, but then settled back down again. She circled silently to his side, sat on a wall bordering the patio, and waited.

Rick had been deep in thought, trying to calm himself from all the issues coursing through his head. If he failed in some way, he'd never forgive himself for the destruction that would follow, either to his small family, his friends, or the world in general. His biggest problem was that he couldn't bring himself to define what failure or success would actually be. Obviously, the greatest failure would be him and Carson on a slab with the Provenger's damned pain machine hooked up while being eviscerated. That was the main thing he was trying to avoid. But obviously, preventing that was not the most ambitious of his goals. Rick knew he had to stop thinking about it. It would drive him insane.

He was just about to go inside, make sure Shainan was really in bed and wasn't up looking for wine, when he realized he wasn't alone. And he knew exactly who he wasn't alone with. He could smell her. She had either gone upwind of him on purpose or by mistake. Either way, he was struck with fear. He knew he couldn't react. His first idea was to try to get some kind of revenge, to kill. For once, he had an advantage. He knew she was there while she believed herself to be concealed. Then he realized a better way to use his advantage. He spent no more than a moment considering this ruse and jumped into it.

"Nwella," Rick said aloud with the most passion he could muster. He waited.

Nwella's mind raced. She was fairly certain he hadn't seen her. She'd scanned him for the tag he had that might disrupt her cloak, and it seemed to be absent. She was sure the cloak had stayed intact. She'd been completely silent. While searching in vain for a response, she was completely off balance.

"I think I love you, Nwella," Rick continued, again with all his heart, punctuating the profession with a woeful look toward the heavens. That should twist her up a little, he thought. I have no idea where I'm going with this, but it's better than doing nothing.

Nwella was immediately relieved as she realized that he'd been thinking aloud. She was simultaneously thankful she hadn't replied. She was about to. Her mouth was open, but no sound was there. What a catastrophe that would have been. Then she thought about how she could use this to her advantage. This human had just professed his love. This sounded like something from samples of the great human literature she browsed with the considerable free time she'd had since they arrived. Maybe this could be another version of her run on the beach with the wild man. She thought about how free she'd felt, how warm and wild that day had been, until it ended so badly.

With that thought, she started feeling warm considering the possibilities right here, now. Could she take him again? Would he have her, here, of his own accord? She thought he might. Had this been what she came for?

Getting caught was now a greater concern. This was not a trip for adventure and she was here on Project funds. Her motions and location could be tracked, though it was unlikely. Then there was the family and the dogs. It was late and they were all inside. She looked around. At the far edge of the yard, another building, she believed for the purposes of keeping animals and their feed. She would lead him there. If things didn't work out, she would stun him and figure out a plan from there.

Come on, you little flesh-eating bitch, Rick thought. What're you gonna do now? Now you think I've fallen for you? You're either going to tuck that away and pull it out some day when you think you can use it, or you'll assume I'm a little more of a whack job than I am. Either way, you'll be wrong. Advantage Rick.

Nwella, still under cloak, walked out in front of Rick about twenty yards away with the barn beyond her at the edge of the yard. While still cloaked, she stepped out of her sandals and slipped out of her gown. What warmth it had provided was now gone, and her skin began to tighten in the cool night temperatures. Her hairless pores tensed with the genetic memory of goose bumps as her body adapted to its exposure to the stony high desert air. She dropped her gauntlet on her gown and stepped out of the mechanism's cloaked perimeter.

She appeared before Rick, wearing nothing but the leisurely breeze that fondled her, standing gracefully on her toes, leg muscles and abdomen flexed, arms slightly separated from her postured torso, elbows and wrists delicately bent, neck straight and slender, chin raised, and eyes wide. It was the pose she'd been taught for seducing and manipulating Provenger males. The low moonlight glared off the left length of her figure, from her bald head to her smooth heal. She presented herself for Rick to take, knowing full well that if he did not act, she would.

Oh shit, Rick thought. The plastic cup of cheap red wine dropped from his hand as he looked upon something that only dreams can conjure. Was it to be a wonderful dream or a nightmare? When she sat on Synster's desk that first day he'd seen her, she looked almost naked and he'd almost lost control. Now she was genuinely naked, and Rick did find himself losing control. He could smell her scent again. The way she was standing, it was obvious what she had in mind. I must be in hell, he thought, again. So much to deal with, so much stress and confusion, and this goddess that I want to hate so badly continues to play with me like a toy.

He found her so attractive, and yet she also appeared evil, with her bare scalp and no eyebrows. It was difficult to get around. It was a strange look. It was exciting. And she appeared so young, probably in her late teens, Rick thought. He realized the absurdity of the statutory rape laws in this situation but still thought it best to cover the issue before things got too serious.

With their Recombinant keeping them looking young, he estimated she was probably sixty years old. He then realized he had absolutely nothing to base this on. His mind raced over the consequences and he figured, what the hell. She raped me first. Now, will I end up making love to her, or will she throw a tag on me? Then I'll wake up on a slab being fileted to the delight of school children. Will she treat me well, or will I get heated up as tomorrow's leftovers?

At this point, Rick didn't care anymore. She was beautiful and she was his if he wanted her, maybe. At that moment, "maybe" was good enough. His rejuvenated body had been trying to deal nobly with Shainan in his bed all these nights, and he was growing tired of restraint. At times, Shainan's beauty and her immediate availability made him feel like he was going to explode. Now Nwella was here, his for the taking, equally as beautiful if not more so, precisely because she was so different, freaky different, glowing in the moonlight.

Looking at things strategically, if he did not respond and she somehow compelled him or punished him, he would relinquish all power. If he did respond, he would also relinquish power but could perhaps make up for that during the sex act. The very act gives the man power, he reasoned. If they became lovers, well, then the door was completely open to whatever opportunities he could arrange, but only if things worked that way with Provenger. Let's face it, he thought, we're treading in uncharted territory.

He slowly rose from his chair and walked toward her. She turned to walk away. Rick could immediately tell she was leading him toward the barn. Good enough place for sex, he thought. Or to kill me and suck the blood from my body, he conceded. She wouldn't go through all this drama to just walk away from me.

That was for sure. Something was going to happen.

She was moving with such poise and elegance. Rick knew she'd probably been trained for all this, no doubt to lure males a lot more intelligent than him to submit to her influence. And she must know she looks good. Damn, Rick thought, mouth slightly agape.

But Rick suddenly realized there was a flaw in her plan. She was unaware that between her and the barn, on the ground in the bone dry desert dust, where the sprinkler didn't reach and no grass grew, were desiccated pieces of the Opuntia Fragilis, or Potato Cactus, an especially nasty succulent whose small fragile sections littered the edge of the yard. They perpetuate and distribute themselves by having their thin and villainous thorns of about an inch long stab into the flesh. They stay there along with a trillion microscopic barbs that don't want to come out and seem to want to inflict pain. The entire cactus pad breaks off from the larger plant and follows the thorn, and the victim, wherever they may go. And with every bump and movement, other additional thorns take root in the flesh. The dogs know where they are and avoid them. They even learn how to carefully pull them off their paws with their teeth; at least, the smart dogs do.

Though completely enraptured, his basic human practicality and compassion took over. "Nwella, don't. Stop! Don't go over there," he said, trying to project a whisper. Rick wasn't sure what to say, as he didn't want to ruin things by giving her the wrong impression. How do you tell a sexy naked alien in mid-seduction that she might step on a cactus? So he didn't. Instead, he added, in another quick whisper, "It's not that I don't want…"

"Eee!" A squeak came from Nwella. To her credit, she continued her graceful waltz toward the barn but with a little less grace, quicker, and with a slight limp. Rick lost her form as it moved out of the moonlight and into the darkness of the outbuilding. He imagined her throwing herself to the ground once she reached the interior, wondering how the hell she was going to save face on this one.

Once inside, he found her reclined, elegantly, in a fresh pile of alfalfa hay, the result of numerous bales broken open, beckoning him with her outspread arms. Rick looked down at her feet, knowing what he would find, but couldn't see in the dim light. Taking in a full draught of the sexual feast before him, he knelt at her feet, held and examined them, and, much to her relief and embarrassment, slowly, carefully, began to pull out the potato cactus.

He could barely see that she had one cactus pad on the bottom of her left foot and a crumpled dried one under the toes on her right. And who knows how many isolated thorns were elsewhere that he couldn't see. It must have been extremely painful, Rick knew. He couldn't take her inside for more light; it would alert the others. Shainan would go berserk. The dogs, because of their natural hatred for the Provenger and Shainan's likely fear or anger, would probably attack Nwella, and Carson would witness an extremely poor example of fatherhood.

Rick took the easy way out. He worked carefully in the dim reflected moonlight, barely able to see. When the large pieces were pulled off and only the deeper thorns remained, he gently blew on her feet, removing the desert dust as best he could.

Rick's hands were hard from his many rigorous outdoor activities and ill-suited to sensing small filaments and thorns in the dark. The mouth, on the other hand, is a remarkable, resilient organ, best suited for and capable of the most delicate work. In the dark, with his lips and tongue, he patiently searched for and found each and every thorn, the large and the small.

He searched the sole of her foot slowly with his lips, around the sides and among the toes. She had soft, delicate, and perfectly-shaped feet. Rick had always been more of a leg man, but this was definitely doing something for him. Once the general location of each thorn was known, he would isolate its location with his tongue and pull it out with his teeth. He never knew foreplay could be so practical.

Nwella was tense at first. This wasn't how she'd intended to seduce him. She wasn't in control. This wasn't her plan. But slowly she relaxed. She stretched out and put her head back, closing her eyes, wriggling her torso to burrow in the hay for warmth. She stretched her hands above her head and swept hay around her.

Nwella could see Rick beginning to shiver in the cool night air. This was a human she could trust. A warmth she'd never felt enveloped her, and caring she'd never known consumed her. An emotion humans called compassion and love overwhelmed her. It had nothing to do with her being just a deviant Provenger. It had everything to do with the seed growing within her, the miraculous product of the passionate rape of an unconscious Rick Thompson, fresh from the regenerative effects of the Recombinant, a machine designed to perfect Provenger DNA. The union that could not happen, the bonding that was never to be, had conceived life in the most unusual of circumstance. The child within her was of the Earth, and all that were of the Earth had souls. And the soul within her womb was powerful, and it was becoming one with her.

Rick and Nwella made love and then talked briefly, then made love again as they spoke of things she hadn't thought possible. Clinging to each other and buried in the warmth of the hay, they shared their heat and their thoughts, fused in body and mind, as though they were two young lovers on the run from angry parents with no one else to trust. With the cold circling beyond them, they shared ideas until the glow of the sun pushed the night away and the reality of worlds colliding called for her to leave. They had talked about the Project, Nwella's impression of humans thousands of years ago, and the troubles her father was having with humans being medicated. They laughed together at Synster, that he had made her Rick's handler.

Rick asked her why she slept with him while he was sedated after the Recombinant. She had no answer; she could not answer. Rick found her to be irresistible, dangerous, and exhilarating. She was a freak, and he could identify with that. He liked it.

As Barnes and Nobelle charged across the lawn for their morning romp, Nwella was in her gravitational bubble, looping back to her cell on the Provenger Nation Ship. She was the first Provenger to have a soul, and she had no idea.

As the dogs ran to the shed, looking for their master, Rick was sitting on a bale, thinking and growing cold. He already missed her warmth. Funny how things work out, he thought. All this hay was just delivered yesterday.

Chapter 26

A very strAnge pArty

It was a Saturday morning and Rick had just come in from some chores. The phone rang and he waited for the machine to pick up. It was Tony.

"Rick, you there? Rick, pick up please..."

"What's going on, you nut?" asked Rick with friendly words and tone while feeling complete irritation, grinding his teeth, enraged that Tony had called him again. "I thought we'd planned to talk later. Doesn't anyone know how to carry on a conversation anymore?" grilled Rick, trying to cryptically convey to Tony without outright calling him an idiot, annoyed with the second breach in their agreed method of contact.

"Rick, my sister...she was in Mexico, they got her... it got her, there was a sinkhole, and I can't reach her. Haven't been able to for days. I'm pretty sure she's gone!" Tony detailed, with a distinctive tone of anger and grief in his voice.

Two days earlier, an entire small town in the Yucatan in Mexico had been swallowed by a collapse of the earth beneath it. Almost no one was recovered. When Rick had seen it on the news, he suspected the Provenger.

"Tony, calm down. I'm sure she's fine," Rick lied. "She'll probably call soon. Keep in mind, there's probably a lot going on down there, and phone lines could be out, towers down."

From sighs and grunts in response to Rick, Tony sounded like he was getting even more wound up.

"Tony, lets meet at the Main Street Brewery. I'll buy and we can talk some things over." Rick decided to throw his clandestine methods out the window this time. Thanks to his relationship with Nwella, he didn't need them anymore.

Rick scheduled the meeting with Tony for later that evening and hung up. He had a long day ahead of him. Rick was going to have some visitors from Washington.

Tony hung up, disappointed again. He hadn't known Rick for long. In fact, the only time he'd really had to get to know him was from their first meeting down in the canyon. The Rick he'd met then was a boiling cauldron of venomous hatred for the Provenger, a guy who'd been put through so much that he could barely hold himself together. What had happened to that energy, that devotion to the cause? Rick had told him about Synster's threats if he didn't cooperate, but they'd agreed that everyone would probably end up getting killed or eaten anyway. Rick seemed to be withdrawing from his original commitment. And Tony's frustration was magnified with the loss of his sister.

Rick is moving too slowly, Tony thought. I need to get him to take action. The longer these Provenger get away with taking people, the bolder their actions will get, the more people they'll take, and the closer we'll get to the end. I must convince Rick that we need to take this to the next level immediately, and maybe even take it public. Get proof somehow, show the world. If everyone is alerted at once, maybe we'd have a fighting chance.

Tony slowly calmed. He thought about his sister and figured he'd better call his mother; she'd probably be worried. As he reached for the phone, it began to ring. He picked it up.

"Tony, its Mom. Have you heard from your sister?"

"No, Ma, but I'm sure she's fine."

"I'm worried, Tony."

"Don't be, Ma. You know things are probably bad there, phone lines down and all..."

"But her cell phone works, she's ca..."

"Ma, you know the towers go to land lines. Those could be out, and the lines could be flooded with other calls. Don't worry. She's gonna be fine. You're gonna get yourself all wound up. You might feel better if you started your anxiety meds again."

"Tony, I already told you I don't need those anymore, I feel fi..."

"Okay, but I'm concerned about your heart. You probably should start taking your Lipitor, Ma."

"I've already told you I don't need it anymore. Cholesterol isn't the issue. Haven't you been reading what I sent you about the Framingham study? What's gotten into you Tony? You sound like a wreck."

"Nothing, Ma. I just want you to be okay," Tony replied.

Mrs. Carrian moved out of defensive mode and back into worry mode. "Let me know first thing when your sister calls. I'm worried sick about her."

"I will, Ma. Love you."

"Love you too, Tony."

"Bye." Tony felt conflicted. If they'd gotten his sister, and if he was killed too, his mother would be devastated. He knew he couldn't think about himself. He needed to think about his sister and his mother, and everyone else who might be taken. He hoped his mother was too old for them to eat.

Tony's attention turned back to Rick again. He would convince him to take some kind of action. If he was worried about the consequences to himself, then they'd work out a plan where Rick wouldn't get exposed. It was just that simple; action had to be taken.

It was 10:00 am and Rick had spoken to Tony not two hours before. He wasn't sure if he'd been able to pacify him. Now, he had to dramatically switch gears. Rick sent Carson out in the Jeep to give Shainan a five-hour tour of the San Juan Range, with orders that under no circumstances was he to allow her contact with anyone, nor bring her back early. Rick would soon host the strangest party he'd ever had.

He caught himself running around the house straightening things. He had the vacuum out, wondering whether or not he should dust the bookshelves in his living room when the reality struck him. He was about to have government bureaucrats snatched from the nation's capital, all bigwigs that he didn't know, except for his brother, who would be among them. Synster was going to grab them and surf them to his living room, where they would be disciplined, brought into the fold, and given their orders. They would be told what government policy they were going to recommend for the foreseeable future.

Who the hell was gonna care what his living room looked like, he wondered? Synster was probably going to scare the shit out of them in some kind of Provenger initiation psycho suite of brainwashing techniques, then send them out with missions. With any luck, Rick wouldn't have to clean feces and vomit off the floor when he was done.

Rick felt foolish for his preparations. It's not as though he needed to decide if he should serve red or white with the pepperoni and cheese appetizer, he thought, joking with himself. He'd just never had people from Washington visit before. With that realization, and the frustration that followed, he opened the sliding glass door and walked outside with the vacuum cleaner. Barnes and Nobelle followed him, sensing his intensity and knowing that something neat was going to happen.

Rick took the vacuum by the handle with both hands and started swinging it while spinning like an Olympic hammer thrower. His release was intended for maximum height and distance. The moment the handle cleared his grip he started for the door to go back inside. He was halfway there before the appliance hit the ground. The dogs chased after as it vaulted through the air, thinking this was terrific fun.

The way things were going, Rick thought, he'd probably be dead before needing the vacuum again. The stress in him was building. His mind was made up to keep his priorities straight. Nobody cared if the damned house was clean.

Back inside, he closed and latched the door, then closed the blinds. The dogs would have to stay out. They could chew on the vacuum to their hearts' content. It had been cast out. They'd never liked that thing, anyway. The age-old rivalry between Barnes and Nobelle, and the vacuum cleaner had entered its final chapter.

Rick sat down and thought about what was going to happen. He needed to be prepared. He reclined on the couch and tried to think, going over scenarios in his mind. He looked at the clock on the wall. Synster would be there in an hour. He had his list prepared. He closed his eyes.

Rick woke abruptly when he heard the now familiar sound of

a low vibration and the soft glare of the milky aura that always accompanied the arrival of someone by Provenger transport. He sat up quickly and then jumped to his feet, trying to look like he hadn't been sleeping, angry he'd been caught off guard. Had he gotten soft now that he was working for the bad guys?

In front of Rick was his brother, David, and four other late middle-aged men. Synster stood next to Rick, a gray briefcase in his hand. David was dressed business casual and looked like he knew this was coming. The other four were a mix, obviously caught unaware. One was in a blue bathrobe and women's fuzzy pink slippers. One was sweating profusely and wearing a t-shirt and gym shorts, looking like he must have been out for a jog. Another was in a dark suit and appeared to be on his way to a funeral. The last man must have still been in bed, wearing pajamas, and appeared ill and disheveled, and since he wreaked of alcohol, possibly recovering from a hangover, Rick speculated. They were all fat, red-faced, and trembling. Their shock was apparent, and they looked around at each other as though they'd just entered a nightmare of biblical proportions. Little did they know that they had.

Rick was extremely apprehensive about what he imagined was about to occur. He had no idea if this would simply resemble a pep rally, or if these people were going to be murdered right there in his living room. Synster was to his right and was going to run this meeting. He'd told his new agent, Nwella, he wanted the satisfaction of personally interrogating them. Rick knew he was there to be introduced as the witness and, possibly, enforcer. He was supposed to keep his mouth shut.

Not surprisingly, the very first thing Synster did was say, "Here, take these." He tossed four tags to the unsuspecting victims. They dutifully caught them and the tags found their way immediately to their wrists. They were Synster's prisoners. His brother David had one on his wrist, having already been initiated.

Rick saw his brother glance at his wrist, observing that Rick didn't wear a tag. Then their eyes met, and Rick noticed a look of surprise and questioning on David's face.

The four men began prying at the bands, trying to get them off. Here we go, thought Rick, with the apprehensive austerity of one who had already felt the soul-tearing pain of the tag.

Synster, dressed in his traditional collar and skirt, gauntlets and sandals, looked just a little bit silly as he gestured for them to sit on Rick's long, leather couch. If they felt the same way about Synster's appearance, they wouldn't think he was silly for long.

As they sat, Hangover panicked and fell to the floor tearing at his new wrist band. Rick and David were embarrassed by his behavior and immediately scolded him, moved in, and got him seated. They wanted to get on with the mess they knew was coming. Finally, they were able to make him sit still, as the others looked on, wide-eyed, observing as though completely separate from the situation.

Rick had been told nothing more by Synster than that this meeting would include top government professionals involved with government health care policy. Once things were calmed, Synster began. "My name is Synster the Provenger." Yada yada yada, Rick thought. Synster gave them the same speech he'd gotten when he was first abducted, all the same threats. The guy who fell on the floor wet his pants, fouling the leather couch. When Rick made a slight movement to get a towel, Synster's quick glance told him to stay. After about ten minutes, they were ready to proceed with the guts of the meeting.

Rick could tell that Synster was enraged about humans being on so much medication, and he could see he wanted to take it out on these poor men. His organic crop had been ruined, and he wanted someone to which he could fix blame. When he was done with his introductory declarations and threats, he didn't even ask them anything. He touched somewhere on his gauntlet and the men were writhing in pain. Rick couldn't look at them as they convulsed on the floor. He knew how utterly ruthless the pain had been, and he refused to imagine how bad it must be for these men. Thinking too much about it actually made him shiver.

Once the agony ceased and they'd climbed back to the couch, Synster began. "You are the men responsible for promoting the health of your people?" Synster asked with a foreboding that even these men knew would lead to more pain. They all looked at each other and immediately didn't want to be responsible for anything. They nodded their heads, knowing that the population of this country was not doing well and expecting now to hear about it. Synster waited a moment and gave them another four-second pulse of pain. He then paced in front of them with his hands behind his back. "And...how do you think you are doing?"

"Not well..."

"Not very good. Sir."

"...Sir." Two of them answered at once. The other two who did not answer immediately dropped to the floor in agony as their tags were activated.

Synster waited for them to get up and sit back down on the couch. "And why do you think your people are not doing well?" he asked looking at Jogger, one of the two that had just been on the floor.

Knowing he must answer, he started, "They..." He glanced around. "We, eat too much, watch too much TV, and don't exercise enough?" Jogger winced, turned his head and tightened his body, preparing for pain.

Looking at all of them, Synster asked, "And what medication should be prescribed to such a person who eats too much, watches TV, and doesn't exercise?"

"Well, none. Medication is for diseases and disorders," responded Suit.

"So are you telling me that the people of your country are not doing well because of diseases and disorders, or are not doing well because of daily habits around the house?"

"Diseases and disorders," they all agreed nodding theirs heads again, apparently in mutual agreement.

"Do they get diseases from not exercising?"

"It's a contributing factor, yes," said another, with confidence building.

"From watching TV?" Synster continued.

"It contributes to weight gain because they're not exercising and probably eating junk while they watch," said another, looking at his colleagues, who appeared to agree.

"Eating too much?"

"Yes, it contributes to weight gain. Eating the wrong things, then complications from there," parroted another, trying to contribute.

"So all the life habits that can be changed are what give most of your people poor health?"

They could suddenly see where he was headed and didn't like

it, but they were trapped. "Yes?" Synster asked and they all nodded agreement reluctantly.

"So what you're telling me, then, is that watching TV, eating too much, and not exercising is caused by a deficiency of pharmaceutical drugs? Because your solution to rid your people of these causes of disease appears to be to add drugs to their systems in the hope that the causes will be driven out."

Synster let the question hover in the air like a vulture watching its victims grope toward a thimble of water in the blazing heat of the Sahara. He wanted them to understand the implications of their decisions and actions. The men squirmed in their seats as David and Rick watched, just glad they weren't a part of this interrogation.

"Why do you think you can interrupt peoples' natural systems with the introduction of simple chemicals and have their health improve?" Synster asked softly. "You don't even understand how intricate their systems are. Do you think you have a more comprehensive grasp of the details of human physiological survival than do millions of years of evolution?" He waited for an answer. "Well, do you?"

No one answered. The four of them gaped while David raised his hand like a middle-school student. Synster did not acknowledge him. He waited for an answer. "Well?" Still no one answered.

He zapped the four on the couch. When they were done writhing on the floor, Synster commanded, "Well?" They all glanced at David and raised their hands. Synster pointed to Pink Slippers, the one closest to David, and commanded, "Answer!"

"We are not smarter than millions of years of evolution. We were just trying to do our best," he replied, then closed both his eyes tightly and slowly opened one, waiting for a possible punishment.

"Then why would you not try to work with the systems of the human body first, giving it all the benefits of a good nutritional and active environment, allowing for natural processes to correct ailments?"

They all looked at each other for an answer. They knew they didn't want to feel the pain of the tag again and four hands went up.

"You." Synster pointed at Hangover.

"We thought the disease process was the natural process, inevitable." He trembled slightly as he looked around nervously and the others looked at him. He realized that maybe he shouldn't speak for the others and corrected himself. "At least, I, thought that might be the case."

Synster didn't react. "But everyone here just agreed that major contributing factors of diseases were a sedentary life and eating too much of the wrong thing, so why is something inevitable if it can be changed? What about you?" he asked pointing to the others. "Do you think the disease process is a natural process?"

They all shook their heads, indicating the negative. Then Suit raised his hand and bravely stated, "Not anymore, we mean, I mean. Obviously you're a man of conviction," he said, trying to cater favor.

"Man! Did you call me a man?" Synster raged. "You are a chimpanzee compared to me!"

Synster zapped Pink Slippers again because he didn't like his clothes and wanted to instill random terror.

"Listen to me, you idiots! Natural selection does not serve its purpose by propagating weakness. Chronic illness is not a natural process. How many millions of wild deer have autoimmune disease? How about zero! And with your tremendous intelligent contributions, how many millions of humans have autoimmune disease. How about hundreds of millions. You have made the grave error of believing that you have some kind of knowledge that rivals your body's knowledge of itself. You add your little compounds to systems and think you are observing the results. Your observations don't even approach the true effects on the entire system. You tinker with relationships that you should completely comprehend by now, but you don't. You investigate the causes of your diseases, and you do it with the elegance of your medieval witch hunts."

These leaders of our nation's health care system gaped at Synster while casting occasional glances at Rick and David, wondering why they were escaping the focus of wrath and interrogation.

"You humans disgust me with your arrogance," Synster

accused, feeling a twinge of hypocrisy with the statement. He paced and thought about all the issues he had with the way humans approach their health. Too many to cover, too many to try to understand. "If a person has an infection," he began, "and their white blood cell count goes up to fight the infection, would you give them a medication that destroys their body's ability to make white blood cells?" Synster glared at them, waiting for an answer.

No one answered until he raised his gauntlet, ready to give them pain. They all seemed confused about such a simple question. They thought it was another trap.

"No, no, we wouldn't," they all answered in almost perfect unison.

"Then if a person is experiencing inflammation and their liver produces cholesterol as a reaction to fight it, would you advocate a medication that inhibits the liver from making that cholesterol?"

Rick knew this was a big sticking point with Synster. It was a medication that too many of his "cattle" took. Too many people took this one drug that damaged the whole system, poisoning their flesh and organs, making them unfit for Provenger consumption. But Rick wasn't really sure what bothered Synster more. Was it the destruction of his crop, or was it the fact that the humans' own research had disproven the lipid hypothesis and was ignored by professionals responsible for this issue?

The captives all looked at him wide eyed and mute. They all knew that cholesterol was the body's lubricant. They all knew that the liver made cholesterol as a response to inflammation, that it protected cells and allowed cellular metabolism to function normally. But they didn't want to admit it because they knew where he was headed, and they didn't want to go there.

"Answer me!" Synster yelled. He gave them another zap. When they got up off the floor again, he told them they had three seconds to answer.

Jogger sheepishly raised his hand and said, "No, I wouldn't want to inhibit the body's production of cholesterol to fight the effects of inflammation."

"Now we're getting somewhere," Synster said as he put Suit under a number of jolts of pain.

When he crawled up off the floor, Suit asked in a whiny panic, "Why did you hit me?"

"Because you didn't answer, and I can't stand pinstripe!" Synster added, "You people don't seem to get it. I want answers."

Rick watched the spectacle before him in silence. He felt for these men, but he thought them very stupid. He'd learned to comply with the tags very quickly. But he only had his immediate obedience at stake; these men had their entire world view at risk. They were being forced to admit the things that they suspected were true but didn't have the intelligence or the guts to pursue.

"So now," Synster continued, "why have you not advocated against the use of drugs that inhibit the liver from making the cholesterol it knows the body needs? Why have you chosen to stop the body's natural protective reaction? As the top health officials in this country, you create policy that recommends what people eat, what drugs are approved, allegedly to 'heal' them." Synster paced a little more. Then he continued. "People think they need to take these drugs when they finally succumb to their lousy diet. You drug them to supposedly correct their condition when you know simple nutritional modifications will prevent any need for such poisons. If I didn't think you all idiots, I'd suspect some sinister plan to fatten them all and make them die early!"

Slowly, Suit put up a hand and offered, "I didn't know nutrition could correct disease. I thought it was genetic."

Synster stared in disbelief. Rick could tell he was trying to enjoy himself while simultaneously venting his frustration that his own plan had gone awry. Synster expected humankind to tend to their own needs, to recognize what was good for them, what was natural for them. They had not done their part, and because of it, Synster's plan was failing.

Rick looked at them in disgust. Their lives had supposedly been devoted to the study of human health. After decades of escalating health problems, it now took an alien with a pain zapper to make them feel negligent in their duties. Now they were being asked to explain themselves.

"Answer me. Why would you want to inhibit the liver's function?" Synster asked in a more relaxed tone.

"We have merely drawn conclusions from studies," answered one. The others all looked very worried.

"So you're telling me you've read all your studies and made your own decisions, or you have read some studies and followed what others have told you? Your own research shows you what the problems are. And yet your government requires doctors to put people on these drugs at the first sign of problems, sometimes before the problems arise, instead of eliminating the cause. Well, things are going to change. And we start with this issue. Gentlemen, you will be changing the way things are done, and I will help you.

"Years ago we assisted in the development of improved high-yield dwarf wheat that we hoped would substantially reduce the cost, enough to make it available to all cultures and feed your starving people, to keep them alive so they could reproduce to provide for our harvest. Well, here we are. We thought this situation would be self-moderating. The higher your percentage of diet that comes from carbohydrates, the sicker you get. The more wheat becomes a part of your regular diet, the sicker you get. It's a fairly simple, linear, and tight causal arrow.

"When we first introduced wheat, we were so concerned that your early ancestors would recognize the pattern of poor health that followed. We went to great lengths to conceal it. Now we've more recently made this grain pervasive across your planet and chronic illness has never been worse. It's staring you in the face and you still cannot see it. Your imbecilic performance in that regard is only surpassed by your methods of treating your ailments. You take symptoms to be causes, you purposefully disrupt your body's natural defense strategies with unnatural chemical intrusions, and you spend fortunes researching how you can intervene in the actions of genes when you fail to allow them to act as they naturally should in the first place. You people are idiots. You are making your planet a hospital ward of poisoned zombies.

"We start with the food pyramid. That will have to change. Nutrient-dense, whole foods only, eliminating wheat and limited in carbohydrates. Then we'll start with those who are on prescription medications. We'll use fines through your government-controlled insurance system to force people to change their diets, and we'll mandate tests to ascertain compliance. Once consumers create the correct, natural intestinal environment with inflammation reduced, the body's endocrine and digestive systems will begin working normally. Without wheat's proteins and starches making your membranes as permeable as a sieve, cellular tight junctions will normalize. There will be less need for antibiotics, psychotropic drugs, anti-inflammatories, and pain medications. Most of your autoimmune conditions will cease to appear, and most will resolve.

"Announcements will be made that the following drugs are ineffective and dangerous: statins, antidepressants, proton pump inhibitors, antipsychotics. With government-mandated compliance to the revised food pyramid confirmed through your health care system, none of them will be necessary anyway."

Rick saw Jogger's hand go up. "Mr. Synster, sir, uh, the food pyramid is with the Department of Agriculture. We're with the Department of Health."

"Really?" Synster was surprised. "So the people who grow the food are the ones putting out information on what people should eat?"

"Yes, sir."

"Well, that explains a lot!" Synster considered the issue for a moment. "Come out with your own food pyramid. I'll give you the information as to what it will be."

Another hand went up from a sheepish supplicant. Hangover asked, "How will we justify these recommendations?" The rest on the couch rolled their eyes at their associate's stupidity. Synster didn't care about justification, they thought.

To their surprise Synster replied, "The justification is in your own research literature. Perhaps you should read it? David Thompson," Synster diverted his gaze as he spoke.

David almost popped out of his chair.

Synster continued, "Our sampling of gall bladders that you've provided from cholecystectomies has been largely unsuccessful. They are too diseased for us to use. Our quality control will apparently require fresh gall bladders. So we'll need to change our strategy. You people already advocate against dietary fat. You claim it is the culprit of many health problems. Since the gall bladder is a vital organ for the digestion of fats, you will represent that its removal aids in the passing of consumed fat without digestion. Explain that this will aid in the reduction of absorbed fat as well as a decrease in blood cholesterol. If your people believed the lipid hypothesis in spite of what your research says, they'll believe this.

"As a requirement for the maintenance of their health insurance at its current cost, all individuals with a body mass index of twenty-five or over must schedule to have their gall bladders removed. They will be fined if they don't get it done."

Suit slowly raised his hand.

"What?" Synster asked.

"We're not allowed to fine them, by law," he said.

"We could call it a tax," suggested Pink Slippers. "A tax for keeping their gall bladders. Everybody crosses state lines. It's a matter of interstate commerce."

They all nodded their heads, agreeing that would probably work.

Synster continued, "With laparoscopic methods on an otherwise asymptomatic person, the surgery should be minimally invasive. The gall bladders will be collected by your government under the auspices of a study and delivered to us. David, you know the method."

David nodded, and all four on the couch stared at him in amazement.

"Use this program of gall bladder removal as an argument for the cessation of statin drug use. They won't need the cholesterol control if they aren't digesting it. I have data here." Synster produced four thick white binders from the case he'd arrived with. "They contain defensible statistics and conclusions from your own studies interpreted in a manner that the argument can be made that experts agree: various health benefits will result from these removals in ninety-two percent of the cases surveyed, eighty-seven percent of the time. Copy it, and get it out to your people."

He gave them to Suit. "Your mission instructions are also enclosed."

Then Synster addressed the group. "I will need from you a weekly list of names of all patients controlled under the government program. From what I understand, that should be everyone under United States jurisdiction, give or take a few holdouts. As your work proceeds, I will need updates as to who is clear of their prescription drugs and what their body mass index is. The list should be ordered with the highest body mass index cleared of drugs at the top, to the lowest body mass index not clear of drugs at the bottom. I'll need addresses for each name.

"We have programmed your tags to inflict level 3 pain for one hour every night at midnight starting one week from today if certain stages of your work are not complete. Your goals with their timelines are included in your instructions. Study them. You will be held accountable.

"You should not try to amputate your arm in an effort to modify our relationship. The tags have recently been adjusted to sense this and notify us immediately, at which time you and your families will be transported to our ship and you will be dealt with according to the manner already prescribed.

"Forget about your current career. It's obviously the most important thing to you, seeing that you apparently haven't let poor job performance get in your way. Your career as you know it is over. You now work for me. You will until you die. Your lives are now merely a struggle to avoid agonizing pain and the total destruction of your lives and families. As a benefit, you will be contacted for a list of those close to you who will be exempt from the harvest. As a reminder, this is pain level two."

Synster touched his gauntlet and immediately their bodies seized in place. They were unable to speak, groan, or move. They began to look a little red and stiff, but otherwise gave no indication of anything wrong. Synster released them.

"Levels two and three have been specially formulated so that it won't be obvious to anyone around you that there is anything wrong. I gave you ten seconds. If you haven't reached your goals, I suggest you go to bed before midnight. Remember your pain will be for one hour at level three. This is something you will all want to avoid. A few sessions an hour long and you run the risk of permanent insanity.

"When you get home, you are likely to believe that all this was just a bad dream. Included in your instructions is contact information for Rick, here," Synster said, gesturing to Rick, "to confirm the veracity of our new relationship. Remember that you may tell no one and only deal with each other. If you decide to commit suicide, your immediate and extended families will be punished as already prescribed."

With that, all five of the visitors dissolved in a hazy white light. Rick and Synster were alone. "Rick, I've got special assignments for you. We need to manipulate certain political situations, and I want you to assassinate a couple people for me. If you get captured, you can signal us and we'll have to terminate everyone in the group that has taken you. So if you care about that, don't let it happen. The targets are two leaders of consumer advocate groups. We want to make it look like a specific corporation was behind the murders, and we don't want our Provenger to risk it. The situation is fluid."

There was a pause. "Okay, who are they?" Rick asked, wondering how or if he'd be able to squirm out of this.

"I'll let you know when it's necessary. You'll get all the information and equipment you need. There is another, unrelated assassination; this one more important. I suggest you start sighting in your best rifle for about three to three hundred, fifty yards. You cannot miss. This is very important." Synster grabbed the case he'd come with and was about to leave.

"Synster, there is something."

"What is it?"

"I need some things. I want my guns, the ones you destroyed. I want replacements. There are some other things. I made a list." Rick took the list out of his pocket and handed it to Synster, who took it.

"I'll look into it. Anything else?"

"No, that's all," Rick said and stepped back. And Synster was gone.

Rick looked at the wet side of his couch and checked his watch. Carson and Shainan would be home in an hour.

After cleaning the urine off the leather as best he could and throwing a towel over it, he stretched out and closed his eyes, glad to have survived one more encounter with Synster.

Exactly one hour later, Rick woke to the sound of barking and keys at the front door. He sat up and rubbed his face. His vision and brain were clearing as Carson and Shainan walked into the living room. They were laughing and sounded like they'd had a good time. Shainan had been making progress with her English. With a combination of sign and simple words, they had started developing a relationship. She seemed a part of the family now.

Sitting on the couch, Rick stared in front of him. In the center of the living room floor, there were three crates about the size of the ones he put his dogs in. If Synster had given him what he'd asked for, each one would be filled with weapons and ammunition, cash in twenties, fifties, and hundreds, and one-ounce gold coins. By Rick's rough estimate, between the gold and the cash, he had anywhere from one hundred to two hundred million dollars sitting in front of him; then again, maybe double that. He wasn't sure. It's a good thing this is a slab floor, he thought, otherwise the crate full of gold might fall right through. Rick now had the resources to hire an army, arm it, and even gild it should he choose. The way Rick saw it, if he could get stuff, get stuff big.

"Carson!" Rick yelled. "Get the tractor, we've got some digging to do! No...wait. Let the dogs in and pull the Charger out front. We're going to town." Rick felt like dinner and shopping. They could risk an evening out with Shainan. He was doing things his way from now on.

Chapter 27

Yootu aRRives home

Nwella arrived at Rick's home one evening without notice. She appeared out of a sphere of milky white light in the center of his living room. He was at the dinner table in the middle of Shainan's English lesson when it happened. Shainan was horror struck while leaping for a kitchen knife, then throwing herself to the floor with her back to the corner. She held the knife pointed in Nwella's direction as though she could see through the cabinets that blocked her view.

Rick was very glad to see Nwella, but she was all business. She ignored Shainan and informed him that another human would be joining them.

"His name is Yootu," she said, "and he is being released from captivity on the Provenger Ship. He has been our guest for the last ten years and our only way to dispose of him is to free him. By law, we are required to return such guests to their home, their spouse, their family, or to a comparable situation. Shainan is part of his tribe." Nwella had become jealous of Shainan living with Rick. "They should probably be married," she added at great personal risk of revealing her motives. "No other location but this one will serve that purpose.

"You will be responsible for Yootu. He has recently sustained an injury. He's been examined and appears to be physically intact, but he may have some psychological issues. He may be dangerous, and you must be cautious with him. Our tests reveal that he is rational and likely not an imminent danger to fellow humans. He has been given the same out-brief as Shainan and should maintain the same dietary restrictions due to his vaccinations. Once we have turned him over, you have complete authority to dispose of him as needed, but we are absolved of all responsibility."

Rick acknowledged that he understood. He wanted to speak to Nwella of other things, but he could see with an almost imperceptible shake of her head and the look in her eyes that she would not have it. She looked nervous. They must be watching, Rick thought. Nwella dissolved in the same sphere of milky white.

A few seconds later another sphere appeared, and there were two huge Provenger clad with armor and knives fully deployed on their left and right gauntlets. They were holding a man between them. They dropped him and he crumpled in a pile on the floor in front of them. They left as they came. There was a long silence. Shainan still cowered in the kitchen behind the cabinets.

Four hours earlier, Yootu had been resting quietly in his enclosure. All was a blur since he'd been told Shainan had been sent back to Earth. He'd lost track of time. He had no will to keep track nor to ask how long it had been. He'd recovered from his rage and the trauma to his body and brain. But somehow he felt very different, as though something in him had awakened. The ancient shaman instinctively knew that a new time was about to begin. It would be either his beginning or his end. He suspected that he now knew why his tribe had called him the Keeper of the Red Moon Spirit. It was now that spirit which gave him life.

They flooded his cell with a gas that made him unconscious. When he woke, he was strapped, arms and legs, to a table in an exam room. Both wrists were fixed with tags. This looked to him like a place where nothing good could happen. He figured this was the end, and he wanted to take a Provenger with him if he could. He waited for a technician to get near. Yootu determined he would have to break his bonds and lunge in one motion to have any chance at contact as the tags were activated. He would try for a fist to the throat. If he could crush it in one blow, he could kill it and leave his life with one small souvenir of defiance. With his last breath, he would tell them, in their own language, how stupid he found them to be and that no matter what they tried, humans of the Earth would never be tamed.

As a Provenger grew near, he summoned all the strength he had, as calmly as he could, expecting the searing pain from the tags that he must ignore. With a burst of force, he tensed every muscle at once from his thighs to his stomach. His arms curled and twisted in a rage that generated a magnified leveraged force against his bonds. They bent and broke easier than he thought as he turned this force into a lunge at the Provenger tending to the examining light above him. His right fist was aimed for the neck, but the wrist straps gave way like strings and his strike flew high and wide, his knuckles grazing the Provenger's skull. Yootu was stunned that he had no pain, and with the absence of it, he was frozen with disbelief. Only a mild buzz ran through his nerves.

He quickly regained his focus, grabbed the Provenger's neck with his hand, and pulled his head down into an accelerating left jab. His fist again hit the Provenger's skull, glancing off the top of his head as the limp body, already unconscious from the first hit, was unexpectedly collapsing to the floor. Yootu popped his leg restraints. They broke easily and he glanced up at the adjacent control room, looking for any resistance to his escape. He saw another technician behind unbreakable glass that he knew he could break.

Watching from behind the glass, the Provenger was terrified. She saw everything from the beginning, but it happened so fast that she was only now reacting. The last thing Yootu saw was her lunge for the control panel, and he felt everything dim as the gas shot from jets positioned around the room immediately invaded every pore of his skin.

Yootu saw colors: red, blue, swirl patterns. He blinked his eyes and felt his head throbbing. He tried to remember where he was and grabbed at a Provenger that was not there. He held his head and rolled to his back. Wherever he was, he wasn't strapped down. He could move, and he wasn't being beaten or cut up. So far, everything was good. He sucked in a deep breath and could tell something was different. He could smell and taste something different in the air. It was life, small and large. It was the smell of things growing. Spores. Molds. There was the sensation of dust and dirt, the scents of wood and smoke, things of the Earth. He wondered for a moment what horrible torment the Provenger might be trying to inflict on him as punishment for his attack.

Yootu heard a shriek, a scream of horror or joy he could not tell, but it was immediately followed by arms that were warm and loving. For a moment, he thought he might be dead and his mother was holding him. Then he realized he was in the arms of Shainan. Before he could open his swollen eyes, they flooded with tears, both for being with her and in fear that she was with him.

If they were on the ship, he knew that he would kill her before he would let the Provenger hurt her. He knew he could do it quickly. He opened his eyes and did not recognize anything. That was a good feeling. She held him tightly, and he realized her cries were of joy. That told him everything. He must be on Earth. He must be home. The rush of being with her gave him a momentary boost. They held each other and looked into the other's face, then remained cheek to cheek. Yootu slowly checked the new environment around him, vigilant for a Provenger. He saw a man and a boy, no threats. He tried to stand with her help but stumbled and fell.

Four hours later, Yootu opened his eyes. Shainan was lying naked next to him on the bed, wiping a cool, wet cloth on his head. She had stripped him, cleaned him off, and put the bison rug over them both. She wanted everything to be as normal as possible when he awoke. She wanted desperately to be his woman in every way. She was undone with joy. But when he woke, she didn't know what to do.

"Shainan," Yootu whispered as he reached out to pull her in. She snuggled her body in tighter to his and positioned her face close as he turned to look her square in the eyes. The presence of humanity that had been so rare for the last ten years flowed into his soul, and he was lost in thoughts of what should have been. He tried to avoid thinking about the moment on the ship that she didn't show for her visit. He wanted to tell her of the imagined day he'd planned, the game he'd killed and brought to her, the fire they would make, and the stories they would tell to their children. Before he'd been told she was gone, he'd planned it all. He wanted to tell her.

"Shainan, I had our day planned," he explained in their dead language. "We had children, and we..." Yootu's chest heaved and he sobbed. So much grief, so much pain for so many years welled up within him, choking out any words, the pain becoming the words he wanted to speak to her. And she knew. She knew exactly what he was going to say. He did not need to speak.

She could not get close enough to him. She wanted only for him to be happy. She wanted only to be with him forever, and yet the fear of being separated again forced great pain into the face of her joy. They both cried until they slept, in each other's arms. And when they slept with the bison hide covering them, they could have been home. They dreamed of things ancient and wild, of their tribe and camp, of children and friends, of fires and hunting, of swimming in their river and loving. They dreamt of paradise.

Shainan was awake for an hour before she stirred enough to disturb Yootu. She hadn't wanted to bother him because he looked so beat up. She remained motionless for as long as she could bear. It was still dark out, and she had no idea when day would come. Finally, her curiosity overcame her, and she started moving about with the express purpose of waking him. She wanted to know why he was there, how long he would stay, what would become of them.

He woke up slowly at first. Then suddenly he was with her, his eyes blinking, his vision competing with the swelling all around his face. He'd assaulted a Provenger, and even though they had determined he was incoherent at the time and would be released anyway after his exit physical, the guards charged with his security had not been easy on him. But now he was free and again on his Earth, something he'd never thought would happen. All he had to do was heal from his minor wounds and he would be complete again. He would be with his love, Shainan.

Yootu rubbed the crust from his eyes and noted a minor headache. He was amazed, considering the drubbing he'd sustained by the guards, recalled only in semiconscious slow motion fragments. He looked at Shainan. There was so much he wanted to do. Had this been the time he'd been preparing himself for? He wondered. What situation would he find himself in?

During his time with the Provenger, Yootu had learned a great deal about what humans would have to overcome in this new world. Eavesdropping during his captivity had taught him many languages as well as providing a fairly comprehensive picture of much of the Provenger technology, all without their knowing. If they had been aware of what he knew, they never would have released him, he thought.

"Shainan, my love," he began in their ancient tongue. "Though I have not always known it, I know now. This is the moment I have been waiting for my whole life. I want more than anything for you to be my woman. I will bring you game and give you children. I will show our tribe..." Yootu realized they no longer had a tribe. "We will found a new tribe, and you shall be the mother of our new nation, and they will honor you always if you will be my woman."

Shainan looked alternately from his right to left eye as she tried to hold back her joy and listened to his words. She knew well that all of this was just too good, and she didn't ever want to lose him. She would be his woman. She caressed his face with both her hands and kissed him slowly, first on the mouth, then on his cheeks, then his nose, working her way all over his battered features. "I will always be yours."

Yootu flipped over on top of her as she encircled him with her legs. Yootu had not been with a human woman for over ten years, and he was overcome with lust and joy, knowing that their union could create a life, a child of their tribe, an heir to their blood, and they would truly be one. He buried his face in her delicious hair, grabbing on both sides of her head. He looked deep into her swimming brown eyes and saw ripples of color reminding him of their river in full flood on the open plains of the Earth, something he had not enjoyed in ages.

Shainan grabbed Yootu by his long hair and wrapped her legs high around his hips, holding him hard. She pressed herself into him, wanting to feel his strength. They loved for themselves and for the life they both instinctively wanted to create, the life they had dreamed of all those years in captivity, the life that would truly make them one and give them, again, the tribe they missed so dearly.

For years, Shainan had beaten back every Provenger advance that she could, but now she had her man with her, a man of her choosing. She took him quickly, as if in fear that he might be taken away. She had so many hopes over the years, so much sorrow and loneliness that she could not expel, a massive void of cold, and now she felt warm, filled with warmth. She reveled in his flesh, his skin, soft, yet hashed with scars. His smell was distinctly human. Shainan loved everything about this moment. She knew that she would be doing this every chance she had.

Suddenly, they were no longer inside, the wind blew, and the scent of cedars filled their nostrils and the air whispered through their limbs. The dark fur of the bison hide under them was becoming warm with the direct glare of the sun. They felt its warmth on their skin and saw around them the hills and forests of their ancient land. Yootu raised his head from her hair and laughed, "Look!" He lifted his weight from her body, and Shainan, seeing only sky, flipped herself over on her stomach and looked out.

She couldn't believe. Not wanting it to end, she moved to her knees, and she pressed herself back at Yootu who returned to her with equal force.

Yootu took the back of her ear between his lips and whispered, "Look at our ancient land."

It was all there. They were atop a cliff and the valley was spread out before them. They could see their village in the distance, its smoke trailing off to the east, the great river just visible through the trees in the distance. Shainan reached back over her shoulders and supported herself by the back of Yootu's neck, pressing her cheek to his lips. She closed her eyes, more content to feel his touch than to look again on her ancient homeland. He held her tightly around the waist and across the chest.

What magic was this? What power was this, she wondered? They both cried and laughed. They were home. Shainan brought her lips to his ear. "You have brought me here, my shaman, my love, my husband."

Shainan lay exhausted in his arms when she noticed the sun was rising, a dim yellow light forming outside the bedroom window. Yootu was also awake and looking straight at the ceiling. He noticed the glow and realized he hadn't seen a sunrise for a very long time. He slipped out of bed and limped to the window. His legs were stiff, but everything seemed to work. He had certainly proven that through the course of the night. Yootu stretched, looking outside at the light coming over the horizon. It seemed like the first sunrise of his life. He felt very much like this was a completely new existence. After their surprise of possibly being back in their homeland during the night, Yootu realized that something very strange had transformed in him. He felt powerful, capable. It was a feeling he knew he didn't yet understand.

Shainan watched him from bed. He rivaled the Provenger in size and strength. His body was crisscrossed with the scars from the injuries he'd suffered at their hands. Shainan noticed for the second time since she had cleaned him that night that his back was painted with the form of a circle with pointed petals extending out from the center. "Why the flower on your back?"

"It's not a flower," replied Yootu. "You are so precious. It's the sun."

She'd remembered stories of his birth told by her friend and cousin, Noanan. The tribal shaman had said that he was of the Sun god and that Noanan had been stolen from her bed and the god had assumed the form of the river to avoid burning her and had put a child into her. Shainan remembered Noanan becoming pregnant with Yootu before she was kidnapped by the Provenger and missed his birth. Noanan had told her that Yootu would be their savior.

Yootu looked out on the Earth from the window of a twenty-first century ranch house in southwestern Colorado. The last he'd seen Earth had been over twelve thousand years before. It is still the same, he thought. Still beautiful, still for me.

Yootu knew that he needed information. He needed to know where and when he was. He'd seen another man last night in this home and he needed to speak to him. "Shainan, who is this man you are with?"

"His name is Rick. He is a good man. He has interactions with the Provenger. I'm not sure what his purpose is, but I do know that he is kind and he is fearful of them. I do not think he is with them. I think he would like to be rid of them."

"This is important." Yootu leaned in very close to her and spoke in her ear with the softest whisper he could manage. "I need to learn everything I can from him. I never told you because I didn't want them to find out, but I can speak all of the languages that the Provenger have spoken in front of me. I have learned them from listening. I have never let on. I know much about them.

They could be here watching us now. Does this Rick have a tag, the pain bracelet?"

"Yes, he does," she whispered back, "but he does not wear it, he is allowed that by the Provenger. He uses it to signal them," said Shainan, even more surprised and impressed with her new man.

Yootu was disturbed by that but knew he should not yet judge the situation. "Good. I need it to be around when we talk. Do you think we can trust him?"

"I've never seen anything to indicate you shouldn't. He seems anguished about the Provenger being here. I believe he is against them."

Yootu thought about this. Everything seemed to him as if he'd truly been released. If he delayed talking to Rick, he would learn little and much time would go by. He'd already experienced what effort and time it took to accumulate information without actively conversing. Yootu decided he would confront Rick directly and let him know he could communicate. He had no idea how much or how little time he had, and he was tired of waiting. He was free now and could take action. He had to trust Shainan on this and trust the human he didn't even know.

"Shainan, remember the thing I stole from the Provenger and told you to hide somewhere safe? Remember how I told you it was the most important thing you could do?

"Yes."

"Did you hide it?"

"Yes." Shainan paused and looked at the floor. "But I'm afraid I've failed you."

"Why is this?"

"I hid it in a clay fat girl statue, the ones we give to girls to warn them not to drink too much ferment."

"Yes?"

"Well, this one hadn't been hardened by fire yet. I meant to go back and get it later, but I never did. Because they took me. If it was put in the fire it would have been burned."

Yootu smiled and comforted her. "No, it was Provenger magic. I think it would survive. I've heard this. Do you remember what the figure looked like? I realize it was many years ago."

"Yes, I think I'd know it if I saw it. There were many of them being made, all the same, so I quickly printed something on the back. I couldn't think of what else to do, so I etched the opposite of a fat woman – a skinny man, like a skeleton."

Yootu smiled and hugged her. They were taking a huge chance by talking like this, even speaking in whispers. There could be a Provenger in the room. The only assurance he had was that he didn't smell their scent. Yootu knew how to use the bolt he had given Shainan to hide. It was a power source for the battle gauntlet the Provenger had used to destroy and shape many things on Earth, like great trees and large rocks. It would be a powerful weapon for them.

"Where is Rick? Take me to him now, please…Wait, I need to know what language he speaks. Tell me something you hear him say."

Shainan thought for a moment. "Carson gitofdos vido ganes an git atside, pikup da dogdert, tame togoto bed, yoo miz yor bus an ime not goint…"

"Okay, okay, I've got it. Sounds like English."

Shainan got out of bed and they both dressed, Shainan in her robe and Yootu in clothes that Rick had left in the room when they carried him in. They barely fit, and Shainan giggled at how he looked. The pants were two inches too short at the ankles, and the shirt was tight and pulled at his neck and armpits. She took his hand and together they went out the door. They walked cautiously down the hall into the living room. Rick was there, sipping his coffee, heard them coming, and was rising to his feet as they entered. He'd been careful to wear his baseball cap for this first meeting.

Yootu, saying nothing, motioned to Rick to come to him. As Rick approached, Yootu spread his arms wide in preparation for a hug. By now Rick was used to the strange gesture and, though very apprehensive, figured this was the appropriate greeting. Yootu and Rick embraced. Yootu put his mouth to Rick's ear and whispered in reasonably good English, "Do no move. We maybe not alone. Do you have tag, the pain wrist? Take me it." Rick almost reacted when he heard him speak. Yootu could tell that he'd managed to restrain himself.

They separated from their hug, both aware now of the other's concerns and capabilities for pretense, and each held the other's forearms, smiling for a moment, making it look good. Rick was a full four inches shorter than Yootu and looked up at him, hoping to never have to cross the man. This guy would make a great professional wrestler, Rick thought. Yootu's forearms felt unusually solid. The parts that should have been muscle felt as hard as bone. He'd only felt this one other time with the same amazement, and it was the forearm of a bear that Rick had hunted in the mountains nearby.

They both separated and Rick went immediately into the kitchen. At the cabinet, he took out three glasses and put them on the kitchen table. Then, taking one in his hand, he went to the freezer. Instead of using the ice dispenser, he accessed the ice by opening the door to the tray. He filled the glass to the top with ice and returned to the table. He used that glass to fill the other two and put it down with them in the form of a triangle.

Yootu wasn't sure what he was doing, but he recognized subtlety when he saw it and certainly understood deception. He played along. Yootu led Shainan to the edge of the kitchen as they spoke of the kinds of foods Rick ate, what the area he lived in was called, and who else lived at the house. By the time Rick was done filling the glasses with orange juice, Yootu had slowly walked over to the table and looked down. The tag was sitting on the table in the center of the three glasses. Rick looked up at Yootu as if to ask, what now?

Yootu looked at the inside of the band for the distinctive surface that looked of soft black leather. It was there. Then he glanced around the kitchen and the adjacent rooms quickly and breathed a sigh of relief. "Tag and Provenger cloak no work close to other. If cloak here now we see them. We still speak soft. You have noise you make?"

Almost before he was finished talking, Rick had spun around and flipped on a radio and turned it up. "How's that?"

"Good."

"Welcome back to Earth."

"It excellent I back," stated Yootu with a huge smile, using the biggest word for something good that he could think of. "I want some clear us." Yootu grabbed Shainan by the arm and pulled her toward him. She willingly came, smiling. "This my woman. You no touch her for sexy time. She my wife."

Rick looked surprised but then realized that what he'd been hearing all night long must have been either a reunion or the honeymoon. He was willing to comply. "She is your wife and I will never touch her for sexy time," he returned, amused by the expression and hoping to God Shainan hadn't mentioned the time he had tried. "But know this," he looked back squarely at Yootu, a man much taller and about sixty pounds of solid muscle heavier. "This is my house, and what I say goes."

Yootu wasn't familiar with the word, "saygoes," but gathered Rick wanted to be in charge in his home. Yootu put his hands out in front of him, palms up, and exclaimed, as if it was extremely important to him, "I respite you house." Two men separated in experience by over twelve thousand years had reached almost complete understanding. Now there was the simple matter of allegiances.

Yootu did not know this man nor how involved he might be with the Provenger, and he was cautious. He'd not tried to take Shainan, and she had good things to say about him, but she didn't understand anything that he said. He could be collaborating with the Provenger. His hair was cut almost to his scalp, and this made Yootu cautious. Maybe he emulated the Provenger. If that was the case, Yootu would have to progress slowly. On the other hand, this man was vital to his ability to orient himself to his current circumstances. This might be a very foreign world. Yootu decided to take it slow.

Rick could sense the caution. He knew that Yootu had just been released from ten years of what must have been a living hell. Shainan had already been able to communicate to him what she thought were the number of years they'd been held. He knew that Yootu must also be extremely suspicious of him but also intensely eager to re-associate himself to human society, that is, if he was really human. But then Rick considered the possibility that maybe Yootu was a Provenger that was Shainan's boyfriend and they'd grown hair on him and sent him down as a test to see if Rick was still onboard. Rick thought he should take it slow.

"I be Yootu," he said, raising his right hand, palm toward Rick.

"My name is Rick," who did the same, then reached out to shake Yootu's hand.

Yootu extended his hand and they shook, as if Yootu had been doing it his entire life.

"Why are you here?" Rick asked.

Yootu thought this might be the first question of someone who was not aligned with the Provenger, and he was glad to hear it.

"Some time," Yootu pointed with his thumb into the air behind him, "Shainan and I were visit. They took her from me. I go…went crazy. They send me here."

Rick decided not to tell him why he lost Shainan. "That seemed to work out well for you. How can you speak English?"

"They teach me when they learn to come here. Maybe they know they bring me here?" Yootu gestured to the room with both hands. Yootu hoped he could get away with the story that he'd been taught. He didn't want Rick to know of his language abilities yet.

"Where do you come from?" Rick asked.

"I do not know how tell this my land called. For many years, wasili," Yootu wobbled his hand back and forth, "me with Provenger. Home tribe in land of hills over plains. Many herds of graze move in land, fish swim river, plants live us everywhere. We hunt, we swim, love tribe, we from this. Shainan know my mother. Shainan one five when I born, and still I more old than her now. This Provenger magic. I speak much. Who you tribe?"

"I must tell you I have some bad news. You're not many years away from your tribe. You are over twelve thousand years away from your tribe." Rick realized twelve thousand may not be a number he could relate to. "Do you understand this number?"

"No, I no think. What is it?"

Rick got up quickly and grabbed the tag as he did. He went to the desk in his kitchen, put the tag down, and tossed some bills on it. He grabbed a piece of paper and a pencil and went back to his seat across from Yootu. "Do you know the number of how many years a person usually lives?"

"Yes, I know this numbers, person live… eight tens years sometime," Yootu estimated, as he looked up into the air and to his right, Rick observed closely.

"Good." Up and right. Recollection, Rick noted. "Do you know what I mean when I say a family generation, like how a father has a son and the son has a son and so on?" Rick asked making horizontal lines across the sheet of paper. "Each son is a new generation."

Yootu nodded, looking Rick directly in the eyes. "Mmm, generation," having no idea what he meant, but knowing he'd figure it out.

Rick believed Yootu's "eight tens" was eighty and was surprised they'd get that old. But for the calculation, Rick assumed most would have children in their late teens through their twenties. Rick considered the number of generations based off of the number of years Synster said the Provenger were on Earth last. "It looks like there have been about seven hundred generations since you have been on Earth. Do you know that number?"

"That hundred, seven times?" Yootu asked, looking down at the paper, a frown prominent on his face.

"Yes, good!" Rick replied as Yootu's eyebrows raised and his brow crinkled. "I'm curious, Yootu. How do you know numbers so well? Did the Provenger teach you?"

Yootu was immediately cautious. The Provenger had taught him nothing, and they believed he learned nothing, so he had to be careful with his response. He held up his hands in front of Rick's face and spread his ten fingers wide. "We need count too, use these ten, over and over for big numbers."

Of course, Rick thought. "How long did you think you were away?"

"I try no think it." Some of the Provenger had talked about time issues, but Yootu wasn't going to let Rick know about his eavesdropping yet. "I suppose I think again I see people my tribe I know." Yootu said with a quick glance to the left.

Left, creative, Rick thought. Then after a long pause, "Shainan loves my dogs, two, they're outside right now," said Rick, trying to act like he was changing the subject to something happier. "How many dogs did you have?"

Yootu was a little annoyed with the question, but after a split second glance high and right, he replied, "I no remember. I have many."

High and right, recollection again. Good, Rick thought. He is actually trying to recall how many dogs he had. At least I think I can be sure he is who he says he is and not a Provenger. Question is, whose side is he on?

Yootu turned to Shainan and took her hands. He spoke to her in their language, and tears welled in her eyes as she listened. They rose, holding each other, and he walked her back to their room, then he came back to talk with Rick. "I need know where my tribe. I too need know I trust you."

Yootu had been considering this carefully. I know Rick is human, I could tell by his stature and his smell when we embraced. What I need to know is whose side he is on. I don't like his short hair. He looks like he is trying to be one of them.

"Why do you work them?" Yootu asked, pointing into his palm.

"I think you're asking why I work with the Provenger, and that's an easy answer," he replied. Rick told him of his abduction and the tag. As best he could, he explained to Yootu the different harvest strategies the Provenger were following as they were explained by Synster. Rick emphasized the differences between Natural Proliferation and Managed Collectivization. He also told Yootu of the threats the Provenger had made against him. When Rick was done, he asked Yootu, "Did you come from the time when they arrived?"

"Yes, but I born after first arrive. My mother almost killed from then. They make her live again."

"Did they bring you grain, wheat, like Synster said, and train you to farm it?"

"We already have wheat, grab it when hunting, put in wet pouch, let it go soft or grow little green. Then collect all and put in large bag, make fun juice. Wheat they give different, bigger. It make me, others, sick, when we crush and eat from dry like they say, fat if too much was eat...en, eaten. Yes, they try," Yootu mumbled in a low tone, "but some we not go that way. I was old ways. Over time they no want us hunt. They kill, take game."

That sounds familiar, Rick thought, thinking of how the west was settled by exterminating the vast herds of bison, depriving the plains Indians of their traditional resources. This guy is for real, Rick determined. "How can I help you trust me?"

"Give what I need and no ask why," Yootu replied. "And don't ask me why," he corrected himself.

"I agree. What do you need?"

"I need talk alone with Shainan, with tag here. I need find where my tribe. I need hunt, soon; I no wait. I need know what you work for Provenger. I need know where water, thirsty, and where I shit."

Rick's eyebrows went up, and he realized Yootu had been there since last night and he hadn't even eaten, let alone attended to the other necessities. "I think we can take care of that," Rick replied, getting up briskly and showing Yootu the bathroom. Rick didn't know what kind of facilities they had on the Provenger ship but thought they must be similar. Yootu was a quick study. One toilet bowl orientation later, and he caught on as quickly as Shainan. How many ways could one take a dump?

But when Yootu objected to defecating in the water, Rick realized that both with his tribe and on a space ship, relieving oneself in perfectly good water would be a bad idea, very wasteful of a precious resource. It was only with sincere assurances that Rick got Yootu to comply. Shainan had only objected once.

Learning from his experience with her, Rick emphasized to Yootu, "the drinking water comes out of the sink faucet, this one here," Rick emphasized, pointing vigorously at the spigot. "The toilet is not for drinking!"

Yootu nodded quickly. Then, with Rick smiling hard at him, he made the association that perhaps Shainan had done this. They both laughed very hard with the image in their minds of poor Shainan drinking from the toilet.

"I joke her on this later," he laughed.

After a zealous fifteen minutes playing with the dogs, a romp in the yard, and Yootu's own personal version of a reunion with Earth, he was ready to sit down to figure out where he came from. One hour later, Rick had completed Yootu's orientation on the computer keyboard and mouse. Rick had him browsing the internet in search of where his tribe might have lived. It posed an interesting problem.

Yootu's language was dead. Terms could only be searched as they might be spelled in English. Yootu had no written language, nor did he know how to write. Rick showed him how to use the mouse to click on things and wrote down as many terms as he could that had to do with early cultures to include terms like, "first, agriculture, civilization, fertile crescent, cradle of civilization, grain, wheat, farming, ancient, Cro-Magnon, first modern human." On a whim, Rick included all the phonetic spellings of Yootu and Shainan's names as well as the most reasonable spellings for all of the place names they remembered. The list became extensive. He set Yootu and Shainan down at the computer to pound out the words as he'd written them, then hit enter and select the "images" to get pictures they could look at.

Rick made food while they "survdanet," as Shainan put it, trying to repeat many of Rick's expressions. Yootu had asked for red meat as his first meal "home." Rick was glad he'd put it that way, and was busy making them all a brunch of broiled steaks and eggs.

Yootu had spent the first hour patiently working with the "technology" in front of him. He repeatedly asked Shainan for help thinking of names of the places they'd known, but it all came to nothing. They saw plenty of pictures of stone structures and wheat fields, muffins and pizza, statues and primitive people, but nothing that they recognized. Every time Yootu called Rick over to read to them the information accompanying the picture, there would be another dead end.

"Shainan, we should search our own names just for fun. Maybe there will be a story on how the two most wonderful people, a handsome man and a beautiful woman, were forced out of paradise," he teased.

Shainan smiled at him and kissed him on the ear. "Why don't we go to the bed for love?"

"Soon. Let me search my name. What is the first way Rick drew it?"

Shainan looked at the paper and found the section where Rick had written their names and circled them. "This one, then this one, then this one again," she said, pointing to the correct keys on the keyboard."

"That's U,T,U," Yootu said, "Say it while you point to it."

Shainan pouted and pointed, "U,T,U, enter!" she said in English, proud of her progress.

The images came up on the screen, and Yootu looked at some of the pictures. "Rick, you come and read this, please."

Rick walked over with some spices in his hands. "Sure, where?"

Yootu pointed.

"Okay," Rick read:

'From the works of Zechariah Sitchin, the god Utu/Shamash as he "rises" from Mt. Mashu to bring the golden dawn. He wears the horned crown of divinity and holds a "pruning saw" in his hand, as the rays of the sun emanate from his shoulder. Mountain, Mountain in the sky, break the god and make him die" is an actual quote from the epic. Gilgamesh and Enkidu chant this as they march toward Huwawa. Huwawa emits this "radiance" that the Sumerians call "melam". It is a blinding light or energy that makes Huwawa almost impossible to confront.'

"That me. I Utu," Yootu said with self-assured confidence. "I shaman my people. I call son of sun at birth!" Yootu exclaimed, motioning toward the sky. "Provenger come with mountain in sky, hot lights burn under."

"Now, just hold on there, Hammurabi. Let's not get ahead of ourselves." Rick Googled, "Utu." And what he read was indeed interesting. It seems Utu was the Sumerian mythological sun god and was part of the myth of Gilgamesh.

Rick took a look at Wikipedia for "Utu". Rick read to them, "the god of the sun, justice, application of law, and the lord of truth. He is usually depicted as wearing a horned helmet and carrying a saw-edged weapon not unlike a pruning saw."

"You must see this me!" Yootu claimed. "My shaman dress has feathers, the sun arms. I fight Layrd Provenger with arm knife. Look like picture. I Utu!"

"Well, I must admit, you do have a point. Frequently mythology develops from actual events through their retelling through the generations." It was clear to Rick that he'd have to help them more. Maybe they could find something that would point to his origins.

Shainan had been attentively watching everything since all the excitement had started.

"Shainan," Utu began. "I think we have found something," he said in their dead language. "It seems that there is a story of an ancient god and his name sounds the same as mine. He is the sun god, and I was born with the title of son of the sun god. My shaman cape was the same as his, and the night I fought the Provenger, before we were taken, I had the gauntlet with the blade, just as they show here! Most of the tribe saw us fight. This internet is a wonderful thing."

"Utu, are you saying I am the wife of a god? Oh, please, great Utu," she said, falling to her knees and bowing her head. "Bless me with your divine manhood," she teased him as she laid her head in his lap and made eyes to go back in their room.

He smiled at her. "Sure, it's nice to be a god, but do you know what this means? We might be able to use this as a clue to find out where our tribe is…was. We could find it!"

Shainan looked up at him with doubt. "I hope, for all of us, but I fear that our history is as dead as our language is."

"You know," Rick suggested to Utu, tracking in the same direction without being able to understand their conversation. "If we research the foundations of this god or of your story," Rick grinned at Utu, "we may just find the area where you lived."

Utu looked at Rick with increasing confidence. He seems a good man. I will keep testing him.

"But first, I think the elk is ready." It had been a long morning. None of them had eaten, and they were hungry. Carson, who had been sleeping late in Rick's room in case there were any complications with their new guest during the night, was called out by Rick and introduced to their new Cro-Magnon.

"Utu, this is Carson. Carson, this is Utu. He is the ancient Sumerian Sun God. If you're good, I'll let you take him to school for show and tell." All of them but Shainan laughed as they sat down to the first red meat Utu had eaten in years. It was everything he remembered.

Utu was amazed by the seasonings Rick had to flavor the meat and demanded a full tour of the cabinet where they were kept. Half way through the meal, Rick realized they weren't going to have enough, and he put three more steaks on the grill. He made extra salad and threw some more spinach, almonds, carrots, kale, and garlic into the wok. They ate and talked for the next four hours. Rick was amazed at the amount of food Utu could shovel.

While waiting for the second set of steaks, Rick let the dogs in, and they went straight to Utu, whining in submission. He'd missed having his dogs these last ten years and was on the floor, much as Shainan had been, talking dog and roughhousing. Rick could see they respected Utu the moment they saw him, and he was always in charge. Rick wondered if the dogs would begin to see him as the pack leader.

After eating, subsequent searches that Utu conducted on the internet proposed the possibility that a Mt. Mashu, near the upper reaches of the Euphrates River, might be an area where they should concentrate further searches. The mountain existed only in mythology, but its location could indicate another clue in their search for an origin.

Also, the myth of Gilgamesh seemed to provide further clues. One part in particular, Rick read, "His slave Enkidu answered him: 'My lord, if today you want to set off into the mountains, Utu should know about it from us. Utu, young Utu, should know about this from us. A decision that concerns the mountains is Utu's business. A decision that concerns the mountains of cedar-felling is the business of young Utu. Utu should know about it from us.'"

Once Utu determined what a cedar was, he realized his home was full of them in the hills. He felt he was close to finding the lost bolt.

That evening Rick was the last one still awake. The newly-weds had retired early, per Shainan's demand, and Rick could hear them. At first they talked briskly, with laughing and some screaming, then laughing again. It seemed to Rick that Utu was teasing Shainan about getting caught drinking from the toilet. Then there was silence, then noise again.

Carson went to his room not long after. Rick put the dogs in their crates, threw on a jacket, and grabbed the keys to the Jeep. He had a date. Rick had given her the coordinates for the Primal Estate. He looked at his watch. 11:30. He snatched a piece of paper from the desk and wrote:

Carson,
I had to go out. Will be at the PE. Might be out all night.

I'll be on my cell if you need me.
Love, Dad.

He left the note for Carson on the kitchen table, in case something happened and he needed him.

Rick drove like a maniac. He was late by about fifteen minutes, and she would get there before him. He didn't want any complications. Rick put the pedal down and took care to be extra vigilant for deer, elk, cows, or horses in the road, continually scanning ahead of him side to side, like he did when he used to fly. Nothing was going to stop him from getting there. Rick looked at his watch again. Twenty minutes of back roads and I'm there, he thought.

One hour later, Rick was lying on his back in the sand, wearing only a smile. The afternoon sun was warming his body and the sultry waves were receding around him from the most recent rush running back down the beach. He sunk his feet into the sand and put his hands behind his head.

He was a little worried about sunburn on his scalp. But that was his only worry. Rick was on a tiny deserted island somewhere in the south Pacific. Nwella was sitting on top of him, also wearing only a smile.

It doesn't get much better than this, Rick thought. He was expecting conversation and a little romance, maybe at a campfire on his plot in Colorado, not a trip around the world. What a date! Nwella said she wanted to go running down the beach later... sounded interesting.

Rick thought about how much his life had changed. He had millions in cash hidden away in various locations, many more millions in gold stashed in so many locations he could afford to forget half of them, and enough weapons and ammunition to start a small army. Nwella had been good for him. She would be an asset to all he had planned.

She leaned down and kissed him on the lips the way he'd taught her. At first she hadn't liked it, but she seemed to be coming around. Then she added her own variations. First, she'd nibble on his lip, then work her way around his mouth with both of her lips, then go in for the full kiss. She had initially been repulsed by kissing. She complained to Rick that it seemed too much like eating, but after a little experimentation she became enthusiastic.

Nwella dismounted and strolled down the beach a short distance. Her sweaty body glistened in the sun. The combination of her feminine curves and her fit muscles on top of impeccable bone structure gave Rick an idea that he tried to suppress. He wanted to have children with her, but he knew that was impossible. They were different species, the politics were life threatening, and he might be dead soon anyway. It just wouldn't work. Does this mean I love you? Rick wondered. He wasn't sure.

As he looked after her, she looked back. She wanted him to follow, he could tell. She glanced back again and with a smile, took off running. Rick jumped up and, with his new body taking him faster than he thought possible, he sprinted after.

Chapter 28

DisappEaring and othEr rEcipEs

Tony felt like his relationship with Rick was getting more pertinent. Each day, the news gave indicators of people disappearing. He knew the time was coming when something had to be done. In fact, he would force it if he had to. He hadn't heard from his sister in two weeks and believed that he never would. His mother was in a depression about it, but even so, Tony still couldn't convince her to get back on her anxiety meds or any others, no matter how hard he tried. She wasn't taking anything right now, and the only reason he didn't seriously fear for her life was that she was old. The Provenger wouldn't target old people. At least, he didn't think they would.

Rick hadn't left a signal for him in two weeks. If there was nothing there for him today, he was going to call again. Tony had a handful of men all dedicated to training as a militia unit. They believed they were organizing according to their rights under the Constitution. And while they all had feelings that their government was overstepping its bounds, they were in no way ready to take up arms against it. People who genuinely were prepared to use violence against their government were truly rare. But they were all good men, and Tony had confidence that if they could be convinced of the existence of the Provenger, they would be the kind that could take action.

Tony felt bad about leading them into a situation where their lives might be at risk, especially for a purpose they had no idea existed. Worse yet, it could be a suicide mission. As he imagined events progressing, he hoped they would have a chance to back out if they chose to. But he wanted them to understand there was a chance they would be collected in a harvest anyway. And these men were the kind who would rather go down fighting.

Tony had seen in the news natural disasters happening everywhere. People disappearing, never to be found, not a body or even a body part. Planes and ships gone. People blamed it on anything they could think of – the weather, terrorists, and even the apocalypse. Some blamed it on a belief that the magnetic poles were starting to reverse. Everyone picked their favorite reason, as people often do. The building anxiety was real. And now he was almost certain that his sister was a victim.

Tony finally saw a signal from Rick at the Walmart, went to the drop where the meeting location was given, and followed its directions. This is where Tony would give Rick the ultimatum.

Tony approached the west edge of the pond at Parque De Vida, a nicely appointed public park near the center of Cortez. It had beautiful open spaces, playing fields, and park benches lining the water, a good place to meet someone while being able to scan the surroundings. Rick was already there, standing next to a bench. They sat down, and neither knew where to begin.

"A lot has happened since we first met, Tony."

"No shit. I've been working my ass off trying to get a crew together. What have you been doing?"

"I've been working some angles. What have you got?"

"I've got almost a dozen guys. They're good, good men. But I've got to warn you, they're not killers. They're interested in doing what's right. They all have military experience. I think if we get them together and tell them what's going on…"

"They'll think we're insane."

"No, they won't. Not if we show them the evidence. They've been watching the news. They've seen the issues with people disappearing, whole groups, whole towns, in natural disasters. That doesn't just happen. Rick, you're gonna hate me for this, but I told them I've been working with you."

"You did what? What kind of a dumb shit move was that?" Rick reacted with a low-toned tirade. "I can't be stuck out like that. What did you tell them we were 'working on', putting together a revolution or something?" Rick thought of the disastrous implications. This changed everything. The only way Rick could feel safe with this relationship was to maintain his anonymity. "Tony, really, I can't believe you. What the fuck were you thinking? All that's gotta happen is one of them says something to the wrong person, and the next thing I know I'm getting dragged out of my office like a criminal. Synster's gonna see the word spread and either frame me as insane, then make me disappear, or just cut to the chase and make me disappear." Rick leaned forward and put his head in his hands. "Shit." Rick could think of only one way out of this mess, and it made him sick.

"They know something's going on. I had to involve you to give it credibility. I didn't mention the NSA. I just told them you had inside information. The government is coming out with the gallbladder thing and the medicine ban proposal. They want to do something. When they do meet you and find out who you work for, they'll be pissed. I had to ease them into it. They've gotta be prepared somehow. You can't just show up. They need to know you're on our side. It's way beyond just a government thing now. They see what's going on in the world. They're not stupid. We're not at the top of the food chain anymore."

"Tony, you don't get it. They'll think we're kooks feeding off the news. They'll think they're being set up. We can't do anything yet anyway." Rick was horrified with Tony's flagrant abuse of their relationship.

"What do you mean can't do anything? We've got to do something. We can't keep letting them do this to us. We've got to show them there will be a cost. I'm not backing down on this, Rick. We're doing something."

"We're not doing anythi…"

"We are."

"Tony, we can't. I'm telling you. We don't have the ability."

"Rick, you don't understand. I've lost my sister. If I lose anyone else, I'm going to start talking."

"Apparently, you've already started talking."

"Unless we do something now, I'm going to go to the papers and tell them about you and your work. I'm going to go to your office and tell them you've been using their computers to check for the alien's probes and passing on if the government knows anything…keeping watch for them. I'll talk to anyone who'll listen." Tony paused trying to think of another threat to tack on. "I'll tell the authorities about your new live-in girlfriend."

Rick shot a glare at Tony, wondering how and what he knew about her.

"Rick, I'm serious here. And I know what you used to do for the military. You told me what you did in Afghanistan. I know what you must be capable of. We can do this. I know you can do this."

"You don't know shit about me!" Rick knew Tony was screwing him. The problem was that Tony knew too little. He really had no idea what Rick was capable of. Tony had received his last warning.

"I told the guys that if something happens to me, they should come looking for you."

Tony watched Rick get red and swollen in the face as he was talking. Maybe I shouldn't have gone this far, Tony thought. He was quickly regretting all he'd said. He'd pushed Rick too far. There was a long pause.

"Okay, Rick, I'm sorry I said all that to them. It was just after I knew I'd lost my sister. I was frustrated and angry. I knew this was going on and I hadn't done anything about it. Well, I'm going to do something now." Tony was glad he'd kept talking. Rick seemed to have calmed down right when it looked like he might blow.

"Tony, you can't do any of those things; it wouldn't be productive. We've got to focus on what will work. The stakes are too high. This isn't about a few years in prison, and this isn't about principle." Rick's volume was growing, and he had to remind himself to tone down. "This is about preventing our planet, humanity, from being the food supply for an alien race. One or two or a dozen or even a thousand people don't matter. We've got to wait until the time is right."

"I understand that, but the sooner we start resistance, the better our position will be. People are going to find out anyway, and soon."

"What you're advocating will lead to the managed collectivization I told you about. Resistance would be improbable or impossible under that situation," Rick tried to reason with him.

"That's where we're going anyway! You're just worried about your own ass, aren't you?

"That's not it."

"Yeah, I think it is. Don't worry. You won't be implicated. We still need you on the inside. We need to kill a bunch of these guys. You need to let us know how, when, and where, and we'll do it. If we make it costly enough for them and make an example, maybe they'll see we're not worth it."

The more Tony tried to convince Rick, the more he became convinced that he would do nothing. This was all bad. All they needed was for some kind of action to be taken. They couldn't keep waiting, Tony thought. But Rick wouldn't listen. The more they talked and the more Tony threatened, the less he was convinced that Rick was committed to the destruction of the Provenger. Now Tony's frustration was coming to a boiling point.

"What have you been doing? Do we have a way to kill them? Can you get us on the ship? I've got access to explosives we can set." Tony didn't want to actually say he had them.

Finally, completely surprising Tony, Rick calmed and acquiesced. "Fine, we'll take action. I've been working on something, and I think it might pan out. I have more information now than I did. I'll contact you next week. I'll have an answer."

Tony felt better but was still disappointed that Rick was so hesitant. He'd been so motivated at first. Had somebody gotten to him? Tony looked at Rick a little closer. "Do you have a sunburn?" Tony asked, looking at his face and then his hands, which also looked sunburned.

"Yeah, I've been doing some work outside," Rick replied.

An hour after he'd left Rick, Tony pulled up to the Cortez pistol and rifle range just east of town. Some of his buddies were already there. He felt a little guilty pressuring and deceiving Rick as he had. His team wasn't exactly composed of the stalwart military men he'd described. The fact was that they were the hodgepodge anti-government group that Rick had always been concerned about. They were prone to conspiracy theories and had negative, fertile imaginations.

Tony had already put them together to execute whatever they thought appropriate once they'd figured out what the NSA was doing in Cortez. Tony's idea was to blow up some equipment. He didn't intend to hurt anyone but simply garner support from like-minded patriots, show that there were people that cared, that were willing to put it all on the line. He wanted to show that aggressive action could be used safely. He imagined that if it was done carefully and professionally, no one would get caught.

To this group he'd added a few more people, mostly comprised of former Army friends who would only go so far as to commiserate with his beliefs and provide vague assurances that they'd be there for him when he needed them, for organizational and training purposes.

Shooting at the range that day was Tom Durham, a small business owner in Mancos, the neighboring town. He had a vendetta regarding the government's recent socialization of medicine. Rob Godfrey, from Durango, was a recently discharged Air Force mechanic and had been pulled over by traffic cops one too many times. His friend Will Jenkins was a former rancher whose family had literally lost the farm and his wife in the debt crisis. They were indeed all former military, but their skills were spotty. When Tony thought about it too much, he doubted everything he was doing.

They were going to shoot for the rest of the day. They would practice a little pistol first, then some long range rifle to check zeros on their scopes, and then have a little competition.

Tony's phone rang. "Yello."

"Tony? Marcus. What's up man."

"Hey, Marcus. How you been?"

"Good. Hey, I'm not gonna make the shoot today...had to stay home with the kids. I..." silence, "I...Count me in for everything else though..." Silence.

"Hello? Marcus? You there?"

"Yeah, I'm here. Hold on."

Tony heard Marcus put the phone down and was irritated. Marcus calls, then puts me on hold! What the...

Crack!! broke the silence. Tony heard a rifle shot on the other end of the line

"Shit! Marcus, you there?" Tony heard fumbling on the line.

"Hello? Hey, sorry 'bout that. I've been trying to get that bastard for weeks now. Finally did. Keeps coming over to my property."

"What the hell are you shooting? Damn! I thought you'd been shot!" Tony exclaimed.

"No...Damn neighbor's dog keeps coming over. Won't be anymore!" replied Marcus.

This is the problem, thought Tony.

Nwella stood just inside the door of the shed at the back of Rick's property, beside the pile of hay. She was scared, more so than she'd ever been. She had planned to meet Rick in ten minutes. She knew he was thinking it would be another date. It wouldn't. She arrived a little early to gain her composure and try to figure out what she was going to do, thinking it would come to her once she arrived, but it hadn't.

She heard the dogs barking and peeked through the shed window to see Rick closing the back door, keeping them inside. He was early, too. She took a deep breath. Whatever happened in the next five minutes would change her life. He walked toward the shed in a space of time that felt both like an eternity and a moment.

"Nwella, I've missed you. What's it been, twelve hours?" Rick joked with a smile

"Yes," Nwella said and was quiet. He knows something is wrong, she thought. They held each other, and she started to shake. Rick quickly pushed back and held her at arm's length.

"What's wrong?" he asked urgently. "Have we been discovered?"

"We might as well be. Rick, I don't know what to tell you, how to tell you," Nwella stuttered, her chest heaving with swallowed breath.

"What?" Rick was starting to panic. His family's lives were on the line.

"I have a child. We have a child. It must have been from the first time."

"We have a child?" Rick stammered, "How can we have a child? Is that possible?" Then Rick paused and his face twitched. "How could things possibly get more complicated? I have a child! You do mean you're pregnant, right? I mean it's not somewhere here already?" Rick glanced around on the floor. "You know, the whole alien thing."

"No, don't be stupid." Nwella bumped him on the chest with her fist. "It's in me. We have them the same way," Nwella explained.

Rick dropped to his knees and hugged her around the hips, burying his face in her stomach. "How are we going to do this? How is this going to work?" Rick asked looking up, nervous and confused, sounding like an inmate in a psychiatric ward. "Do I call Synster 'Dad'? Will he kill me? You know you took me first." Rick gasped and laughed. "How can this be? Does he know? Are you sure?"

"Yes," Nwella replied.

"Yes to he knows, or yes to being sure?"

"Yes, I'm sure."

"You're sure he knows, or that you're pregnant?"

"I'm sure that I'm pregnant, you dope! I already said, it must have happened that first time, when I took you after your treatment by the Recombinant. The treatment must have done something to make it possible. It shouldn't have happened."

Rick was still babbling on his knees, apparently not knowing what to do, and Nwella could sense it.

"Don't worry, my love. Because of my condition, I have immunity, and so do you."

"Immunity against what?" Rick asked.

"Against anything," Nwella responded.

"What's anything?" Rick asked rising to his feet again, still holding her close.

"Recriminations cannot be brought against us. It is the law," Nwella explained.

"Well, we have laws, too, and they only extend to our species, sometimes just to citizens and sometimes not even them. Do your laws extend to humans?"

"This law would have to. Its impetus emanates from the life within me, and only in that respect, affects us. We are the sources of this life. We are responsible for this life," Nwella explained. "The law protects us only to protect the life within me. The lives of our children are of primary importance to us. My real violation is my aberrant sexual behavior. We have a strange unofficial rule regarding that. It can be done; just don't get caught. But there is no hiding a pregnancy."

"That sounds reasonable," said Rick, thinking hard and fast. There was a long pause. "Nwella, I want you to know I won't abandon you. I want to keep Carson safe, but other than that, I only care about you. Against all logic, I love you, Nwella. I think I have since that first day I saw you."

Nwella looked at Rick, wondering if he could handle the next few bombs she was about to drop.

"What will you do?" Rick asked

"I will be cast out," Nwella whispered. "They won't hurt us, but I will be cast out. If there was nowhere habitable to put me, I would be forced to remain on the ship, and I would be made to wear certain attire that would show everyone that they were not to speak to me. That would be for fifty years. It would be torture. I wouldn't recover. No one ever has. But since we have access to Earth, I could choose to come here, especially since you are the father." Nwella knew that humans sometimes terminated pregnancies. That had never been a Provenger way and never would be, as far as Nwella was concerned. Even if she did, it would have shown up on her next Recombinant scan anyway. She would then not only be an outcast but be subject to worse penalties for having terminated the pregnancy.

"Like I said, I'm here for you. I'm not sure what the implications of you being cast out are, but if it's possible, I want you to come live with me. Utu can overcome his anger. Shainan can get around her fear. We can retrain the dogs."

Nwella stroked Rick's cheek and decided that now was the time to tell him.

"Rick, I need to tell you something else."

With trepidation Rick readied for the worst. He looked at her, dead in the eyes, "There's more? Go ahead."

"Until recently, I was doing this for the thrill, nothing else. But, I guess since I've become pregnant, something has happened. It's a feeling I've never had."

Rick was silent for a moment and then confessed, "The same for me. Until recently, I was also in it for the thrill, as well as the added security of having you involved with me. I was using you."

"Okay, I understand that, and I was doing all that, too." Nwella paused. "I think you knew that. I raped you while you slept, after all." Nwella looked at the ground. "But I also mean something else." Back to his eyes. "Rick, two nights ago, I had a dream." Nwella stared at Rick, waiting for a response.

Rick looked at her. "So what was the dream?"

"I don't remember. I woke up in a panic. I wasn't sure of what happened. I had to research it before I was sure. I found the studies done on Shainan."

"I'm sorry. I don't understand," Rick confessed.

"Rick, we don't dream. Provenger don't dream."

"That's right, I forgot. What does it mean?"

"I'm not sure, but when the dream studies were done on Shainan, our scientists were looking for something. They were looking to discover our history related to dreaming. Apparently, there were considerable resources being put into secret studies of this type, and since our last war, that research has been lost. Only fragments remain, so I have no idea what it means. But it's obviously got to have something to do with the pregnancy."

Nwella paused then, even more serious than before. She said, "Rick, there's something more you should know. It's bad, really bad. I'm afraid you'll hate me when I tell you."

Chapter 29

The mAmmoth hunt

"I'm Steinman Blake with CNN, reporting. Recently, turmoil has erupted in the medical community in the wake of new government recommendations regarding some of the most commonly-used pharmaceuticals. According to government experts with the Department of Health and Human Services, an updated meta-analysis, which combine the results of many research studies, have led government experts to the conclusion that most of the pharmaceuticals we take are not only damaging to our health but unnecessary, provided that humans follow the correct diet for our species. They've produced studies that indicate the vast majority of chronic disease and autoimmune disorders are epigenetic in nature, meaning they arise from the environment we create in our bodies from the foods we consume. They admit that genetics play a role in predisposition to particular ailments, but state that the environment created in the living cell is what makes this predisposition expressive. This renders us either susceptible to many infectious diseases or inclined to develop chronic maladies such as autoimmune disorders. Pharmaceutical companies are outraged and are complaining that their tested and approved medications are being sidelined to something as superficial as nutrition."

"Steinman, let's not make the mistake that the government has turned holistic on us. The health care community has also recently been blindsided by 'Gallbladdergate,' the new initiative to compel all statistically overweight people to, at least, schedule to have their gallbladders removed in a noble effort to reduce cholesterol. Detractors are calling for congressional hearings regarding the delivery of those gallbladders to the government for research purposes. Steinman?"

"That's right, Bob. This is starting to create a pattern of outrageous moves on the part of the Department of Health – moves that seem to defy everything they've been saying for the last fifty

Utu turned the volume all the way down. Listening to the television had helped him to improve his English considerably in the last few days. Every word that he heard used in context was confirmed. The patterns of syntax rapidly congealed in his mind, and English speech became a part of him with almost no effort. Rick told him it was good that he didn't sound like Tarzan anymore. When Utu searched "Tarzan" on the internet, he found pictures of muscular men wearing animal skins. He suspected that perhaps he should feel insulted.

Utu had been glued to the computer every spare moment that he wasn't enjoying himself at his new earthbound home. He'd learned much since he was first shown how to use it. His unique ability to learn language appeared to overlap into written communication, and he was already reading and writing at a rudimentary level. He was getting access to more than just pictures. The isolation he'd suffered during his captivity resulted in a ravenous appetite for knowledge of his new world, and Utu was amazed that he could learn just about anything he wanted if he knew some basic words concerning the subject and searched the correct terms on the internet.

The loud squeak of the door to the back patio slowly opening and closing gave Utu the impression of either someone who was deep in thought entering, or a deaf person trying to sneak up on him. It compelled him to look. Rick was standing there with an ashen face.

"We need to talk, Utu," Rick said. "Are you ready to trust me?"

"Maybe," he replied stoically. For a moment, Utu thought Rick had come across the two mule deer carcasses that he'd hunted and had hanging in a large cedar tree about a hundred yards behind the house. He'd cleaned them and had managed to eat most of one among himself, Shainan, and Rick's two German Shepherds, which were now his best friends.

Utu couldn't avoid the temptation. He had searched the house and found the rifle Rick had shown him one evening. Rick had demonstrated to him briefly how it worked and how to sight it. Utu had been exposed by the Provenger to many technological wonders since a boy, when he thought they were magic. He'd also experienced and heard about many amazing machines on board the Provenger ship. He wasn't your typical Cro-Magnon. He expected these miracles to work. He took technology in stride, especially if it could be used to hunt.

During the week when he wasn't searching the internet or making love to Shainan on the small patch of turf in the back yard, he hunted the woods behind the house when Rick was at work. It was a beautiful tool, he thought. He'd taken more meat with less effort than ever in all his life. And he had done it alone. It had been heaven. His only complaint was that it was so loud that it made his ears ring. Now he'd been discovered. He knew he probably hadn't earned the right to hunt this territory. But he had told Rick he needed to hunt, and Rick seemed to agree. He had been warned.

"Let's sit at the kitchen table." Rick beckoned him to sit. As Utu assessed Rick's serious demeanor, it appeared that he had experienced some kind of momentous revelation. Utu dispelled his first impression regarding the discovery of the carcasses and suspected this had something to do with the Provenger. Utu believed that Rick now knew some of what he'd been waiting to tell him.

"I've just become aware of what is going on with this harvest, how it is likely to be done, and where we'll stand after it happens. I've left you alone for these last few days. I wanted to build trust between us. I think we're part of the way there." Rick got two glasses out of the cabinet, the wine out of the refrigerator, and put them down on the table. They both sat down. Up to now, when they ate, Utu had refused alcohol.

"It's our custom that when two friends come to an agreement, they have a drink together. Will you consider it?" Rick hoped some wine would loosen his lips.

Utu looked at the wine. Alcohol had destroyed his people

after it had become readily available, and he viewed it as spiritual poison. But he knew that each new situation deserved new consideration. "I'll consider it."

"I just found out that the current harvests are merely preliminary trials of some type, that the harvests will increase rapidly for people in the harvest age, somewhere between twenty-five and thirty-five, until such time that it becomes so obvious that everyone can't ignore it and things start going to hell." Rick paused to get his thoughts together.

"Synster is stalling to get people off drugs; they need their meat organic. When that happens, all remaining humans who have been designated for the harvest will be taken all at once, or at least as fast as they can process everyone. Once most are taken, the Provenger will come down in massive numbers, shut down our power plants, remove toxic waste, reduce our buildings to dust, and eradicate our history and technology. The few pockets of people that remain around the world will literally be reduced to the Stone Age. No offense."

"None taken," Utu replied without missing a beat.

Rick continued. "I can only suppose that you and I will be among those lucky few, along with everyone in this town and anyone else on a no-kill list, who will remain alive. That is, if you can call it lucky. We'll be allowed to start over, building population and civilization again."

"Where did you learn this information?" Utu asked.

"Well, that's another thing I need to talk to you about. I'm having an affair with Nwella. She's a Provenger." Rick saw a black stare come back at him and added for context, "She is *my* woman."

Utu raised an eyebrow. "Sexy, aren't they? Not as good as Earth women, if you ask me," commented Utu, keeping his cool remarkably well, considering his landlord was now sleeping with the enemy. Nothing surprises me anymore, thought Utu. I did it myself. But can I trust him? Let's see where this goes.

"She's Synster's daughter," Rick added to the already interesting scenario, "and she's pregnant."

Utu made a variety of painful faces at the flood of unpleasant disclosures, puffed air out of his lungs, pushed back from the table, and shook his head. "Couldn't be. I've slept with many,

many, Provenger women. None of them ever got pregnant. And Synster's daughter?" Utu put his hands behind his head. "He is going to tear you apart. She's making it up. Gotta be…lying to you…the pregnant part."

Rick was growing agitated. "From what you could tell, do they obey their laws?"

"What do you mean?"

"Do they obey all of their laws all the time? For instance, in my…our society, we have laws, but we frequently ignore them and do the thing anyway," Rick explained.

"Oh, yes, they always obey their laws… almost all the time."

"Almost?" Rick asked, the pitch in his voice going up an octave.

"Yes, almost. As long as they have something to lose in their society, they obey their laws. If they are cast out, for some reason, usually morality issues, then they disobey. They are "rufqwrinst." It means like a pirate, living outside the law. They would be very dangerous then. But I only heard of that happening a couple times. If you want to know what I think, I think she is lying to you, for some advantage. I never got a Provenger female pregnant; how could you? Look at us." Utu motioned, pointing back and forth between the two of them. In his world of biology, the bigger the man, the more virile he was.

Rick sat back and crossed his arms. "She said it happened just after I went through the Recombinant. Would that make a difference?"

"You went through the Recombinant? How did you get them to put you through?"

"Carson was injured and sick. I asked and they said it would give him a better chance at survival. Also, I didn't want to subject him to something like that alone. I guess Synster needed me badly enough or had some other motive. If it was the Recombinant that allowed this to be possible, I don't think they knew it could happen. They haven't put many humans through, so they told me."

"My mother was put through before I was born. So was my father, I think. But now you'll have a nice healthy baby, maybe as strong as me. Do we know if it's a boy or a girl?" Utu smiled at him. "You know the Provenger have a way of knowing that."

"Yeah, we do, too. So do you still think she's lying? She also said she had a dream."

"Maybe not," Utu paused. "And Provenger don't dream."

"Well, she said she did, and looked up the study they did on Shainan's dreaming...said they were looking to fill in some knowledge gaps in their history."

"I don't know anything about that," Utu lied. In fact, he knew quite a bit. Dreams were indicators of spiritual energy, both good and evil. Provenger didn't have dreams. To Utu this could mean only one thing. They had no spirits; they had no souls. He'd overheard rumors that long ago they'd considered the possibility of researching a type of energy that humans would consider souls. For some reason it was never pursued, maybe because of the war.

"Well, do you think Nwella lied about the harvest?" Rick asked.

Utu stared at Rick for a long time. Rick waited. Utu stared some more. Finally, Utu spoke, "I don't think so, if she is pregnant. I think you can trust what a pregnant Provenger female tells you. It has been my experience that when they need to deceive, they avoid you before they would lie. It's offensive to lie. That isn't something they're really likely to do when pregnant. Regarding the harvest, I think that's how they're going to do it, or something close. They will return this world to where it was and probably do the whole cycle all over again. With their ability to move forward in time, it is not long for them, these thousands of years we need to fill Earth. It is only years for them. The problem they have with an intelligent population is that they always advance. That's why they have to ensure they don't advance too fast. Did you ever wonder how many times they've already done this to us?"

"Maybe..." Rick then asked, "If you've been thinking all this, then why didn't you tell me?"

"You work for the Provenger, Rick. Why should I tell you anything?"

"You should understand why I do. They threatened to kill me, everyone in my family, and everyone I know in the most horrific way."

"Well," Utu paused, collecting his memories on Provenger laws and protocols, "they can kill you for the sake of the project, I think, but they can't just go around and kill everyone else, not for punishment or revenge. I think that would be against their law. Probably all those that they would have killed for your punishment would die in the harvest anyway."

"Hopefully, the Provenger will honor their deal. Someone needs to survive to perpetuate the species. I've been able to exempt family and friends, take them off the harvest list," Rick explained further. "Also, by working with them, I can position myself to know them, learn their weaknesses."

"I see," Utu said, processing the word "exempt" in its context for the first time. Utu continued, "But also, and I've got to say this, most of my knowledge of the Provenger is from hearing them speak to each other. I couldn't ask questions," Utu explained. "I need to tell you now, Rick. Obviously you've figured it out. I'm good with languages, like the Provenger. I can speak their language, yours, and all the others, to some degree, from the interaction I've had with them. One of their favorite things to do was to help themselves learn by trying to teach me. Of course, I couldn't learn a thing," Utu smiled. "I never let it be known that I knew their language or any of the others. If I had, I would be a threat to them, and they wouldn't have let me go. This is my secret. If you let it go, I will die. They will kill me. You haven't told Nwella I can communicate with you?"

"No, of course not. But if she becomes an outcast, she will come to live with us, in our own little Stone Age tribe."

"That would be awkward," Utu admitted. "We can't let her know we talk to each other. And if we do, I'll have to act simple, stupid."

Rick looked up at him with doubt.

Utu continued, "That's how they know me. At least, until we know we can trust her, if that would ever be possible." Utu paused. "Does it scare you, losing all your technology?"

"Yes, I suppose it does."

"Your technology, it is all a thin veil of civility concealing the brutishness beneath. It is not real."

"Yes, I suppose it is. That's very profound you know," Rick admitted, impressed by the thirty-seven-year-old shaman.

"I read it last night on the internet. I think Shainan is getting jealous of it. She wants me in bed." The two hunters, twelve thousand years and a kitchen table apart, smiled at each other and decided to have a drink.

Shainan had gone to bed early, hoping Utu would follow, but she instead awoke to the noises of men talking in the kitchen. The sounds comforted her as she remembered them from when she was a girl. The men would drink their ferment, when they had it, through reeds from the single skin in which it was made. They would tell their stories, bragging and fighting, usually not hurting each other. In the good years, it was almost always in fun. She would lift her head from the buffalo hide and strain with both ears to listen in on the stories. She wanted to hear them now.

Shainan rose from her bed and sat on the floor, opening the door a crack to listen. She was glad to identify the voices of the three of them, Carson, Rick, and her sun god. She could hear they were telling stories of bear, horses, deer, bison, mammoth, and elk, not because she understood the words but because she understood the sounds – the laughter, the exaggerated tones, the inflections. It warmed her heart. It gave her the feeling of safety to have a tribe again. As insignificant as it was, it gave her hope that perhaps they could one day be free of the Provenger. Life could return to normal.

She flattened herself on the floor, ear next to the crack in the door, and closed her eyes. She was back in time, a girl of the tribe, sleeping in her tent with her mother and sisters, the boys and the men outside by the fire, talking of their hunts to provide for their tribe. She would need that tribe if the child growing within her were to have any chance of a future. She listened.

"Get the...yes, yes, so when we get close we give all the spears to the smallest your age Carson so we'll have our hands free, we'd never do it with less than ten we taught the dogs to stay with us so we would always have a solid ring around the beast the dogs would be running back and forth they'd make a fantastic roar and confusion where did you spear first well all over really some for the eyes head some would try for the tendons on the back of the legs one time we threw all our spears and the mammoth was over them and wouldn't move so we had to get her to move to another spot no shit to get and the spears under her the first spears that went in she would always pull out with her trunk if she could reach them, then once we can put more spears in her than she can pull out and maybe a tendon or two horrible business so the boys just keep handing us spears yes and just as fast as we can when we get an opening and when tired we rest and collect spears that she's pulled out and thrown and the boys get a chance enough blood loss and she goes down...As many spears we could with sharp bone tips, some with very sharp stone, best spears are heavy to go deep hit blood they fall out we throw again they can't be too thick so they'll go in by long thin hardened shaft to a point at the end of thick shaft I got hit by a trunk once thrown onto Risto...

The talking stopped, and Shainan's eyes popped open when she heard and recognized the name of her cousin. Risto was Utu's uncle but was more like a father to him. She knew why Utu had stopped. He was telling a story of hunting and said his name. She should go to him, she thought.

Shainan walked into the kitchen where the men were sitting. They all had a glass in front of them and two empty bottles in the middle. She hadn't bothered to put any clothes on, again, and Carson and Rick were glad to see her beautiful form. They'd gotten used to the unshaved legs and underarms. They didn't even see that anymore.

She looked down at her Utu. His face was buried in his folded arms crossed on the table. He was crying for the memory of Risto. "Come, my god. Risto hears you. The stories are over," she commanded in the language only they could understand. She leaned over and held him, crushing her full bare breasts into his back. She strained to help lift his massive heap of a body to his feet, and they walked into their room together. She was determined to make the most of what night they had left. She would use her passion for him as a knife. She would skin the grief from his body and soul.

"Well," said Rick, turning to Carson, "I bet nobody in the world for the last ten thousand years has done that."

"Done what?" asked Carson.

"Sat around and got a first person account of a mammoth hunt. The guys at the hunting club are gonna be jealous. You'd better get some sleep. It's almost morning."

"Night, Dad. Thanks."

"Goodnight, Carson. Love you."

"You, too. Ha, Utu." And Carson shuffled off to his room.

Rick sat down on the side of the couch that hadn't been peed on and looked at what was left of the fire in the stove. It was almost out. Just a bed of glowing coals remained under the ash. He would have to add more wood. He'd also have to open the ash cleaning door, at the base, to allow a huge amount of air in to get the wood burning hot. First, he'd see sparks and then flames. Then he'd hear the roar of a fire that could grow too hot, too fast, if he let it. The expanding metal of the cast iron stove would make clinking sounds as it heated. Joints could break if it heated too fast. The soot in the chimney could catch on fire. The night could be ruined if he wasn't there to close the ash cleaning door and cut off the source of excess air. He had to set the inferno into action. Only he could stop it. Only he could control it.

On a pad of paper on the table next to the couch he wrote:

11/24, 1630 favorite hunting spot parking area. Bring whole group-I have equipment-everything needed-going hunting.

Rick put the paper in his pocket, ready to leave it at their drop point in the morning. "I have to step things up," he said aloud. He had to meet with Nwella one more time before this meeting. He had only days left.

Chapter 30

Fortune to the highest bidder

Sitting on the couch, sleep overwhelmed Rick as the adrenaline that had been surging through his veins was worked out of his system by his slightly distracted liver. That very night he'd learned he would be a father to a human alien hybrid and that he'd probably have to start planning for college expenses again. That is, only if he could save the human race from an imminent harvest to become food for aliens led by his new kid's grandfather. And how would he tell Carson he'd no longer be an only child…and that he'd have a new step-mom?

Rick had learned many more interesting things from his all-nighter with Utu. He'd learned that the Provenger power system that ran everything, from their transports to and from the ship, to their distance and time travel, wasn't so volatile after all. The way Synster had described the two orbiting neutron stars, or binary star, at the center of their ship made it sound like the ship's containment system was all that protected the entire solar system from destruction.

Though his information was from numerous sources over a long period of time and Utu still wasn't completely sure, he had a strong belief that the energy of the stars was brought to the ship through the same method that the ship used to travel, or that the stars were "there, but also not there". These are the two different versions he'd overheard described.

Utu synthesized these two versions with what he heard about the shutdown capabilities of the ship. The stars could be "put away" at certain times to allow maintenance or repairs to the physical portions of the containment system. When this happened, the circular shape of the ship accommodated the creation of artificial gravity by spinning. While the ship was under these conditions, the Provenger used a power source that sounded to Rick like standard nuclear technology. All this made it seem like, except for their very advanced main power system, they weren't all that much more advanced than humans.

After talking with Utu about it for some time, Rick concluded that if the containment system were removed or destroyed, the stars would simply be gone and irretrievable, without appearing locally and without the resultant destruction of the solar system. This kind of containment also made sense with regard to size. Normal-sized neutron stars, Rick had reasoned, regardless of the massive size of the Provenger ship, would be much too large to be contained at its center.

It was resolved between them that the destruction of the ship would not result in the destruction of the solar system, which was Rick's main concern. It was assuming a great deal, but it at least pointed toward an opportunity.

Rick also learned that you need at least a dozen people and at least as many dogs to hunt a mammoth. The mammoth needs to be panicked enough to forget its herding instincts and the protection it affords to reduce it to confusion and exhaustion. Bows will work to take out eyes, but to effectively bleed the animal, there is no substitute for heavy spears. You need lots of them, and you need to isolate the mammoth so you can get the spears into it. You've got to bleed it to death. There is no such thing as a killing blow. A heavy, flexible spear, as Utu described it, is best because it needs a lot of inertia behind it to penetrate deeply, but not so heavy that it can't be thrown with the throwing stick. Once the animal has tired, then the solid, very heavy spears with a long, sharp ivory or stone head thrown or thrust by hand make for a quicker kill. It is a long, messy, brutal process that takes time and patience.

Rick also learned that it was "vital" that he obtain one of the Provenger's working fighting gauntlets. Utu stressed that it was the only way humans could have a chance at fighting them.

"How vital?" Rick asked. Utu knew something.

"As vital as having enough spears," Utu advised. "Having the gauntlet would be equal to putting a thousand spears into a mammoth. Not having it..." Utu held up the spoon in front of him. "Try killing a mammoth with this. There are just some things I cannot tell you, Rick. I need to get a gauntlet."

That's pretty vital, Rick thought. I must meet with Nwella again.

Chapter 31

Tony's rebellion

Rick knew a little about anatomy. The human head is an amazing system. The skull, the main structure of the head, encases, like armor, the most important organ of survival to the human being – the brain. While other animals have claws, fangs, bone crushing strength, lightning speed, flight, incomparable sense of smell or eyesight, humans really have only their brains to help them survive. While different people can have all the aforementioned attributes to a certain degree when compared to other humans, animals have taken these traits to a higher level. It is only the human brain and a person's ability to use it that give them any chance at survival. Humans have certainly taken this to a higher level. The skull is the strange exoskeleton of a normally endoskeletal beast that protects this vital tool, this interesting cluster of predominantly omega 3 fatty acids.

The rest of the body seems only as an afterthought, a device by which the brain can be moved from place to place, to impose itself on the world. The locomotion and the senses of the body seem merely the means by which the brain might be protected through the sensing, and defense against, or removal from, danger.

If one were to put two hundred pounds directly on top of the head, the pressure would stress the many plates of the skull and their synarthrodial joints. Some flexing would occur, as would some compression of the spinal column and a very high pitched ringing in the ears of the person beneath would begin, alerting him to a problem. One would have to add much more weight before the skull would be crushed. Alternately, given a medium size stone with an impact to the temple, a similar sound may be heard. But in each case, the mighty skull, with so many different bones that even the experts can't decide their number, will remain intact.

The skull doesn't have to break to bring death to a person. Violent motion can cause trauma to the brain as it moves inside the skull, colliding with the dull and sharp structures that hold it in place. But still the skull will remain intact. Heating the skull would kill a person long before the skull would eventually roast hot enough to either boil the brain and pop a section out under pressure, or crack the bone through the effect of the heat.

But take a very small piece of lead and propel it at high speed toward the skull, and it has no problem penetrating and transferring all its remaining energy to the soft brain tissue within. Use a larger piece of lead, and the brain will be launched out the opposite side, clustered with bone. No time for ears ringing there, nothing but complete, instant removal of consciousness, a step into the void.

Tony Carrian paced the distance from his SUV to the cliff edge and back again, multiple times, collecting burs on the cuffs of his pants from the weeds that littered the sand. It was a clear, cold evening, and the sun was just under the horizon. It was getting dark fast. Rick was there, reclined in his Jeep, looking like he was sleeping, patient, while all of Tony's friends were arriving. Rick had refused to talk to anyone about any plan or even show himself to be introduced until they'd all been gathered as a unit. All he would say to Tony was that he'd conferred with his contact and that everything was ready. His Jeep appeared to be packed with equipment.

Tony felt nervous about the meeting. He didn't even know if this was just a planning meeting or if they were actually going to do something. Maybe he'd rushed Rick too much, pushed him too far. He was beginning to have second thoughts. The weight of responsibility for the safety of his group began to press on his conscience.

Tom Durham was in the bed of his truck trying to organize some gear, and Tony walked over to him. "Tom," he called out.

"Yeah, hey, Tony. Hey listen. Can we talk?"

Tony nodded as he walked up. "Sure, that's why I came over."

"Okay, let me put this away. I'll meet you over by that thick cedar, over there." Tom pointed. He stuffed his things into the box in the back of his truck, closed the lid, locked it, and vaulted to the ground as Tony sauntered to the tree, deep in thought.

Tom walked up. "Tony, I don't like this. I don't know this guy, and you said he's NSA, and the only reason I'm here is to support you, and the fact that if the feds roll up, we've never really talked about anything except being pissed about the way the government's run and socialized medicine. I'm pretty sure nothing's going on out here, so whatever this guy comes up with, I'll have time to decide what I'm gonna do," Tom rambled on nervously, Tony nodding all the way.

"Yeah Tom. You know, I've been thinking and I'm sorry I brought you into this." Tony paused to think. "Tell you what. Hear what we've got to say and then you decide. You don't have to say anything. Just hear what we've got to say." Tony looked him in the eyes, asking Tom to trust him.

"Okay, Tony, but if this guy is a whack job, I'm outta here."

"Understood, and I don't blame you. But I think you'll find what we have to say interesting," Tony said, thinking, this guy is going to crap his pants when he learns the reality.

It was a half hour beyond the meeting time and, not including Tony, there were nine of them there ready to hear what Rick had to say. Tony was watching him from a distance. Rick stirred, checked the watch on his wrist, and remained still. With a burst of movement Rick got out of the Jeep and headed for Tony. He was dressed in desert fatigues with a 1911 on his hip. "Everybody here?" Rick asked, sounding agitated and impatient.

"Yeah, everybody's here. We're all just waiting on you," Tony lied. It was Marcus again. He was late. He'd said he'd be there, but Tony didn't want to wait any longer. Chances were Marcus would call in a half hour and cancel anyway. "So what's the surprise in the Jeep?" Tony asked, now just hoping for a training session with some kind of new weapon.

"Soon enough," Rick said. "Why don't you get them all together over here and we'll get started?"

Tony called them over and introduced Rick by name only. Rick was about to speak but then stopped. He glanced at Tony.

"Tony, I got to say something to you in private. Just one second?" Rick gestured that they step away together. After a few paces, Rick stopped and they turned, face-to-face.

"Tony, you're a good man. I want to thank you for supporting me, all the way from helping me out of the canyon that first day to motivating me to get moving with a plan to fight these things. When all is said and done, I'm sure the day will come when you get the recognition for being…" Rick stopped for a moment, a little choked and thinking, "…for doing all that you've done. I hope I don't let you down." Rick finished, his voice quivering a little, and he stuck out his hand.

Tony shook it. "Thanks, Rick. I really appreciate that. I'm sure you won't." They stood still, looking at each other for a moment. "Is that all?" Tony asked.

"Yeah, that's all," Rick replied. The image of a small piece of paper with writing on it flashed in Rick's mind. On the piece of paper was written, "I am the Lion."

They turned to walk back to the group. As they did, Rick drew his 1911 pistol and carefully and deliberately put it to the back of Tony's head. He pulled the trigger. The sound of the near contact shot was perceptibly muffled by the proximity of the muzzle to Tony's scalp. The .45 caliber automatic Colt pistol round, 230 grains of copper jacketed lead that entered the back of Tony's head was moving at about 950 feet per second. It penetrated the skull and entered the brain before any of the surrounding tissue even had a chance to register the impact. The shock of the energy wave moving through Tony's mind thoroughly scrambled his brain into a goo that followed the mushrooming round. Bone and skin fragments from half of Tony's face flew from his forehead in the direction he was walking. They hit the ground a moment after Tony's limp body did. He hadn't felt a thing. That's the way Rick wanted it. There would be no open casket. In fact, there would be no casket at all. The Provenger would gladly take the bodies.

Tom Durham stared with the others and could not believe what he had just seen. The nightmare they had just entered began in slow motion from that point forward. They gawked at Tony's lifeless body in front of them. Looking around at each other, they realized they were not alone.

Will Jenkins had been watching Rick closely and saw him drawing his pistol. He drew as quickly as he could and had his pistol out and ready, trying to confirm with his mind what his eyes had just seen. When they all turned to see the monsters behind them, Will acted. He managed to fire one poorly aimed shot at a Provenger, and the bullet stopped short of him with a buzzing sound surrounded by a small glowing circle. It dropped to the ground. They all tried to assimilate the image of the four Provenger standing immediately behind them.

They forgot about the murder they had just witnessed and jumped back to draw their weapons, but they had none. By now, any pistols the men had with them disintegrated on their bodies. Will looked with disbelief at the powder in his hand.

Rick fell to his knees, Tony's body face down in the dirt before him, and watched in horror. Two men ran for the trees. Two Provenger reached them within three strides, running them through the torso with the two long blades of their gauntlets. They turned back on the group as both men continued to run away, mortally wounded. Now there were seven left. The two Provenger that stayed with the group had immediately cut down the two in front of them, and the rest followed with blinding speed that Rick could not have imagined. The Provenger wore excited grimaces and were obviously enjoying themselves. Rick saw moments where the Provenger had an open path to slit a throat but instead struck for a limb, increasing the gore and prolonging the terror of their victims. Every swipe of their gauntlet knives struck the men's flesh. Then every slash to a throat sent blood pumping through the air and another body to the ground.

My work. My murders, Rick thought. He had known this day would come, almost from the beginning of this nightmare, when he would have to betray his kind. He had now done the worst. He'd broken a trust and a bond. "God help me if this is not for the greater good."

The Provenger collected all the bodies in a heap and sent them, transported somewhere to be processed. They then disintegrated the vehicles and all the blood in the sand. They left no trace. It took them about three minutes.

When Marcus Holliday pulled up, there was no one at the meeting place. He was only an hour late and nothing was there, only one set of tire tracks to be seen by his headlights. He tried to call Tony but there was no service. He shook his head and drove home, cursing his friends for either having fooled him or making other plans without telling him. No one was left that knew of the meeting, no one but Marcus and Rick.

Chapter 32

A thousand spEars

Utu had just come in the back door with a chunk of meat from the second deer carcass he had hanging in the tree. He'd been gorging himself every day and loving it. The temperature outside was perfect for the meat. The combination of cold nights and cool days with the dry air helped the meat keep wonderfully, the flavor intensifying every day, although he could tell now by the smell that he'd have to start cooking the meat a little hotter and longer with a few more spices from Rick's huge collection.

Utu heard Barnes and Nobelle outside and could tell by their barking that someone must be starting up the driveway. It must be Rick, he thought. He wasn't expected home until later. Utu quickly stuck the meat in a pot, added some water and a stick of butter, put on the lid, and turned on the heat. He listened. Still coming up the driveway, driving awfully slowly, he thought.

Utu grabbed some granulated garlic, curry, paprika, oregano, and salt out of the cabinet and dumped a copious amount of each into the pot, closed the lid, and listened again. Utu heard the gravel, then silence where the Jeep would be driving over the concrete pad in front of the garage, then... crash! The sound was unmistakable. Rick was in trouble.

Carson was in his room listening to music and Shainan was on the internet looking for home. She heard the impact and looked up at Utu, worried. He instinctively pointed to his own eyes and twirled his finger in front of him, as if pointing to the entire room, silently signaling for her to stay put, watch, and be ready. Committing one of those errors people make when new to a language, Utu called out as calmly as he could, "Carson, your Dad just drove into the garage."

With the calm that indicated only the interest of his father returning for the evening, Carson let his song end and casually closed out his computer.

Utu dashed through the mud room and into the garage to find the Jeep had missed it by about three feet, and impacted the left side of the door opening, creating a lot less damage than he'd thought from the sound. Rick was slumped over the steering wheel. Utu helped him out of the Jeep and guided him into the house.

Carson came into the kitchen right as Rick entered. "Dad, where have you been?" Carson could immediately tell something was wrong. Rick was babbling incoherently and falling down. He was obviously drunk and ultimately shaken from the impact.

Utu grabbed Rick under the arm, almost lifting him off his feet. Shainan approached to help, but Carson waved her off. "I've got this," he said, taking his father under the other arm. "Let's get him to bed. Something bad must have happened. He's never done this."

As they carried Rick to bed, Utu looked him over for injuries or any sign of blood. He found none. "I'm going out to the Jeep to see what's happened."

"I don't know what that was all about," Carson said to Shainan when he returned to the kitchen.

"He..." Shainan put her fist to her mouth and tossed her head back.

"Yes, drinking," Carson said.

"Trinking," Shainan repeated, nodding in agreement.

"Drinking," Carson said slower.

"Trinking."

"No, d,rinking, drinking."

"Drinking," Shainan said carefully, with a smile, proud of herself.

Utu was back in the kitchen almost before they'd realized he'd left. He had an astonished look on his face. It was a combination of being a witness to a disaster and a little boy on Christmas morning. "Look what I found in the Jeep." Utu threw a Provenger battle gauntlet, without the knives, onto the kitchen table. They stood looking in silence.

Early the next morning, with a terrible headache preventing him from sleeping, Rick sat at the kitchen table staring into space. Carson and Utu were sitting with him. Shainan was coming in from feeding the dogs. Rick's face was pale, and he looked terribly ill. "I'm such a fool. I can't believe I had that much to drink last night. I actually stopped at the liquor store on the way home and drank from the bottle while I was driving."

Utu stared at him without speaking.

"Utu said it ruined his people," Carson said.

"Carson? Could you go play videogames with Shainan, please?"

Carson looked back at his father in disbelief. "Sure, Dad."

After Carson had taken Shainan off by the hand to the other room, Rick took a long look at Utu. "Last night I killed ten men on the off chance that it would help me get that thing," Rick confessed, nodding to the gauntlet that Utu had in front of him.

"Well, now you have it," said Utu, surprised at Rick's confession. What made Rick such a killer, he wondered? Utu checked again to ensure that the tag was on the counter so they could talk without being watched. "This will enable you to cloak yourself. It even has a transport mechanism on it. Anywhere on Earth." Utu looked up at Rick. "How did you get such a thing?"

"Synster gave it to me. Because..." Rick paused and swallowed, "I delivered to him a group of people that were going to tell everyone they were here, harvesting, then try to kill as many Provenger as they could. Nwella helped with the decision. My new assignment is to hunt down and terminate resistance groups, identify and eliminate anyone who may know or does know and may tell. The Provenger will harvest who I've targeted, or if it serves a purpose, they will have me kill them. Can you imagine? I think Synster believes I'm enjoying myself."

"Rick, you took an incredible risk to get this. I think you have done an incredibly stupid, horrible, and great thing. With this," Utu leaned in closer to Rick, "I think we may be able to rid ourselves of the Provenger."

"How?" Rick was confused. "It only cloaks and transports."

"Synster must have his hands full to be so careless to give you such a thing," said Utu, shaking his head.

"How can we fight them with it? It doesn't have any function as a weapon."

"Leave that to me. We must find where I lived before we run out of time. I left something there that I need. Rick, we can defeat them."

Rick looked back at Utu with doubt. There was much more that Rick didn't feel he should share with Utu just yet. Synster had given him an assignment that seemed to indicate desperation regarding the Project and one that Rick didn't know if he'd survive. Utu had said that the Provenger only broke their own laws when they went rogue. He didn't mention anything about having others do their dirty work for them.

Rick recalled his last communication with Synster. It seemed that both Synster and Rick had a problem with a certain Provenger. That Provenger had caused the grievous injury to Carson in the belief that he was injuring Rick. Synster had informed Rick that Ryvil had attempted to kill him to remove him from the Project, and to make the U.S. government officials more difficult to manage. Ryvil needed the injury to look natural to his fellow Provenger and authorities on Earth, while making it seem suspicious to those humans who knew of Rick's work with the Provenger.

"You see," Synster had explained, "if you turn up dead, your brother will panic and believe that his life is in immediate jeopardy. The others in your government that I've contacted will believe the same. The only thing that keeps everyone working together is some hope that they can save themselves, that they have some kind of future. The fear of imminent death would likely cause them to panic and divulge everything they know. If they all did that at once and supported each other's story…now that would be difficult to undo. That would take us one step closer to Managed Collectivization."

"Can't you run this attempt to kill me through your algorithm to see how it happened, or can happen?"

"Unfortunately, no. All such assessments are strictly regulated. It would leave a record. There would be no other logical explanation for this event. Ryvil was trying to kill you. After failing with this stunt, I can't imagine he'd try the same thing again. But he will continue to thwart this project at every opportunity. He has demonstrated that. He must be neutralized. And this is something I cannot do."

Rick thought about the prospect of successfully killing a Provenger, and, while highly preferable to killing a person, he doubted his efforts could bring success.

Chapter 33

The last of the CaRRian gang

The disappearance of Tony Carrian and nine other men of the area, labelled by the media as the Carrian Gang, created considerable consternation among the populations in town and the surrounding counties. Vigils were held, rumors were traded, and theories were thrown about.

Marcus Holliday, a notoriously unpredictable character, did one of the most responsible things he could have done under the circumstances. He went to the county sheriff's office and told them what he knew about the incident. He started off belligerent about locking up the pistol he had on his belt and ended up spilling his guts. Obviously, he changed the story a little to make it seem innocent. He'd told them of the planned meeting "to go shooting" and related that it seemed to him that none of them had ever arrived at the designated time and place. He also mentioned that his friend, Tony, had said that if anything bad happened to him, that it probably had something to do with Rick Thompson. He insisted they confront Thompson immediately. When they didn't indicate that they would, Holliday tried to start interrogating the deputy taking his information, questioning their motives for resolving the disappearance and threatening to go to the media.

What Holliday didn't mention was that Tony had said that Thompson was with the NSA. Holliday wanted to implicate Thompson, but he didn't want to sound like an antigovernment kook doing it.

It was a Wednesday evening when a Montezuma County Sheriff's Deputy rolled up the long driveway to Rick's place. Detective John Robby had spent the last week running down leads on the case, and this lead seemed to have the most interesting prospects. He knew from talk in the office that Rick's wife in Denver had recently disappeared and wondered if there was any connection. But then again, there appeared to be a great number of people disappearing lately, all over the world. Now it had come to Cortez.

Robby had come alone for two reasons. The first was that resources in the county were stretched thin and detectives usually worked their cases alone. The second reason was that he didn't expect to delve too deeply with this interview. He was there to find out what Thompson's association with Carrian was and assess its relevance and importance. If there seemed to be anything there, he would keep it to himself, act disinterested, go away, and come back with reinforcements.

He'd already done his homework on Thompson: no record, good credit, everything looked standard. He lived in a nice home that appeared to be well kept. A number of deputies in the department knew and liked him. They'd told Robby about his ex-wife. Foul play was not suspected as she was an alcoholic and had been getting herself into trouble lately. Her condition had worsened since she'd lost her son to Thompson, and more recently she'd lost her job. The real intriguing thing about the Thompson angle was that a link to Carrian was made when his home had been searched. Certain paraphernalia at the house indicated that anti-government sentiments were a general theme. Also, documents, a hand-written log, and a map were found that looked like Carrian had been following Thompson. Robby needed to get this worked out.

Marcus Holliday, the source of the information, on the other hand, was questionable. He had a record; a couple assault charges, no convictions, a DUI reduced to a misdemeanor, a poor credit history, and, according to the deputy that he spoke to, very bad breath. Holliday was known around the county as a self-proclaimed gun slinger. He had the credentials to back it up. He'd won the Four Corners Cowboy Action Quick Draw Championships the last three years in a row. This competition was fired with single action army revolvers and included a variety of stages where the draw and numerous shots were fired at a variety of targets, all usually within a second or two. His significant abilities with this weapon, his habit of carrying it with him everywhere, and his propensity to be a hothead, potentially made Holliday a very dangerous man. In Robby's mind, these conditions, together with Holliday's accusation, almost made Holliday the better suspect.

Rick saw the unmarked Crown Victoria rounding a curve about a mile away. He'd been working out front fixing a latch on his gate. He put down his tools and casually walked inside. He found Carson and Utu at the computer reading intently about some place in Turkey. They seemed excited. Shainan wasn't there. She'd been sleeping late since she started getting morning sickness a couple days ago. Utu had told Rick the day prior to her illness that he could tell she was pregnant.

Rick quickly got their attention. "Guys, police coming up the drive: plan A."

They acknowledged plan A and turned back to their reading. Rick walked back outside and continued working on the latch. It was getting colder as the sun was setting. The cruiser rolled to a stop and, after making a radio call, the Deputy emerged from the car.

Rick put down his tools and walked over, slowly, expecting either to get grilled about his wife or about Tony Carrian. Here goes, he thought.

"Evening, I hope you have good news about my ex," he said with some actual sincerity.

"No, sir," the detective said shaking his head while walking up to Rick. "Actually, no news. I did hear about that, and I'm sorry she hasn't been located yet." He stuck out his hand and they shook. "I'm Detective John Robby, Montezuma County."

"Rick Thompson. Pleased to meet you."

"I wish I had some good news for you but I'm actually not here for that." Robby paused, like a good investigator, waiting for Rick to volunteer whatever might be on a guilty mind.

"What can I help you with?" Rick inquired.

"How do you know Tony Carrian?" Robby began abruptly, carefully observing Rick's reaction.

"Oh yeah," Rick responded, without much emotion. "Not well. Is this about his disappearance? I saw it on the news and heard people talking."

"Yes. How do you know him?"

"We've spoken a few times. Has he turned up?"

"Possibly," replied Detective Robby, watching closely for any reaction from Rick, who gave none. "What was the extent of your relationship?"

Rick was expecting some technique to be thrown at him and was ready for anything. He could tell that Robby would be persistent. "Let's see, I met him the first time out by a plot I own west of 491, about a month ago. He was changing a tire and I stopped to help him, but he didn't need help. After that, he must have looked me up. I like to be listed. It's a matter of principle. He called a couple times and wanted me to get involved with his shooting club. I declined. We bumped into each other and had lunch at the Main Street Brewery once, many weeks ago. That's about it, I think. I may have seen him in town a couple times. I only have a few friends around here. I don't need many. And because of my work, I don't particularly like it when people I don't know approach me." Rick threw out the bait.

"What's your work?"

"I'm a systems analyst. We contract for the NSA, keeping various communication systems running. Security is an issue, so I don't like it when I get approached. I'm a little paranoid I guess, but that doesn't mean people aren't after me," Rick added with a smile. "I usually just represent myself as an IT consultant, so I'd appreciate it if you keep it confidential. It's not top secret crap, but this is the West, and we do have some folks out here who hate the feds."

"Sure, I understand. Where were you that night?"

"Let's see." Rick looked high and left, where he looks when he's trying to remember something. "That was on the twenty fifth, right?"

"No, the twenty fourth," replied Robby.

Rick looked left again, "Okay. Well, I'm pretty sure I was here all day. Carson wasn't feeling well, so I stuck around and got some chores done."

"Alright." Robby was now starting to get the picture. Somehow Carrian knew about Thompson's work and was following him. Holliday was part of Carrian's group and probably wanted to throw suspicion on the NSA. One last test, thought Robby. "Did you know any of his friends?"

Rick was about to say "no" then stopped himself. Relieved, he realized he could have just fallen into a trap. If he'd denied knowing Tony's friends without asking who they were first, it would seem that he was trying too hard to distance himself from the situation.

"I don't know. Who were his friends?" Rick asked, smooth as silk, relieved he'd dispensed with the north-eastern fast-talking habits of his youth.

Detective Robby listed the names of all the men who had disappeared. Rick acknowledged that he'd read the names in the paper and had been curious about the disappearance, but said he didn't know any of them.

"How about Marcus Holliday, how do you know him?" asked Robby.

Rick thought for a moment. He genuinely didn't know the man. "I don't know him. Well, maybe I've heard that name." Rick sensed an opportunity. "I seem to recall Tony mentioning a Marcus that he was upset with. I don't know if it was the same guy, but this Marcus shot his neighbor's dog when it wandered onto his property. Class act, eh?" There was a pause and Rick realized there was a question he must ask. "Detective, why are you asking me all these questions?"

"Just canvassing, really. Talking to everyone who we've found out knew them. Do you know of any reason why anyone would want to hurt Mr. Carrian?"

"Well, like I said, I don't really know him. He seems like a nice guy." Rick was relieved that "seems" came out, instead of "seemed".

Robby was satisfied that he didn't need any more for now. He was going to ask Thompson why he thought Carrian might be following him, but figured that answer had already come out. He could always ask later. "Can I just see some ID to verify your employment?" asked Robby. "And I won't have to bother you anymore."

"Sure. You want to come inside?" Rick inquired. "It'll just take a second," hoping to God this man didn't speak Armenian. It was the only potential flaw to their cover.

"No, thanks. I'll wait out here. I don't want to intrude anymore," said Robby, much to Rick's relief.

Rick got his "Contractor" credentials from inside, returned, and presented them to the deputy as well as offering to give him his supervisor's phone number for verification.

"No, that won't be necessary. I'll contact you if I need anything else," replied Robby, reviewing the credentials and driver's license.

Rick noticed a gold ring with a crest on it that he didn't recognize. "Interesting ring," Rick observed, trying to be personable.

"It's Armenian. I got it visiting family there last year. My dad changed our name from Robhanisyan when he immigrated. Can you believe he made me study Armenian most of my life just in preparation for that one trip? What a waste, eh? I should have been learning Spanish."

"Yeah, isn't that something," Rick laughed nervously, the blood pressure draining from his head.

As the deputy drove away, satisfied with the interview, Rick was left very relieved but a little paranoid about him declining to come inside. Was he suspicious? Did he buy it? Would he come back? Except for not being able to speak Armenian, everyone inside had been ready. Carson and Utu had their back stories down cold, and Shainan didn't need to speak because she would play deaf. And, thanks to the Provenger, the two Cro-Magnons had their papers as well as their shots.

Rick walked inside. "Utu?"

"What?"

"I want you speaking fluent Armenian with a perfect accent in two weeks."

"Okay. We'll need that Rosetta Stone thing."

"Order it." The caveman was coming along nicely, Rick thought.

Weeks passed without hearing from the deputy again and things seemed to be calming down. Rick was anxious for his chance at Ryvil and wondered when Nwella would confess her sins to the Provenger, begin her banishment, and move in with him. At that point, Rick would find out how his relationship with Synster would evolve.

With Christmas coming, Rick didn't know who to get presents and stockings for. Certainly Carson. He didn't want Utu and Shainan to feel left out. Maybe Nwella? Definitely Barnes and Nobelle. Problem was, Christmas wasn't the only holiday he wasn't prepared for. It was the calm before the storm.

Chapter 34

The introdUctions

Nwella appeared one evening on Rick's back patio in a manner similar to which she had that first time, except without the intent for romance. It was too cold for Rick to be out, but he was sitting by the fire pit anyway trying to keep warm and think, as usual. She arrived with information that would put their lives into high gear.

"Rick, I have a health scan in three days. I can't avoid being discovered. I must confess my situation as soon as possible. Also, Synster has ordered me to tell you that your special project should be initiated. I don't know what that is, but I have encrypted coordinates to give you for transport. It must be at the exact place and time indicated on your gauntlet. All that he told me is that it would be tomorrow. He said I was not to ask for details. Rick, I don't know if I can bear the next few days."

Rick held her and tried to give some comfort.

"Good," he said. "It's time something starts happening." Project Ryvil, he thought. He'd been looking forward to this – killing a Provenger with the approval of Synster and avenging the assault on his son at the same time. He already had all the other information from Synster, the local conditions, the weapon, and the circumstances. It sounded pretty easy.

"I'm scared for you," Nwella said.

"Let's take things one at a time. You'll join us when you confess." Rick didn't want to say "banished". It sounded too negative. "That is resolved, right?"

"Yes."

"And no one will come after us for revenge, especially Synster. Right?"

"Yes. That is not our way. I'm fairly certain," Nwella responded, the word "fairly" weakening Rick's hope for the future. "During my formal confession, I will be sure to say that I was the one who took you while you slept. Synster will read that report. With what he knows about me, he'll certainly believe it."

"I'll take all that as a yes. So what we need to do now is introduce you to the people you'll be living with. Then you'll tell whatever authorities you need to of your situation, you'll leave your life there, and start your life here."

With that, Nwella burst into tears and collapsed in Rick's arms, sobbing uncontrollably.

"I didn't realize a life with me was such a horrible prospect," he joked, trying to raise her spirits.

"I'm sorry. It's not you. It's just that so much is happening so fast. I don't know if I can adjust. But I'll do what I can. As long as I have a chance to confess, I'll be allowed some preparation for this world. If they discover my condition without my confession, the banishment would be immediate with no preparation. And I need to do it when Father is away. I don't want to face him. He'll be at Kylamity Base with some council members for the next two days, so now would be a good time." They looked into each other's eyes for a moment. "You need to be ready tomorrow afternoon. Do you know what you need?" Nwella asked.

"Oh yes, I've been ready for some time now," Rick said, barely able to contain his enthusiasm at the prospect of killing Ryvil. Synster must be with the council members as an alibi, Rick thought. "Let's start getting you acclimated right now. Everybody is inside. You need to meet them all. We'll do it in stages. I've got it all planned. Utu already knows about you. He's managed to learn some English, so I've told him. And of course you can speak his language. You'll meet him first, then Carson. While you meet Carson, Utu will brief Shainan on what is going on. She actually listens to him."

Rick paused, then continued. "I know this sounds strange, but you'll have to get your scent on Utu so he can play with the dogs and they'll smell you. That way, the dogs will receive you better. Meanwhile you can meet Shainan. You should get her scent on you, once again for the dogs. But we'll see how that goes. I'll go in first. Ready?"

Rick had been planning for this moment for a long time. He had it all thought out. He had begun to see them all as a team, a team that might be capable of saving the situation. He had two people from the distant past who seemed to have capabilities that he could not even comprehend, particularly Utu. Then there was Nwella, his unlikely love, now carrying his child and making them both immune from adversarial action by the Provenger. She had knowledge of Provenger technology and methods that he could use for defense, or survival, if the worst should come. Nwella assured him that random violence against Carson or those he cared about was against their law. He felt they had a chance.

"Rick, my head is spinning. I don't understand much of what you are saying or why. Would you please protect me through this?"

"Always."

Rick was the first one in. Utu, as usual this time of night, was at the computer, researching. Shainan, conveniently, was in her room, and Carson was reading something for school in the living room. Perfect, Rick thought.

"Carson, could you please put Barnes and Nobelle in the garage? We have a visitor I need to introduce you to."

Carson looked up and rolled his eyes. "Dad, what now?"

"Just do it. We're all safe."

Utu looked up with a serious look of hatred on his face.

While Carson was getting the dogs into the garage, Rick addressed Utu. "I know this will be difficult. But if you have any sense of long-term goals, you'll listen to what I have to say. Nwella will be joining us soon. Not only is she having my child, but I love her, no matter how crazy that may seem to you. She's different now, I think. At heart, she's not really a Provenger anymore. You should consider her that way."

Utu stared at him patiently but with a tone of judgment.

"She is carrying my child, a Human/Provenger hybrid. I don't know what will come of that, but I think the concept is intriguing. She makes us, her and me, at least, immune from Provenger violence, and she has comprehensive knowledge of their technology and culture. She is an asset to our team. You need to receive her as such." Rick looked for confirmation. He didn't get any. "I need your assurance that you'll restrain your anger against her while you fully assess the situation. You need to understand her value and what she means to me." Rick was fully aware that if Utu wanted, he could do anything, and Rick wouldn't be able to stop him.

"Rick, I understand. I know she can be an asset. That doesn't mean I won't hate her. I'll be nice," he said simply. "When everything goes to hell, and if she's the cause of it, I'll kill her first. In the meantime, I'll play along."

Rick looked up and Carson was standing at the edge of the room, having just walked in, looking with doubt at these two men, judging them as having serious issues.

"Utu, we don't want her to know yet that you can communicate well. Speak simply, like when you first got here, or worse even. Or don't talk at all."

Even though Utu understood this, it was annoying for him to accept. He was tired of playing the fool in front of these beasts. "Rick, I can do better than that. Most of what I say I'll speak in my language, and she can translate it to you in English. This way we can both know immediately if she's being honest with us. And I'll play the fool for a while, Rick, but not for long."

"So when do we get to meet her?" Carson asked.

"Right now," replied Rick. He opened the door and let her in.

She wasn't nearly as threatening an image as either of them had imagined. She looked beaten down. She was wearing what looked to be human clothing, but the style was just a little off – colors, cut, shoes. To Carson, she looked like she might be from Europe. She wore a gray long sleeve shirt, brown pants, and black shoes. And there was the bald thing. If she was to stay long-term, it was something that would have to be changed, somehow. Carson thought, maybe we can pencil in eyebrows and throw a wig on her.

She held her head down and stared at the floor, looking very meek. Then she briefly glanced up, first at Utu, then at Carson, then back at the floor.

"Hello," she said.

"Utu, Carson, this is Nwella...She'll be one of the family," Rick added to make her feel accepted and convey his sincerity to everyone. She glanced up at him. "Starting in a few days, she'll be living with us." Rick waited, looking back and forth at Utu and Carson.

"Hello," said Nwella again, still looking at the floor.

"Hello, Nwella," said Carson, wondering when the surprises would stop. "Welcome."

Rick glared at Utu.

"Hello, Nwella," Utu droned.

Rick turned to Nwella, took her hands in his and looked deeply into her eyes. "You will be my wife."

Nwella was confused and wasn't sure what to say. She glanced at Carson, who was rolling his eyes, and then at Utu who was staring off into space. "Yes?" she responded.

"Carson, this will be your new step-mother."

"Dad! She looks my age!" Carson replied, exasperated.

"Nwella, how old are you?" Rick asked her.

"Thirty-seven years of Earth," she answered.

"Carson, it's the Recombinant. It makes them all look much younger. And Carson, she's pregnant. We're having a baby."

Carson looked back at his father with no expression. Now, he had no idea how to feel.

"Me check," Utu said in English, as he stood and carefully walked to Nwella. "May I?" he asked in his own language, as he stuck out his hand toward her abdomen.

As Nwella slowly nodded, Rick was starting to panic. If Utu got close, he could kill her in an instant. What if he somehow could tell if she was pregnant or not? What if she wasn't, and he knew she was lying and decided to take his revenge now? Why didn't he warn me he was going to do this? Before Rick could think of how to react, Utu had his hand on her.

After a few seconds, he backed up with a surprised look on his face. "Rick," Utu said as he nodded.

"Nwella, could you please explain to Utu that Shainan needs to know about you, and we also need to introduce the dogs to you," Rick asked, trying to hurry the process before Shainan happened to walk in.

311

Nwella, using Utu's ancient language, now explained what Rick had asked her to convey.

"Right," Utu said to Rick. "I get." He turned and walked out of the room to find Shainan.

There was an awkward moment where no one knew what to say. Rick and Carson stood, alternating glances at each other and Nwella, as she stood looking only at the floor. They heard some screaming in the room down the hall, muffled excerpts of which only Nwella could understand. Something about "flesh eating bitch," "never again sleep at night," and "dogs will tear her apart!"

Utu and Shainan walked into the room a minute later. They were both stoic and composed. Rick made the introductions, and Shainan looked her square in the face and in her own language said, "Nwella, welcome to our home. Please let me know if there is anything I can do to make you more comfortable. How long will you be staying?"

Nwella glanced up at Shainan and said, "Hello". Then added, "Shainan, I'm afraid this will soon be the only place I'll have. I sincerely hope you'll be able to forgive me for the part I've played in the abuse of your people."

Shainan was surprised at this show of humility. "Huhf!" was her only reply. It was difficult for Shainan to forget that she had once been scheduled as the main course at the banquet attended by Nwella.

Rick sensed that they were somehow done and wanted desperately to proceed to the next step.

"Nwella, what we need to do now won't be easy for any of us. And quite frankly, it may be dangerous. Nwella, we need to introduce you to the dogs. We all need to get your scent on us, then go play with them, give them a few treats that you've held, then maybe things will go smoother. Utu has your scent on his hand. Carson, could you please approach Nwella and give her a hug, or hold her forearms or something?"

"Sure, Dad." Carson walked right up to his future step-mother. He was about to hug her, as she did look like an attractive sixteen-year-old, but then he remembered she was pregnant by his father and a hug might be weird. Carson held out his forearms and they held each other's arms for a moment, and to avoid the awkwardness, they began to shake their arms up and down, as with a handshake, making it even more awkward.

Utu thought for a moment. He wasn't going to touch this Provenger again, just to get her scent. Then he had an idea. He could get the job done better and get a little payback at the same time. It would also test her, to see if her humility was genuine. Utu had her scent on his hand so he pointed to it, looked at Rick and said, "Here."

Then Utu turned to Nwella and told her to translate to Rick exactly what he said. "I know dogs, and the best way to have them meet you is to have them smell your clothing. Give me your shirt." Utu stuck out his hand, waiting.

Nwella translated this to English as closely as possible for Rick. Rick glared at Utu and wondered what he was up to. It was obvious she had nothing on under her shirt.

Nwella felt humiliated. It wasn't that she would be bare chested in front of these people. That was a Provenger fashion, after all. What bothered her was that she would have to turn her clothing over to this human that was demanding it. But any pride that she had was already beaten from her. Nwella peeled off her shirt and gave it to Utu before Rick could think of anything to say. They were all immediately distracted by her beauty, every line, every curve, her skin tone and posture, perfect.

Utu was surprised she complied so readily. He was going to use the shirt to wipe under his arms with the pretext of applying his scent, but Nwella's pitiful demeanor and simultaneous beauty tempered his distain. Rick was annoyed with Utu and felt only compassion for Nwella. Carson was thrilled and bothered. His new stepmother was gorgeous. Shainan was jealous, with all her men obviously admiring the Provenger's half-naked body.

"Okay, well. There we go. Let's get this done," Rick said, motioning to Utu and Carson.

"Um, should I stay here?" asked Carson, "to keep an eye on her, I mean things, I mean Shainan?"

"No. She can handle herself just fine, I'm sure. Now grab some food for the dogs, put it in Nwella's hands for a moment, and follow us," Rick commanded.

Shainan stared at Nwella and Nwella stared at the floor. Nwella seem genuinely penitent, Shainan thought. They both waited in silence while they listened to the antics in the garage. At first, there was barking, then whining, then low growling, then barking again. They heard the muffled sounds of Rick giving the dogs commands, then silence, then praise. This seemed to go on for an eternity as Shainan and Nwella stood there waiting. Shainan noticed that Nwella's breathing was rapid and thought she could see her heart beat between her breasts. Shainan began to feel some pity for this female that was losing everything and being tested and processed for inclusion into her new alien home. She felt a small urge to show her some genuine kindness   She was about to ask Nwella if she would like to sit when the men came back in from the garage.

Rick walked to Nwella and gave Carson the signal to let the dogs in. They ran into the living room and moved in on Nwella as Rick stood next to her, entwining his arm with hers. Rick had chunks of meat in his other hand and told the dogs to sit, which they did only after giving Nwella a quick and cautious sniff. Once the dogs made the slightest effort to sit, Rick immediately rewarded them with the meat, knowing that his opportunity to reward their good behavior might be fleeting. He wasn't sure if this was the best way to introduce Nwella, but it was the best he could think of. He couldn't have his dogs being aggressive toward her in his house.

Barnes and Nobelle circled Nwella thoughtfully, sniffing, watching. The dogs smelled the alien's scent but also the scents of Rick, Utu, and Carson. The rest of their pack had already examined this animal and found her, sniff, yes her, to be no danger. From her breath wafting down with each exhale, from her skin and the chemicals of her perspiration, the two German Shepherds could tell that this animal before them was not human but only slightly different from one. They could discern from the chemistry of her perspiration and the odor from her crotch that she ate mostly meat which, as long as she was part of the pack, would mean they might share some of it. She appeared, then, to be one of them. They could also tell that she had never born cubs before but might be with one now. And that must mean acceptance by Rick, who was leader. She seemed to be no threat.

Nwella began to tremble, and Rick put both arms around her. Utu tossed her shirt back, which she immediately put on. They all noticed a swath of dog slobber down the front, as Nwella's chest started to heave as tearless sobs came percolating silently to the surface. She was truly a pitiful sight.

"I think we've all had enough for one evening," Rick said, as he turned her to walk her back outside.

Nwella stopped and looked back at them all. "Thank you," she said, as if they'd done something nice for her. Then they walked out the back door and onto the patio.

"Well that was pretty weird," Carson said confidently.

"Carson, that reminds me. You haven't talked to your dad about what Shainan found yet, have you? Because I'd like to talk to him about it tomorrow."

"Na, I didn't say anything."

"Okay, because I'll let him know tomorrow. He's got a lot on his mind tonight." Utu knew he needed to act immediately. With Nwella's confession to the Provenger, there could follow a cascade of events that might destroy his current opportunity.

Earlier in the day, Shainan had found the figurine where she had hidden the bolt that Utu had given her over twelve thousand, eight hundred years before. It was a miracle really. Utu had expected they would need to find a general location and then get some kind of scanning technology to find it under the earth. But earlier that day when Shainan was looking through the contents of museums in Turkey, she found the figurine. It had survived. It was of a class of figurines called a "Venus" figure. The site described it as having the etching of a skinny male on the back. Shainan seemed sure this was the exact one. And now it was within Utu's grasp. With the gauntlet they had, he could transport himself there, grab it, and be back within a matter of minutes. When the bolt was inserted into the gauntlet, it would give him the power to transport himself all the way to the Provenger ship, something the gauntlet alone could not do. He would destroy as much of the ship as he could and come back to Earth. He knew the bolt had a limit to its energy, but regardless of the amount, he had to try.

With this disaster of Nwella's pending banishment, things were about to get unpredictable. Utu wasn't sure if they'd let her go. They might kill everyone in Rick's household the second they learned of the situation. Whatever might happen, Utu needed to be prepared. He would get this bolt that night, no matter what, and very soon destroy as much of the Provenger ship as he could.

Chapter 35

Confounding variableS and other delicacieS

The next morning, the weather was clear and the air was crisp and cold. Rick was making some last-minute preparations for his appointment with Ryvil later in the day. He'd been assured by Synster that the difficulty and danger of the task would be minimal. Rick had asked if Ryvil would be cloaked or have his shield deployed. He had learned their shields could block bullets on the day they ambushed Tony and his men. Synster explained that those Provenger were prepared for trouble. That kind of shield uses a lot of energy and would not be deployed under normal work conditions. To do so would unnecessarily deplete energy reserves.

Putting together his gear for a hunt was one of Rick's favorite things to do. He'd play a little bagpipe music while he gathered everything in one spot, make sure it was all serviceable, and then weed out the unnecessary, keeping only the barest essentials. For this mission, the first thing he did was clean, load, and strap on his favorite pistol, the old Les Baer 1911 Hardball that his father had bought him when he was just 18, the same one he'd used to kill Tony.

Rick didn't need much gear. He knew he would transport in with the gauntlet, take the shot at about three hundred yards, and get out...sounded easy enough. Rick chose his Remington 700 VTR in .260 Remington. There would be no way even a Provenger would be able to survive a center mass hit with that caliber. Complete with bipod and Leupold Mark 8, 3.5-25x56mm scope, it was as perfect a package as anything to reach out and touch Ryvil at long range in any light condition. Rick had taken down two elk with that rifle at just about that range, and both the rounds had gone exactly where he'd wanted them, right behind the ear. Rick had just checked the zero three days ago, and it was ready.

As the day wore on, it was beginning to warm. Carson, being a teenager, was, of course, still in bed. Shainan and Utu had been sleeping late as they sometimes did, but Rick could hear them stirring at about noon when he was finalizing his preparations. As he was on his way out to the Jeep to grab his "go bag" to check for some extra things he might need, he heard a motorcycle in the distance. On this remote road he didn't have any friends or neighbors who owned one, and so it was an unfamiliar sound in the area. It caught his attention. As he neared his Jeep parked a distance from the garage, the biker made a turn onto his driveway. He hoped it was someone who was lost and looking for directions, but the closer the bike got, the more he doubted he'd be that lucky.

When it stopped ten yards away and the rider got off, he knew with certainty he was not lucky. Rick got that "aw shit" feeling that he had felt when he was walking up to Synster that first time in the canyon. The biker was about average height and slightly overweight, with a protruding wheat belly. Definitely human. He was wearing all black leather to include a skull cap doo rag. Among the buckles and zippers of the outfit was a belt that caught Rick's attention. On that belt was a holster carrying a Single Action Army revolver. It was a little forward on his hip, in a slight cross-draw position. The holster was worn but not worn out. The revolver was shiny black, about a five inch barrel from what Rick could tell, and had the look of being loved by its owner.

Rick was a gun nut and liked to see people exercising their rights, but having a stranger roll up in such a manner didn't sit well with him. Colorado was open carry, but normally people who did it were out in public, not calling on people they didn't know. The biker stood there for a moment and just looked at him. Rick didn't have a good feeling.

"You Rick Thompson?" the biker bellowed.

"You came to my place, friend. Who's asking?"

"Name's Marcus Holliday. Tony Carrian was a friend of mine. Do you know him, Thompson?"

"Yeah, I know him. Listen, I don't know what you've come here for, but I don't know where Tony is. I told the deputy everything I know. I don't want any trouble with you."

"Too late, Thompson. You got trouble."

There was something about the way this Holliday said "Too late Thompson" that sounded to Rick like it was a little slurred. The last thing Rick needed just before his mission of revenge on Ryvil was a vigilante who'd overindulged in liquid courage. Rick began to formulate an impression of the man; up all night drinking, pissed about his friend missing, thinking he knows exactly who's responsible, determined by daybreak to do something about it, judgment severely impaired after hours of delusions of grandeur.

"Listen, either you leave here now, or I'm going to have to call the police. Like I said, I don't want any trouble."

"Where's Tony? He told me that if anything happened to him, it would be because of you."

"Yeah? Well…the world isn't that cut 'n-dried," retorted Rick.

Holliday bladed his left shoulder toward Rick. He was looking pretty confident. He had both his hands unnaturally positioned just above his navel. Rick was no cowboy action fanatic, but he'd watched his share of quick-draw shooters online and knew the speed and accuracy they were capable of. The way Holliday had his holster positioned, his right hand was ready to draw and press the trigger while the left hand was right there over the cylinder, capable of snapping that hammer back simultaneous to the draw. Rick knew it could all happen faster than he would be able to see it. With the exception of actually being there picking a fight, this guy seemed to have all the signs of knowing what he was doing. If Holliday moved for his gun first, it would all happen before Rick would be able to even flinch, let alone make it half way to the 1911 on his hip. Rick knew this guy must be able to see that he was armed. What the hell was he thinking?

A series of images raced through Rick's mind. If he was killed, Carson and Nwella would be screwed. If he was injured, he wouldn't be able to kill Ryvil as scheduled, and the investigation into his involvement with Tony would deepen. It might turn up something more on his involvement with the Carrian Gang disappearance. All this seemed to be getting complicated pretty quickly. And all roads seemed to lead to Carson, Nwella, and his coming baby being alone, and the world being at the mercy of Managed Collectivization. All of a sudden, the life of this man in his driveway dwindled in importance, except for the fact he was an obstruction.

Rick was getting pissed. His mind raced. He'd thought about a moment like this many times. For his own safety, Rick had to believe this man was going to back his words with action. He quickly recalled the rules of a gunfight. Bring a friend and a lot of guns. Too late. He thought of another rule. Cheat. Okay, cheat. I still have time for that.

"If you don't tell me where Tony is, there's gonna be more trouble than you can handle, mister."

Rick thought, if this guy gives me the countdown, I'm going to have to shoot him! Don't do it, don't do the countdown! In a flash, Rick devised a plan. Action beats reaction. Shoot fast while moving to cover, and shoot some more from cover of the Jeep.

Holliday continued, "You've got five sec..."

Rick immediately drew as fast as he could and fired, both hands on the weapon locked out hard and crouched and pointed in Holliday's general direction. Rick thought he saw his front sight a little low on Holliday as the first round broke. Rick simultaneously lurched and shot, dashing toward the Jeep to his right.

Holliday had been bluffing. He wasn't going to draw on anyone. He was just trying to scare Thompson, make him talk. Who ends up in a gunfight these days? His mind flashed, he must be guilty!

But he had bluffed the wrong man. When he saw Rick draw, much to his amazement, he reacted. Rick had his first shot out, putting one in Holliday's gut by the time his revolver was emerging from the holster. Holliday's first shot was lightning fast and aimed right at Rick's chest, or at least where it had been a quarter second ago, before Rick moved. Holliday's second shot followed the first one before he had time to track Rick's movement. Both had zinged by Rick's left shoulder.

About this moment, Rick's second and third shots missed Holliday, flying to the right.

Holliday's third shot almost caught Rick, tracking just behind, and the fourth round overshot, tracking just in front of Rick's chest as he ran for the cover of his Jeep. Holiday's lightning speed and dead eye accuracy left him nowhere with a moving target. Rick made it to the back of his Jeep and continued to the opposite side. Staying low, he delivered three more quick shots as a panicked, wounded, and exposed Holliday was delivering his revolver's last two rounds into the grill of Rick's Jeep.

Rick's second and final hit took Holliday right in the bladder. It smashed through his soft tissue, and 230 grains of mushrooming Golden Saber .45 ACP tore over his enlarged prostate, crashing into the back of his pelvis, and collapsing him like a toothpick scaffold, to the dirt, paralyzed from the waist down.

"Thompson, please! I wasn't gonna shoot. Christ!" Marcus winced with pain. "I can't move my legs! This all got outta hand; please help me!"

Rick thought he'd shot every round in his gun, but the slide hadn't locked back. This time he got Holliday in his sights, centered right on the downed man's chest. Slowly Rick came out from behind the Jeep. Holliday had dropped his empty revolver. It lay in front of him in the dust.

"Please! Rick, right? Please, Rick. Help me. Call 911. I'm shot, please," Marcus pleaded. "I've got two kids."

"Shut up." Rick didn't want to hear it, fuming at the man for making this happen. Rick, even if he could legally explain his actions, couldn't afford to be in custody tonight. They would still arrest him until things got sorted out. He had a Provenger to kill.

Marcus crabbed backwards on his elbows as Rick approached. "No, no, goddammit, you sonofabitch!" Marcus saw the look on Rick's face. "For Christ's sake!"

"Christ has nothing to do with it." Rick moved his aim to the bridge of Holliday's nose, and just before the shot broke, Rick changed his focus from the front sight to Holliday's face. He saw a man pleading for his life, then the recoil of his 1911. Rick's slide locked back. He instinctively dropped the magazine from his weapon and swept his belt for a magazine that wasn't there. He yelled at the corpse, "You don't challenge a man with a weapon and expect the fight to be anything but final, idiot!" Then he instantly calmed. "People watch too many movies," he muttered.

Rick looked back at the house and saw Utu standing there. Then Carson ran out, panicked and screaming.

Rick wasn't sure what to do. They had to get rid of the body and the bike. They could have a hole dug in a half hour. Rick released his slide, holstered, and checked his watch. Plenty of time. "Carson, get the tractor," Rick ordered, wanting to give the boy something to do. But Carson kept screaming. Rick motioned to Utu to quiet the boy. Utu quickly grabbed him with a hand over the mouth, picked him up, and walked him inside.

Rick watched them go in, hoping the few neighbors he had around wouldn't hear the screaming. Gunfire around there was normal. But the sound of a gunfight with screaming following wasn't. They needed to clean things up and get everything in the back yard fast. Rick ran for his tractor.

One hour later, Rick and Utu were standing over a large hole with Marcus Holliday and a gently used Harley in the bottom of it. Carson was inside the house with Shainan trying to calm him down. Rick was tempted to keep the revolver, but knew it could only lead to trouble.

"I didn't expect to be doing this a couple hours before my duties today. I'm already exhausted." Rick patted Utu on the back. "You're pretty good with that backhoe. Let's fill'er in."

"Rick, I need to tell you something." Utu wanted to sound serious but not too serious. He wanted to avoid more drama. He felt that Rick was able to kill too easily and it bothered him. Utu hadn't expected to tell Rick just after he'd executed someone, but Rick had to know, and soon.

"What is it?"

"Rick, last night I used the gauntlet. I went to Turkey."

"You went where?"

"Turkey, it's a country on the eastern edge…"

"I know where Turkey is!"

"Then why did you ask me…"

"Why did you go to Turkey?"

"We found the bolt that powers the gauntlet. Shainan did, looking through pictures from our searches. It was at a museum in Ankara. I went in, broke it open, and left. I had the cloak on the whole time. I was in and out in seconds. No one saw anything."

"Holy shit! Where is it?"

"In the house."

"Show me."

Utu stared at Rick before they started toward the house. "Don't we want to cover him up?"

Rick stopped, turned, and considered Marcus for a second. "No, he'll keep. I want to see this thing."

Rick and Utu walked briskly toward the house. Because of the escalation of events in the last hour, Utu had made some decisions. He knew he needed to use the power of the gauntlet as soon as possible. He would use it now. He had determined that morning that he was going to transport himself to the Provenger ship and destroy as much of it as he could, but then Rick's gunfight with Marcus had delayed things. He was going to stay only until Marcus was taken care of, but now it seemed as if Rick didn't care much about getting him buried. He didn't really need him anyway; he had the tractor.

They walked silently to the house, and Utu went immediately to his room, where they kept the gauntlet, figuring if the Provenger tried to take it back, Utu would be more capable of fighting them off. Utu quietly put the gauntlet on and felt for where he'd hidden the bolt the night before. He lifted the mattress and pulled it out. On the way back to the living room, Utu poked his head into Carson's room.

"You guys okay?"

Shainan, spooning Carson on his bed and stroking his hair, looked up and nodded. He hadn't told her he would be leaving for the Provenger ship. He didn't want to alarm her, especially in her condition.

Rick looked at it in amazement. It was a solid black cylinder, just as Nwella had described, about the size and shape of an old 35 millimeter film can, perhaps a little shorter. It looked puny in Utu's palm, and yet it held so much power, the potential for multiple transports across the solar system, independent of any outside power source. In weapon mode, which is what he assumed this cylinder facilitated, Nwella told him a single bolted gauntlet could lay waste to cities.

"It weighs almost nothing. It goes in here," Utu pointed to a shallow hole of the same size on the top of the gauntlet on his arm. "Then I can destroy just about anything I have a mind to. Rick, I'm going to destroy the Provenger ship. I'm convinced I need to go immediately. I was going to do it this morning, first thing, but I delayed because Shainan wasn't well. Then you got involved with the man in the hole…"

"Utu, you can't go now. Nwella is still there!"

"Rick, your thinking on this is clouded. When she confesses, they might immediately come for us. The fact is, we have no idea what they might do. That's exactly the reason we need to act now. For your sake, I hope she can make it back. But you need to think of Carson first."

"Utu, Nwella said we have immunity because of the baby. They won't come after us. You even felt she was telling the truth."

"What if she's wrong? What if they do? What if she loses the baby? Any way you look at it, we need to destroy them as soon as possible. We have the capability right here, right now. The longer we wait, the more likely we are to lose this capability. They are very careful with these things. The only reason this one exists is because they thought it was destroyed thousands of years ago. For some reason, they missed it. What if their scanners are capable of seeing it somehow? What if they see it here? They'll come get it, and we will lose our chance. We'd be lucky if they didn't kill us."

"You can't go until Nwella gets back."

"Rick, that might be too late. I can't afford that."

Rick realized that Utu was determined and also probably correct about the need to do it now. But Rick wasn't willing to lose Nwella. He believed what she'd said about their immunity and believed she'd be an asset to any future issues they might have with the Provenger. And he loved her. Nwella had told him that at this very moment Synster was on Earth, as was Ryvil. Who knew how many other Provenger were on Earth? Rick would need her help dealing with them.

Rick also realized that Utu was probably twice as fast and three times stronger than he was. Utu could really do anything he wanted, and he wouldn't be able to stop him. Rick casually took a couple steps away from him.

Utu quickly put the bolt in the gauntlet. Rick drew his 1911 and held it on Utu, not believing the course of events unfolding. Utu was his friend, his ally, and now, in a moment, they were ready to sacrifice everything for what they believed should be the next step.

"Don't move!" Rick growled, determined to save everyone. He believed he was right concerning keeping Nwella alive, as an ally. Yet, he felt the same about Utu. And still, Rick sensed he might shoot the brother he'd always wanted.

Utu froze. He was looking at the controls on the gauntlet. The colors on the controls changed once he put the bolt in, and he had to figure out which ones would take him to the ship and which combination was the weapon. He'd seen it done a long time ago and needed to be sure. He hesitated.

"Don't move. Dammit, Utu. You can't do this to me. You can't do this to us! Let me see if I can signal her. I can call her off the ship."

Utu considered this. As his mind raced through the possible issues involved, fingers poised over the controls, ready to press, both men heard a tapping at the back door. They looked at the same time. It was Nwella.

"That was fast," said Utu.

They both exhaled in relief. She looked strange, but no other Provenger was with her. Rick lowered his pistol, backed up to the door, and let her in.

"Who's the dead man in the hole?" Nwella asked.

Rick holstered and threw his arms around her. "Why are you back so soon?"

"It's done. I'm banished," she stated with a stoic resolve.

"Are you alone?" Rick asked. "Why is your head red...and your eyes?" She appeared to have a horrible rash, with her scalp and the skin around her eyes swollen and red.

"Syrjon was leaving for Earth with Ryvil this morning. I confessed and was sentenced last night, and he offered to give me a hair cell implant procedure. I'll be growing hair," reported Nwella with a forced sense of enthusiasm. "What is going on here? Why were you pointing your weapon at Utu?"

"Utu has a bolt, I think you call it, in the gauntlet. He was going to your ship."

Nwella's first reaction was disbelief. Then it changed to horror. She was almost panicked in her agitation. "No, oh no." The men sensed her alarm and somehow knew it wasn't for the safety of the ship. She hurried up to Utu, without even thinking that it might be dangerous to approach him. She grabbed the gauntlet with her fumbling, shaking hands, and turned it to see the top, the bolt sticking out of it. She verified it was real. "Oh no!" she cried.

"What? What's wrong?" Rick asked.

"The Guard, they'll be coming. They're the caretakers of the Essence. The bolt activates it. They'll come to destroy this and all of us. The bolt activates a signal. The scanners. It's the only thing they do, to prevent its theft. That is what powers the bolt," blurted Nwella, panicked.

Rick and Utu understood enough of what she said to know they were in trouble and looked at each other in horror. "How long do we have?" asked Rick.

"How long has it been in the gauntlet?" Nwella questioned

Forgetting to act the fool, Utu replied in perfect English, "I just put it in, maybe a minute ago. I lost track of time when Rick pulled his gun on me." Utu glared at Rick.

"Then we may have time. What were you going to do?"

"I was going to transport to the ship and destroy as much of it as I could."

"You would have failed." Nwella threw a pinched look at Utu. "How can you talk so well?"

"I'm much smarter than you ever imagined," retorted Utu, forgetting everything he'd ever dreamed about how he'd reveal himself at this moment. The imagined satisfaction drained from him.

Nwella cocked her head. "Forget that. No time. None of the outer ring of the ship can be modified by gravitation waves. It's built that way. But, if you do this correctly, there may be a way to save us. I'm not sure how long we have, but there is some delay before the gauntlet signal will be decoded and interpreted by any of our scanners, somewhere between five and ten minutes, I think, or maybe less. Not only will the Guard move to recover it, but they'll be able to track it from its origin once they get the signal. So ditching it won't do any good. We'd all be in danger regardless of where it was. If you promise not to kill any Provenger, then I'll show you how you can shut down the scanners and disable the ship by taking out its main power source. This will strand it in orbit and prevent the Guard from finding us. Do you promise not to kill any Provenger?"

Utu didn't like the idea of not destroying the ship, but he sensed that she was being honest about not being able to. If he could eliminate the ship's ability to travel, retain the gauntlet, and avoid being discovered by the Guard, whatever they were, what Nwella was saying sounded like a good option. "If I can truly disable the ship and strand it in orbit, I promise not to kill a Provenger. On this trip," Utu added.

Nwella knew time was very short. If Utu didn't disable the ship within a few minutes, they would be identified and swarmed with Guard that would annihilate them. She wasn't going to quibble over context. "Done."

The Provenger Nation Ship was composed of two rings or wheels, one inside of another held by spokes between them. The inside ring support structure that carries the Essence and holds the binary star would have to be collapsed.

Nwella pressed the controls on the gauntlet to produce the exact type of disruption beam he would need, and she showed him how to aim and activate it. She then modified the settings to deliver Utu to a receiving station on a spoke adjacent to the inside ring. Due to the zero gravity in that area, no one lived or worked on the inside ring or the spokes. Those structures were merely the binary star containment system and storage areas.

"Think of the ship as a wheel within a wheel, connected by spokes. You must destroy a section of the inside ring, then a section of the spoke just beyond it. The section of the inside ring and the piece of the spoke that is connected to it should then start drifting toward the center. Before it drifts too far, you must then at least crack the second spoke. That should start a chain reaction that will break all the spokes around the smaller wheel that is the containment system. This should result in the ship's loss of the binary star. With the charge that exists on this bolt..." Nwella turned it to look, "you might have enough power for a transport back. Do you understand?"

Utu's face was blank. He'd heard most of what she said, but part of his mind was stuck on the statement that he just made about being smarter than she ever imagined, and regretting it.

Nwella glared at him, "Do you understand?" As she spoke Nwella could feel valuable time ticking by. The urgency of the need for immediate action was pounding her.

"Um, what's a spoke? I mean, I know what a wheel is, but all the ones I've seen don't come with spokes."

Nwella rolled her eyes, completely exasperated. Rick realized Utu lived in a pre-wheel society and the modern technology of the Provenger didn't use wheels. And most wheels on Earth didn't have spokes anymore. "He's a Cro-Magnon. No wheels!" Rick yelled at Nwella, pointing vigorously at Utu.

"Oh, right!" she yelled back. "So a spoke is a support which connects the outside of the wheel to the center," she said, violently making circles and lines in the air with her hands.

"Okay, okay, I get it!" Utu reassured, then paused. "Um, where is the second spoke from where I am?" Utu asked, trying to concentrate.

"You're on a spoke. The second spoke would be on either side of you, depending on where you arrive on the station, beyond the first spoke. You make the choice. It could be either side, either of two spokes!" Nwella responded quickly.

"Either side of what?"

"Either side of the spoke you're on!"

Utu's face became twisted. "So I'm not shooting any of the spoke I'm on, right?"

"No, that's right. Don't shoot your spoke!"

"Maybe we should draw a picture. I'll get a pen," Rick suggested, hurrying over to the desk at the edge of his kitchen. He grabbed the only pen he saw and an envelope on the desk and hurried it over to the living room table.

"Here!" He thrust it at Nwella, and they all leaned over the table to watch.

Nwella tried to draw a circle, but the pen simply made a dry impression. She looked at Rick. Rick grabbed the pen and scribbled back and forth across the paper, quickly. It started to write, and he slapped it down into Nwella's waiting palm. She tried again to draw a circle but still, no ink. Rick leapt toward the desk for another pen as Carson walked into the room. The moment he spoke, everyone jumped, thinking the Guard were there.

"What the hell is going on here? Is that guy buried yet?"

"Carson! Watch your language! Do you have a pen?" Rick asked as he hurriedly shuffled across the surface of the desk with his hands groping for anything that resembled a writing implement.

Carson walked over to the table next to Nwella, picked up a felt tip pen, popped the top off, and handed it to her. She drew the big circle, the spokes, the small circle, and showed Utu where he would be and what sections to destroy, telling him, moments before he vanished, that he would be able to see his targets through windows and to hit the green panel on the gauntlet to come home.

Utu nodded his comprehension. "Tell Shainan I love her." And he was gone.

Rick realized that their very lives and the future of humanity depended on the effectiveness of a rushed set of instructions communicated in a non-native language from an advanced alien female to an ancient Cro-Magnon male. He needed to shoot at something called a spoke, a thing of which he had never previously conceived. Rick recalled the couple times he'd tried to get directions from his ex-wife. "We're doomed," he muttered.

Meanwhile, in South America...

Ryvil and Syrjon were scheduled to survey an area in the Bolivian Andes for human populations that might be appropriate for immediate harvest. They were also tasked to assess the area for other mammalian species that might be easily harvested in volume.

Synster must be getting desperate, Ryvil figured. This assignment to survey for species not perpetuated by Provenger programs was approaching a violation of their renewable resource directive. Ryvil knew that the second assignment would be futile. He'd been to this area before and no such animals existed in any kind of volume that would allow for efficient harvest. He knew the area because he'd visited an ancient Provenger base there, one of five on Earth that had been established by the Provenger long before their recent war. So far as he was aware, he and Syrjon were the only living Provenger that knew of them. They were still intact, effectively shielded from all scans, and well-provisioned. The Old Ones had planned well, Ryvil thought.

Ryvil and Syrjon arrived on a rocky hill in a thicket above a small village, one target of many for their survey. It was a potential whole community harvest that could be concealed with a landslide. Initial scans by Syrjon seemed to indicate the area was of low value for landslide potential, although the inhabitants of the village were perfect.

It seems that the native Inca of the area had relied on quinoa as a staple food for generations. Decades ago it became popular in other areas around the world as an alternative carbohydrate when many recognized their problems with wheat. This brought money to the Andean farmers who owned their farms. It allowed them to afford more imported products, to include highly processed foods. For those workers who were merely paid a wage to labor on these farms, the increased cost of quinoa now made it inaccessible. For both groups, the increased use of grain starches to include inexpensive wheat had fattened these communities nicely. They hadn't yet developed a significant medical industry capable of dispensing drugs for the chronic illnesses that followed. The population of almost two thousand in this village area alone were both fat and organic, perfect for harvest. Syrjon scheduled them for processing.

On the Provenger Nation Ship...

Utu arrived in a massive white corridor lined with windows all around. Above, he saw what looked to him like the night sky. He immediately panicked and thrashed about for something to grab as his body told him, with a hollow feeling in his gut, that he was falling. He blinked hard as he tried to perceive the walls around him move, but they remained still. They should have been racing by, he thought. He should hit the floor that he saw beneath him. He felt like he was falling, but he was not. This was very strange. If he ignored the feeling of falling, he next realized that he was drifting, moving about as if in water but still falling and going nowhere. Utu couldn't understand what was happening to him or where he would go at the end of his fall.

The whole ship must be falling with me. I'm in a falling ship. When will it hit, he wondered? Utu thought that perhaps the entire Provenger ship was somehow in trouble, and that if it was falling, perhaps he wouldn't need to destroy anything. In fact, he needed to get out of the ship before it hit. He had his finger over the green control, ready to transport back, when he wondered whether or not the fall would destroy the ship.

He thought of the last mammoth he ever saw go down during a hunt. It fell to the ground and everyone cheered. They thought it was dead because it didn't move. Some made the mistake of stopping the attack. They got in too close and were killed.

Perhaps it would not be destroyed. Maybe he should continue the plan to make sure the ship was damaged, and between disabling the ship's power source and the impact, the ship would be smashed.

Utu decided to continue as planned but to proceed as quickly as possible. He looked out the nearest window and saw, perhaps, only a quarter of the ship. It was truly massive. He had no comparison. The ship filled the entire view straight out the window. It was only when he looked up that he saw the stars. "Those things must be the spoke," he said aloud, looking back at the massive structure directly out the side window. Grabbing a railing under the window, he crushed his face to the pane. Looking to one side, he followed its length as far as he could.

"That must be the big wheel," he observed of the massive arch that curved away from him in the distance.

Then he turned his head and looked in the opposite direction.

"That must be the small wheel," he said of the arch that looked to be at the center of the larger outside arch. "Destroy a section of the small wheel."

Utu pointed the gauntlet in the direction of the small wheel and activated the beam. Nwella had set the range for distance, and Utu was glad to see that it didn't damage the wall in front of him, but he could tell something was being destroyed. He could see and hear his corridor vibrating. He pressed his face to the glass again and looked as far as he could in the direction he'd fired. He thought he saw material moving free of the rest of the ship.

Utu then looked directly out the window, at the spoke immediately to his front. It seemed very distant, but it was difficult to tell. Utu again steadied himself on the rail so he wouldn't float around, took aim, and again activated the beam. The spoke in front of him looked blurry for a moment, and then the section receiving the beam burst into a cloud of crumbled pieces.

"Oh, yes!" Utu said with excitement. He waited a moment to determine if he could see the inner wheel and the spoke it was connected to start to move. Everything was so massive he couldn't be sure if he saw movement. He could see the next spoke through the gap in the section he had just destroyed and decided to proceed with a shot at the second one. With these three sections destroyed and the ship still falling, certainly the whole thing would break apart, he thought. Utu took the third shot and marveled as the next spoke blew to pieces even more violently than the first.

"Hasta la vista, baby!" Utu quoted from a movie he'd enjoyed. He touched the green control and found himself standing in Rick's living room.

Deep in the mountains of Idaho...

Synster and his entourage had been at Kylamity Base for two days giving a tour to members of the Project Council. He'd brought his sixteen-year-old son, Beyn, with him for educational purposes, as well as his two trusted associates, Layrd and Streyn. When Rick disposed of that troublesome Ryvil, Synster didn't want any of his best Provenger to be suspected.

The tour consisted of a half-day presentation on the progress of the Project. It highlighted the adaptations made to the harvest strategy to accommodate the additional time and resources that were needed to compensate for the inorganic development of the subject species. The council members understood that something unexpected almost always happens with these projects, especially when dealing with living entities. It was the superior project director who successfully overcame those issues. It appeared that the quotas were being met and the Project was on track.

The group had attempted a hunting trip in the mountains of New Mexico, as it was too cold in Idaho that time of year, but they had been stymied by foul weather. They were getting a tour of the full capabilities of Kylamity Base when they learned they would be there longer than they'd planned.

They all simultaneously received an alarm on their com-monitors. The message was simple. A catastrophic structural failure of unknown origin had caused considerable damage to the Provenger Nation Ship. According to protocol, to reduce power usage, all transports between ship and planet were indefinitely suspended pending further notice. They were reminded that if they were in an area not yet neutralized or in any region of Earth conducting field work, they were to immediately activate their cloak for the next hour and their shield for the next five hours.

"Damn," Synster said out loud, to the surprise of everyone present. They were all equally disturbed by this development, but Synster's outburst seemed to them unprofessional. Even though they had conducted drills for this type of thing, it had never actually happened, and they were all on edge.

"Father, do we have to cloak and shield ourselves?" Beyn asked.

"No, son. We're in a neutralized area. Only those conducting field work need to do it." Synster turned to the others. "Provenger, we should probably go to the main deck and wait for further information," Synster commanded as he turned quickly and strode away from them. "Ryvil," he seethed under his breath.

Back at Rick's house in Cortez...

Utu smiled at Rick and Nwella. They had been patiently waiting for him, pacing the room. Carson was sitting on the couch, still trying to figure out what was going on. Because of the minimal time dilation of Utu's transport, his absence seemed a little bit longer for Rick and Nwella.

"How did it go?" asked Rick, feeling encouraged.

Nwella rushed to his gauntlet to see how much power he had remaining and stepped back. "A little," she said. She was going to remove it but feared Utu might suspect her of something.

"Take it out," she said.

Removing the bolt from the gauntlet, Utu began to brief them. "When I got there, the ship was already falling, so I figured they were in trouble from something already. The damage I did would only add to it," Utu reported.

"What do you mean they were falling?" Nwella asked.

"The ship was falling, the whole thing, with me in it."

Not quite understanding what Utu was talking about, Rick quickly asked him, "Did you take the shots that you needed?"

"Yes, of course, but I hurried a bit. I didn't want to be in the ship when it hit."

"Hit what?" Rick and Nwella asked in unison.

"The ground?" Utu asked, sheepishly.

Nwella started shaking her head. "This is my fault."

"Utu, there is no ground. The ship is in space. You don't fall anywhere in space."

"I felt like I was falling."

"Did you take the shots you needed?" Rick asked, frustrated.

"Yes, of course."

"Did you see destruction?"

"Oh, yes! What's wrong?"

"Utu, the falling feeling you had wasn't you and the ship falling," Rick explained recalling the sensation of skydiving and rapid descent in aircraft. "It was zero gravity."

"He's never experienced it before. It's my fault. I was rushed, and I forgot to tell him," Nwella confessed.

"Oh, Hell! I almost left before taking any shots. I figured, what could survive a fall that far?"

Everyone collapsed in the chair nearest them. "If he'd come back then, there wouldn't have been enough energy in the bolt to complete the job," informed Nwella.

Rick's nerves were shot. Now, he had to complete the assignment Synster had given him, he reminded himself. Shouldn't winning a gunfight, digging a grave, almost shooting a friend, and disabling an interstellar space ship be enough for one day?

"I need to start thinking about this thing I'm doing later," Rick said, glancing at his watch. "Nwella, how do we know he got the job done? What I mean is, how do we know the ship is disabled?"

"Well, really, the only way we'll know is if they don't come after us. If it was successful, all scanners would have shut down automatically. If they had done that, they wouldn't have had the time to detect this bolted battle gauntlet. Also, Rick, by protocol they would order the suspension of all transports between the ship and Earth, to save energy, and have Provenger remain in place, for safety," Nwella explained.

Well that should make it easier to get to Ryvil, Rick thought. "Nwella, how do we know when or if your father has heard about all this? I mean both your situation as well as the ship?"

It finally sunk in for Nwella where her father was. "Oh, Rick, Synster is here on Earth. Things happened so fast, I'd forgotten."

"Yes, I know. That's why I still have to go through with my assignment. This project of yours is still ongoing. I guess they won't be harvesting, right? ...without the power to transport all those people? Right?"

"Well, yes, I suppose," Nwella responded, fairly certain of herself. "With that power source gone now, they'll be conserving all energy sources just to keep basic systems running. Except for the use of the bolted battle gauntlets, all ship-to-planet transports are powered by the primary source, which we think Utu just destroyed."

"Oh, yes. Don't worry. I destroyed it. Don't doubt me just because I thought the ship was falling," Utu said, feeling a little inept, "or because I wasn't up to speed on the whole spoke wheel thing."

"So they can still come here with the battle gauntlets?" asked Rick.

"Yes, as long as it has a bolt. There are plenty of those. They won't want to use them, though. Now they'll need them to power systems on the ship. The important thing is to keep that bolt," Nwella emphasized, pointing to Utu, "out of that gauntlet. We never know when they might recover their ability to see it. As long as their main power source has been destroyed, they will have lost their opportunity to find us. We should be safe."

"Be that as it may, I don't want to risk it. Everybody, pack up what you need for a few days. Carson, take everyone to Denver. You know that town. It's pretty big. Maybe you can hide there better, and the Provenger might be less likely to make a scene coming after you. I'll stay for this other assignment. You've got three minutes. Let's go."

Rick also wasn't completely sure he'd be successful, and if he wasn't, they'd all be safer somewhere else.

Everyone was working frantically at stowing some things for the trip. Shainan was roused and feeling better. She was talking quickly, mostly to Utu in whatever language it was that they spoke. Utu occasionally said something to Nwella in the same language. Maybe this will all work out, Rick thought. He made a note to himself to ask the name of the language. It was pleasant to listen to. Since they all spoke it, he thought maybe he should try to learn it. It would be their own little tribe's private language.

Rick was in his room grabbing some things for Nwella to wear when he realized they could buy whatever they needed along the way. Then he heard the door creak. Looking up, he expected to see her. But it was Utu.

"Do you have a second?" Utu asked.

"Sure. Sorry about almost shooting you. I really didn't want to do it. I don't know if I would have." Rick added with all sincerity, "You are like a brother to me."

"You had your reasons. It was a difficult moment. Hopefully we'll never be in such a situation again. Sorry about the whole wheel and spoke panic. I felt really stupid," Utu admitted.

"No worries. It was something we couldn't have anticipated."

Utu sat on the edge of the bed. "I need to tell you something. I've known about it for some time now but didn't know how to tell you. I think it might be an asset to our cause."

"Is it something that can help me in about an hour?" asked Rick, thinking about his approaching revenge against Ryvil.

"I don't know, but it's something you should be aware of. I realized it when you pulled your gun on me. If you'd shot me without knowing, well then, you never would have known."

Rick was starting to get interested.

Utu continued, "When Shainan and I made love for the first time, that's when it happened."

"Yes, I know. You're a stud in bed. But I don't think that will be enough to scare away the Provenger."

Utu smiled and shook his head. "No, it doesn't have to do with the sex, but I think our emotional state had something to do with it. I'll cut to the facts. We found ourselves in the past." Utu waited for Rick to respond.

"What?"

"Yes, we found ourselves back near our village. We saw our village and our tribe. We've done it many times since that first time. I'm just not sure if we were really there, because I didn't recognize anyone and they wouldn't speak to us when we tried to talk to them. I'd like your help trying to figure this out."

"You probably dreamed it. Are you sure you were awake? Did you both have the same dream?"

"We know it wasn't a dream; it was too real. I think we were really there. Since we've done it, we've never had anyone here to watch to see if we're gone. Am I being clear?"

"Yeah, you're wondering if your bodies disappear or something."

"Yes, exactly. If I really am going back in time, I think we could use this to our advantage. But since I couldn't speak to anyone, I'm just not sure if it was real or if it would have any value."

"Utu, it probably was just a dream, maybe what's called a waking dream. Maybe you and Shainan have some kind of connection where you can share these memories and they seem real. I don't know. We'll have to look into it. When I get back."

"Rick, I think I could take you."

"We don't have to have sex, do we?" Rick faked a little nervous laughter, and Utu chuckled with him.

"No. Shainan and I have done this without sleeping together. Just short trips. We were always worried about getting stuck there. We didn't know anyone," Utu said with a shrug. "It seems like our tribe is here now. Thank you, Rick. I just wanted to tell you."

Rick finished burying Marcus, the Harley, and his revolver; a simple matter of pushing the pile of dirt, created from digging the hole, back over him with the front end loader. Rick thought about the possibility of disintegrating the whole mess later using Provenger technology, possibly with the gauntlet.

337

He went inside to put on his gear. Already fully outfitted in his green camouflage utilities, the rest of his equipment was waiting on the kitchen table. Rick had gone over the plan in his head, wondering whether or not he should tell Nwella what he was about to do, wondering if that would make her an accomplice and subject to any Provenger discipline. It was difficult trying to work out all these issues. What he needed was a consultation with a Provenger lawyer. Fortunately, none had hung their shingles in Cortez yet. He was glad he hadn't told her. Now that they were gone, he could focus.

He'd said goodbye to all of them in a rush, explaining to Carson exactly where to stay in a very nice hotel downtown. Rick pulled his son aside. "Carson, I don't know exactly how long I'll be gone. I want you to stay gone for the next three days. Leave your phone off. Don't turn it on to call me unless it's life or death. They might be able to track you. After three days, come home. I'm going to keep the dogs here, at the house. If I'm not here when you come back, depending on how they act or don't act, you'll know how bad it might be. Send Utu up to check. First, drive by the house. If everything is okay, I'll leave a shirt hanging over the front gate. Remember who you have in the car. Two ancient humans, one with authority issues that can talk circles around most people, except regarding wheels and things like that. Just keep in mind he's smart but he doesn't know a lot about a lot of things. And then Shainan who can't talk at all and is supposed to be from Armenia and deaf. Neither of them have really ever been out of the house except Shainan that one time with you. They'll both be very interested in everything they see, and you'll have to keep a close eye on them. Understand?"

"Sure, Dad. Keep track of them. I understand."

"You also have an alien who currently looks like she's been through a nuclear accident. So please, drive slowly. Make sure she wears her hat. You really don't want to get pulled over." Rick gave Carson five thousand in cash and made sure the others had their ID and another thousand dollars each. He also stowed a few pounds of gold under the liner in the trunk.

Nwella had been lucky in her timing. The Provenger, in addition to allowing her the surgery to enable her to grow hair, had also created an identity for her to include birth certificate and other identification. Nwella and Rick were both unsure if they'd had time to make the documents valid on Earth.

Rick sent them away in a flurry of confusion and tears. He promised to be careful and see them again.

An hour later, Rick had used the gauntlet to transport himself to a hill above a small mountain town in the Andes. He instinctively took cover behind a boulder and surveyed the area. The rolling countryside was sparsely treed yet still green enough to make his camouflage appropriate. He should have been placed no further than three hundred and fifty yards and uphill from Ryvil's location. All he had to do was find him.

Rick immediately recognized that the terrain was very similar to the areas where he would predator hunt in canyon country. This was his most important predator hunt yet. He couldn't afford to fail now, especially after all they'd been through and all the luck they'd had. He was hoping it hadn't run out.

Rick had arrived cloaked and quickly realized he didn't need to be concerned about being seen. He lifted the binoculars hanging from his neck and scanned the area downhill. Perfect, he thought. He immediately picked up two figures on the terrain below him, approximately three hundred yards away in a boulder field. He immediately recognized one of them as Syrjon. Rick was glad he didn't have to kill him. The other he knew to be Ryvil. Rick's gauntlet had been programmed by Synster to bring him this distance from Ryvil, and Rick recognized him from a picture he'd been shown. There was no doubt.

"This is going to be easier than I thought."

His view of them seemed to squirm a bit, as though there was a heat shimmer mirage between him and the target. Rick knew heat wasn't the problem. It was rather cool out and a little overcast. The rocks around him weren't hot, and he doubted others were further down the slope. Rick hadn't used the cloak while looking through optics before but guessed that might have something to do with it. He touched his gauntlet and deactivated the cloak. He grabbed his Remington, assumed a prone position over a small boulder, and put it to his shoulder while checking to ensure the muzzle area was clear. In a moment he found them again. With the cloak off, they were perfectly clear. The smaller figure, Syrjon, stooped and disappeared behind a boulder.

Considering all the environmental conditions, Rick knew this would be a simple shot. His scope was zeroed for exactly this range, there was no wind, slightly downhill. Easy. Rick had already carefully chambered a round before he left the house. He moved his thumb to the safety and pushed it forward to the "fire" position. He suspended his breathing and relaxed the core of his torso. He then focused on only two points, the reticle of the scope on Ryvil's chest and the growing pressure between the pad of his index finger and the surface of his trigger. He maintained those two points, having no idea when the shot might come.

The shot cracked before Rick thought it would while the center of the reticle was perfectly positioned high on Ryvil's chest. Right where all the goodies connect, Rick thought. He should be down.

Rick instantly cycled the bolt action and reacquired his target. Ryvil was still standing. Without thinking, Rick positioned the reticle on the same spot on Ryvil's chest, built pressure on the trigger, and another shot cracked from the rifle. It happened so automatically that when Rick delivered the second shot, it felt like merely an echo from the first. Rick cycled the bolt again and reacquired, but Ryvil wasn't there! Something was very wrong.

Rick quickly checked to ensure there was no obstruction forward of the muzzle, something he thought he'd already done. There was nothing in front of him. It had been a clear shot. A feeling of terror overwhelmed him. What if Ryvil had his shield up? Shit!

Rick scanned the area for his target. He could find nothing. Then he realized that even if he could find him, he still couldn't shoot through the shield. He'd failed.

Rick instinctively flipped the safety off "fire" with his thumb and was placing the rifle down in front of him to push himself up when he felt crushed by a boot between his shoulder blades and the full weight of a body above it. He immediately knew someone had been closing on his position while he'd been preoccupied with his task. Two eight-inch-long knives slid past both sides of his neck and stuck into the rocky soil, pinning him. It was Syrjon!

"Not a very nice way to thank us for everything we've done!" he said in a polite but forceful tone.

Rick didn't know what to say. He felt like an ass, and he knew this time he was really a dead man. Everything was ruined. He just hoped they wouldn't kill Carson and was glad he'd sent them to Denver. Maybe they would still have a chance.

"I wasn't shooting at you. By the way, did you get our thank you note?"

Syrjon smiled, remembering Rick's general good humor in stressful situations. "No, it must be in the mail," Syrjon laughed. "We must wait here for a moment. Ryvil is coming up the hill and he might have a few things to say to you before we finish our business here. I'd advise you not to move. I wouldn't want you to get cut on my blades."

In fact, Rick couldn't move, pinned as he was. He thought about making a lunge for his pistol but knew the angle was wrong to get a quick grab at it. In that moment of hesitation, Syrjon removed the temptation by pulling the pistol from its holster with his free hand.

"You won't be needing this."

Rick heard movement below and knew Ryvil must be approaching.

"So this is our shooter!" bellowed Ryvil.

"Rick Thompson, our Candidate Species," stated Syrjon.

"Are we to thank you also for the destruction to our ship?" Ryvil inquired, but sounding as if he already knew.

Rick figured he'd better not admit to anything other than what he knew they were sure of. He asked, "Regarding this little shooting incident, I don't suppose we could chalk this up as just following orders and forget about the whole thing?"

"No, I'm afraid we can't do that. Your action has changed everything. As your kind says, that bell cannot be un-rung," Ryvil responded. He picked up the rifle and, admiring it, put it back down a considerable distance from Rick's reach. He nodded to Syrjon, who pulled the gauntlet blades out of the ground, releasing Rick's neck. "You see, we now have the opportunity to know, with all certainty, who put you up to this. Synster?"

Rick sensed he had no options left. If these guys could get distracted from him and his family by fighting each other, all the better. "Yes, Synster."

Rick, with his face partially in the dirt, could only sense that they were either signaling or somehow communicating to each other. He felt some of the weight lift from his back.

"We aren't going to kill you. Or harm you in any way," said Ryvil. "You are very valuable to us. You must consider us allies, both to you and your entire race."

Syrjon's foot lifted entirely from Rick's back. Rick rolled over slowly, not believing what he was hearing, though every indication was that he would live. "What?"

"We were alerted that the ship has been compromised," Syrjon explained. "Its main power source has been lost, irretrievably. Luckily, following protocol, we had our shields up, and you were not able to hit Ryvil. Regarding the ship, it will never phase again, at least not without help. Its ability to travel is severely impaired. If it were to come here as fast as it could, it would take many, many years."

"There is much we cannot tell you in case you are suspected and questioned," Ryvil added, "but we will offer as evidence of our honesty only that we let you live after trying to kill us. Another Provenger ship may come. Knowing this, Synster will be intent on continuing his project. You must continue in your current capacity."

Rick sat up. Syrjon unloaded Rick's 1911, dropping the magazine and locking the slide to the rear. He handed it back to him, not completely convinced he was now calm.

"Though our goals," Ryvil nodded at Syrjon, "and yours are not exactly the same, they are similar in that the survival of the human race is desirable. We will be able to help you on occasion, but not in any way that can be made obvious. You may already realize that with the reduced power capabilities of the ship, harvests will not continue. But Synster will pursue the correction of human diets for the elimination of drugs and unnatural additives. He wants his harvest organic. All this can only help the human race, in the short run."

"If you're against him, then why are you surveying villages for harvest?" Rick asked.

"Why are you trying to kill me and supporting agendas that serve his project?" Ryvil countered. "We are all occasionally forced into service that we do not support. It is our burden. We must bear it only so long as we have to."

"What should I tell Synster about whether or not I shot you?"

"I would certainly like him to think I am dead, especially now that we are all stranded on this planet, but he knows that the ship's signal would have prompted me to activate my shield. He would know that your attempt would fail. You must say that you were able to transport home moments before you were caught. You must be angry with him for not warning you."

Rick's mind was spinning. I must be the luckiest man alive, he thought. All he wanted to do was go home and be with his family, raise Carson, marry Nwella, have babies in the house, and forget about Marcus in the back yard. There were probably a million questions he had for Syrjon and Ryvil, none of which he could think of and none of which they were likely to answer.

"If we're allies, then why did you try to kill me and instead hurt Carson?"

"Rick, you really need to give me more credit. If I'd wanted to kill you, do you really think I would have failed? The answer to your question is in the results of the action that I took. That is all I will say," responded Ryvil.

Rick had his instructions, and he was alive. For now, that was enough. As he pressed the controls that would take him home, Syrjon and Ryvil were walking away from him, starting up the vast mountainside that had loomed behind them. They assured him they had the means by which to continue their project.

Three days later, Carson, Nwella, Utu, and Shainan were all back from their trip, settling down and getting some much needed rest. Apparently, they'd enjoyed quite an adventure. When Carson and the others poured themselves out of the Charger when they first got home, nobody wanted to talk. They all looked exhausted and dirty.

Rick asked, "What happened? You guys look like you've been through the mill." They had brown stains on their clothing that looked like dried blood.

Carson pulled a blood stained samurai sword out of the car and assured him, "We're okay, Dad. Nobody really wants to talk right now. Some stuff happened, but we're good now. We didn't leave any evidence…to speak of, and Utu made sure we weren't followed."

Nwella, Shainan, and Utu all nodded agreement, as Utu tucked another sword into his belt and shuffled toward the front door. Carson paused as he followed the others, as if in deep thought.

Rick was about to stop him and demand answers, but he was interrupted by Carson's statement. "You might want to check the trunk, I think you'll like what you see…some of it, anyways. We're developing quite a little arsenal."

Rick walked to the trunk and popped it open. There were two plastic garbage bags tucked as far back into the rear as they would go. Rick grabbed the nearest one and pulled it open…the remains of the leg of some kind of hooved animal. Utu. That makes sense, Rick thought, remembering the two deer carcasses he found a week ago hanging in the trees out back.

He grabbed the next bag and pulled it open. Four Provenger gauntlets. Rick quickly checked for bolts. None. He was about to yell to Nwella, who had just entered the house, to ask if it was safe to have them. Then he realized that if they weren't, she probably would have done something about it.

Rick didn't ask for details for a number of days. He had been through a mission where he'd returned covered with blood, and he understood. Everyone seemed to just want to sleep for the next twenty-four hours. By the way they looked, Rick suspected they'd been on the go for much of their trip. They'd obviously had a run-in with the Provenger and must have killed them. Provenger don't just leave those gauntlets lying around. And after what he'd been through, he just didn't care. As long as everyone was home safe, that was all that mattered. Carson would tell him when he was ready.

The next evening, Rick wanted to get things back to normal. Utu and Shainan were in their room either making love, taking one of their dream trips down memory lane, or talking about their developing baby. Carson was healthy, thanks to the Recombinant, getting caught up on some homework, and getting over the thought of a local man being buried in the back yard.

344

Rick and Nwella were expecting Synster to arrive and he didn't make them wait long. It was an unusually mild evening, so Rick and Nwella were on the patio sitting by the fire wrapped in bison hides. Barnes and Nobelle were inside. He appeared in a startling manner, directly in front of them. Synster tried to ignore Nwella. She was banished, after all. He had read the report, and had only narrowly decided to let Rick live.

They spoke about his recent mission. "I tried to get to you regarding the complications with your last assignment, but I couldn't get away. It was a shame the assignment was a failure. I wanted that done. It may be impossible now that he's gone. He cannot be found," Synster said, divulging the fact that Ryvil had absconded.

Synster believed that neither Rick nor Nwella knew anything of the Provenger Nation Ship being compromised. He believed that perhaps Ryvil had gone mad and committed sabotage. Perhaps Ryvil expected the new ship to arrive at any time and would benefit from the delays caused by the disabled ship. Synster was still working on a theory, but resources for an investigation were stretched thin. He would be lucky to be able to operate at a minimal level while stuck on Earth.

"We will, nevertheless, continue with the Project. Rick, I will be contacting you regarding the progress of our initiatives and your government's policy changes."

To Rick and Nwella's great surprise, he turned to Nwella and said to her with all sincerity. "I am grieved that we should come to this. Take care of yourself. Don't eat any of the candidate species. It would be poison to your system. Wheat is in everything on Earth." And with that, he was gone.

Nwella turned her head toward Rick and gave him a dumb stare. After what she had been through the last three days, she had begged for death with that poison in her system. She would never be the same. Her body had taken the brunt of the toxins so that her baby would survive. She felt she had been weakened to almost human strength.

Rick thought about what Synster said. The candidate species. "Hmm, that's funny. On this last assignment, I saw Syrjon, and he referred to me as their 'candidate species'. I remember. He said, 'Rick Thompson, our candidate species', just like that."

"You must be mistaken, Rick," Nwella said. "The candidate species is the one we genetically alter for our purposes. For this project it was wheat."

"No, I'm pretty sure that's what he said."

"Rick, you must be confused. Let's talk about our baby. Do you have any names in mind?"

"Well, there's a lot to consider. There's the boy/girl issue. Then there's the human/alien thing." Rick gave her a wink. "How about Ryan if it's a boy and Gwen if it's a girl?"

As the fire burned low, Rick and Nwella spoke of simple things that people in a stable world with common interests might concern themselves. Rick felt he deserved a break. The world was, for now, safe from the harvest. They had time to think, to plan, and to hope. Meanwhile, the universe around them swirled with complexities that neither of them could, or desired, to understand.

End of book one: The Candidate Species

Appendix A

Recipes
...an obligatory addition for diet books and serious novels

Shainan's red meat cooked in ash
1. Build big fire
2. Let fire burn down to coals
3. Put meat in fire
4. Wait until village dogs lose interest and walk away
5. Flip meat and leave for same amount of time
6. Remove meat, brush off large coals and season with salt, if you have it.

Utu's whole fish cooked in ash
1. Build big fire
2. Let fire burn down to coals
3. Put gutted fish in fire
4. Wait until village dogs lose interest and walk away
5. Roll fish over and leave for same amount of time
6. Remove fish, brush off large coals and season with salt, if you have it.

Appendix B

Nwella's Provenger Nation Ship diagram
30 second attack plan

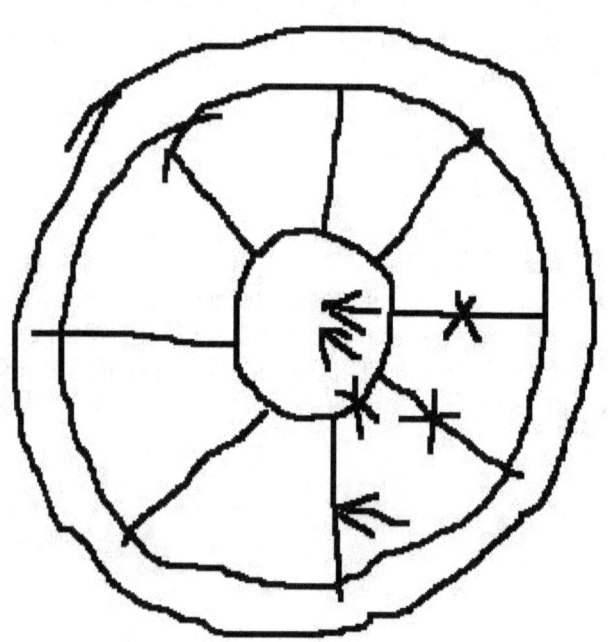

Appendix C

Meeting of the 3-237 Perpetuant Cycle Project
Planning Committee

****

Preparations for Contact

TRANSCRIBED RECORD

Meeting of the
3-237 Perpetuant Cycle Project
Planning Committee
Vote for the Approval
Candidate Species: Yngorn
Subject Species: Carnate

Project Minister:
 Listen and be heard, this twenty-fourth meeting of the 3-237 Perpetuant Cycle Project Planning Committee, all who have Interest be here withheld of all selfish undoing, and maintain the good of the Nation for all and forever.

Science Director Synster:
 As you've already been informed in your brief, our objective of populating this planet through the advancement of their agricultural technology has been fully vetted by the Algorithm. A delicate balance must be struck between the subject species' population growth and their technological impairment. The goal is to provide us with a maximum population increase over time without their posing a technological threat upon our return. As has been well-established, any intelligent organism, provided with the

efficiencies of agriculture, will have the time and the incentive to develop and accumulate technology. A hunting/gathering society, on the other hand, has the time but not necessarily the incentive or means to do the same.

If we merely provide the carnate with a wholesome, reliable, and nutrient rich source of food to generate the population numbers we need, the Algorithm has calculated that they will reach a technological advancement comparable to ours within a period of approximately five thousand years. We will be absent from this planet well beyond this time as the Union schedule demands. There is every indicator that we would return to a superior society technologically capable of defending itself. This would obviously be counterproductive. We are therefore compelled to include various progressive deleterious effects to our agricultural product introduction. These qualities are designed to obstruct health and productivity in their post-harvest years.

Our goal is that they be reasonably healthy and of proper carcass mass index during harvest age, without being advanced enough to defend themselves against us. Our return to this planet is scheduled for nine years, eight months, our time. Allowing for Accelerated Gravitational Time Dilation, we will return in approximately twelve thousand, eight hundred and ninety-three years planet time. We have the charter to proceed as necessary to generate a viable product. We must be aggressive. Let's just say, any enemies we make now, won't be around to trouble us later.

General Reaction:
Laughter, Agreement, scale 6.5 out of 10

Synster:
Prior experience has shown that it is imprudent to rely on a single mechanism to achieve our ends, and we are best rewarded by implementing multiple strategies. We are fortunate in regard to this planet, as we have a grass that grows throughout a great variety of regions that is highly receptive to genetic modification. We can amend its qualities to suit our needs. This enables us to implement not a single, but a multi-pronged approach with this one species to achieve our goals. There is other vegetation that offers potential, and it will be made available for agricultural

development. But it is only this one grass that produces a grain, largely poisonous and unpalatable to the human population, which we will modify to enhance its beneficial properties for the purposes of achieving production goals.

This grain, Yngorn, named after the Provenger that discovered it, is currently of minor use to the subject species population, particularly in its non-germinated form, due to a great variety of deleterious effects it inflicts on human physiology. When these populations do find it in quantities that allow for its collection, they are only able to make use of its limited nourishment through soaking it long enough to sprout or have it ferment. In its un-sprouted grain form it is hard on their teeth, dry in their mouths and almost void of flavor. It requires significant effort to access and collect, and considerable processing to be consumed. It is the last thing the subject species would perceive as food. Despite these efforts it is still detrimental as food, as it is small and course, imbued with toxins and proteins damaging to their digestive systems, and relatively deficient in nutrients even when processed. We will introduce strains that will eliminate the high degree of these negative aspects. The resulting plant will retain certain elements of its poisonous characteristics. These effects are by design. They bring us numerous benefits to help meet our goals. These benefits involve the deterioration of subject species health at a measured rate, with the majority of degenerative effects occurring after the subject species' reproductive and harvest age. This will reduce individuals' contributions to their society later in life when they are most knowledgeable and experienced, ensuring slow technological progress while simultaneously maintaining the level of civilization necessary for perpetuated population growth. We can count on this grain to provide general nutrient scarcity, impaired nutrient absorption, innate and adaptive immune system responses, and addictive tendencies.

PAUSE

Let me elaborate. Our improvements to the grain will allow it to be accepted as a common food by these primitives. Its characteristics will achieve the desired results of providing suitable caloric nutrition to provide energy for labor and reproduction, while simultaneously eliciting long-term physiological effects that will: one, increase carcass weight and fat marbling of tissues and organs during the harvest age, two, promote accelerated mortality for those in their post reproductive years, removing them from resource competition with the youth of the species, and finally, three, as the Algorithm has exposed, the accelerated mortality will also limit the productive life of those intelligent enough to push technological frontiers. This will force subsequent generations to either relearn, retrain, or rediscover their accomplishments and abilities, rather than benefitting firsthand from the innovators' continued efforts over an extended lifetime. This is vital to the prevention of any problems with an uncooperative and highly advanced population on our return. This will provide us with fat stock that dies off quickly after the reproductive and harvest age, an almost ideal situation.

PAUSE

There are numerous qualities of this grain that make it favorable to our needs. We have designed a slightly larger grain, making it cost-effective for the carnate to collect. We have retained the grain's ability to remain dormant under dry conditions through the actions of phytic acid in the grain. This acid acts as a natural preservative, in that it inhibits germination, allowing it to be stored for long periods. It will therefore be available during famine when natural phenomena limit traditional food sources. These times of famine have regularly afflicted and reduced the subject species. Throughout these periods of great need, carnate will come to see this grain as a savior, something which supports the body of their society when it might otherwise stumble and fall, a staff of life, if you will. This is a major mechanism by which it will be gradually adopted by societies that have not undergone the Contact Protocol. It will eventually be perceived by all related societies as a source of energy that is plentiful, reliable, and intrinsic to their culture.

The biological effects on the species' health are especially important. As I've already stated, this quality is vital. During our absence, in the vast amount of time it takes for them to populate the planet, we must have a mechanism to impede their technological development. Limiting the productive length of their later lives is the best method. There are many characteristics of Yngorn that help us accomplish this.

First there are the effects that deprive them of the dense nutrition upon which their species has become dependent throughout their evolution. The qualities of this relatively nutrient deficient grain will actually inhibit nutrient absorption of other foods that are eaten by carnate through the following mechanisms.

Substitution: the grain will regularly be substituted for their relatively nutrient dense foods; the game and vegetation that they collect during the course of their day. This will result in a deficit of the variety of nutrients necessary for proper cellular metabolism, especially the fatty acids and trace minerals they require for all metabolic functions.

Chemically inhibited absorption: phytic acid that preserves the grain for storage does so by binding minerals. Phytates will also bind minerals offered by all foods during digestion and prevent vital trace minerals from being absorbed through the intestinal lining, further inhibiting healthy cellular metabolism.

Gut Irritation: both the proteins in the grain, and harmful bacterial overgrowth promoted by the overabundance of starch, will create intestinal lining irritation. The starches in the grain will promote the growth of non-contributory bacteria in the digestive system. These bacteria will provide three important deleterious services. One: as already stated, the bad bacteria overgrowth will irritate the mucus membranes causing an overabundance of mucus, thereby blocking some absorption of nutrients by these membranes. Two: through competition for space and resources, these bad bacteria will inhibit the growth of productive bacteria that would have aided in the digestion of nutrients, leading to decreased nutrient absorption. And three: they will aid in the activation of the immune system in the area of the intestinal lining that is overpopulated with the invasive bacteria. This reaction will contribute to the destruction of nutrient absorbing tissues on the intestine wall.

Immune system reaction: The intestine will now be coated with the unusually adhesive grain proteins. They will irritate the absorptive lining and will initiate an immune system reaction, resulting in destruction of the absorptive tissue. This process sounds similar to the immune system reaction to the bacteria, but is actually quite different. The proteins of the grain have unique qualities to make the intestinal lining more permeable.

PAUSE

All the aforementioned mechanisms combine to result in an organism that thinks it is eating well, but having the nutrient absorption and health of one that is not. Much of what is being eaten is rendered unusable by the body. There is one exception regarding these obstructions to absorption. Starches and sugars will pass to the body in abundance. After approximately twenty-four years of this process, the human body will begin to feel these negative effects, right around harvest age. For the next ten years, on average, the effects will slowly take hold. At approximately thirty-five years the carnate will be well marbled and replete with the fat that we desire.

The nature of the grain's powerful starch, amylopectin, which is quickly digested, even under the aforementioned circumstances, will provide them with a great deal of immediate energy when eaten. This effect, as well as chemical effects on the brain, will be mildly addictive. It will also induce a considerable insulin spike which the species' body is not designed to handle. This will promote general inflammation and fat deposition. The accumulation of fat will accelerate later in life as inflammation takes hold. As the species eats more of this grain it is increasingly starved of nutrients, signaling the brain with a need for more nutrients. This will result in the desire to eat more grain, resulting in greater fat deposition through insulin spikes and continued nutrient deficiency. And so on, and so on. It is a self-enforcing cycle. Beyond the age of most efficient reproduction, this cumulative effect will drive the physiology of the species toward weakness without immediately affecting the quality of their flesh and organs. The first nutrients to be targeted by this decreased capacity for absorption will be the trace minerals that are vital for cellular metabolism. Due to the aforementioned factors, regardless of the nutrient levels of all the foods carnate eat, the presence of a high starch diet will inhibit their ability to use many of these nutrients. Their deficiency of iron, in particular, will be beneficial to the end product, as there will be a slight reduction in that metallic flavor some Provenger experienced during the taste trials.

Over all, the trace mineral deficiency will gradually lead to aberrant gene expression within the species' cells, the cumulative effect of which will manifest itself in a variety of different disorders, depending on the individuals' genetic makeup, that will dramatically weaken the individual, eventually resulting in mental and physical decline, and ultimately, premature death. But prior to that ultimate event, this process will promote the deposition of fat both in the body in general as well as surrounding the primary commodity organs.

Their current diet varies considerably through the seasons as they move about, take advantage of animal migrations, reproductive cycles, and seasonal plant availability. Though most of this species suffer from parasites, this seasonal nutritional change, as well as their continual relocation, tends to contribute to a seasonal intestinal biome diversity. Over the short-term, this has inhibitory effects on the proliferation of any one particular bad bacteria or parasitic infestation that would otherwise benefit from any one perpetual food source. With the adoption of agriculture and the resulting sedentary lifestyle, bacteria and parasites of specific types would be more capable of gaining a foothold in the consistently conducive environment. This makes the adoption of infectious disease mitigating habits by humans all the more important. Otherwise, infestations would become so chronic as to impact our long-term population goals. These habits will be part of our Contact Protocol. Obviously these are issues we don't generally need to deal with in our world, and so are typically overlooked.

For those with the individual genotypes that are especially resilient to the mal-absorptive path of degeneration, there are some naturally occurring proteins within Yngorn specifically that achieve a necessary degeneration through a completely different pathway. I've touched on this briefly already. The original potency of this effect has, once again, been reduced by our modifications to make the grain more acceptable as a food.

Using the mechanism that currently regulates cellular tight junctions, or permeability, of epithelial tissue in humans, we can naturally destroy their longevity. We can do it both organically and without the administration of toxins that could affect the end product. We will do this by simply opening their intestinal lining as well as other organs consisting of epithelial tissue, to allow the invasion of undigested proteins throughout their bodies. We have found that proteins in this grain naturally affect their permeability mechanism. These proteins, when collocated with human epithelial tissues, initiate a signaling process which makes the tissue become more permeable by loosening the tight junctions between the cells. All living tissues require this mechanism, of course, as all life needs to maintain a balance, called homeostasis, between what it keeps out, and what it lets in. By increasing what is let in, the immune system is activated in some very detrimental ways.

During the digestion of this grain, the gut lining becomes overly permeable to undigested particles, as well as irritated. The bloodstream will then become exposed to the contents of the intestines through a leaking intestinal lining, potentially throughout significant portions of the digestive system. In addition, once these proteins make it into the bloodstream, they will have the opportunity to affect all other membranes' permeability in all systems of the body. The intestinal lining, vital organs, vascular system, the nervous system, even the brain itself will not be spared. With this increased permeability, the grain proteins will invoke an innate immune system reaction resulting in a general increase in inflammation, and an adaptive immune system attack on various internal organs to which these proteins resemble or attach.

Depending on the genetic makeup of the individual, their past history of disease exposure, and their current nutrient deficiencies due to the other deleterious effects, the carnate will exhibit different debilitating conditions. Internal organs will be attacked through an autoimmune reaction leading to their eventual compromise. Keep in mind, this will all be occurring in a body that is experiencing high inflammation and nutrient deficiencies that are inhibiting all normal and productive hormonal signaling. In fact, some of their accelerating disorders will actually originate from hormonal imbalances due to these nutrient deficiencies. Ironically, even if they recognize this, and eat nutrient rich foods, as long as they keep eating this grain, or suffer from the intestinal damage already sustained, they will be unable to recover. Conversely, even if they stop eating the grain for substantial periods, the immune system, already activated, can continue its attack for significant periods of time. It would require long periods of abstinence to calm this mechanism; not likely, due to

Yngorn's addictive properties. This will make identification of the problem exceedingly difficult, even as their technology increases.

Once again, the potency of these effects have been carefully calibrated through our genetic alteration of Yngorn, to reach a critical point of maximum effect beginning with the post reproductive years, after certain hormonal changes in the species have been reached.

The Algorithm has considered every variable, and has determined this is the only way we can meet our simultaneous needs: population increase, fattening during harvest age, and physical and mental decline consistent with our need for intellectual and technological growth retardants. In my personal opinion, this grain provides us with a tool to further our objectives beyond anything we could have dreamed. We are truly quite lucky. It is genuinely a multipurpose tool for the Natural Proliferation management technique. For our purposes this grain, along with others in its genus generally called wheat, is truly a super-food.

The importance of the adoption of wheat requires some assurance that it not be abandoned in favor of some other emerging food source; something the Algorithm has difficulty predicting. Therefore, some of the proteins in wheat have been modified to bind with certain receptors in the species' brain that influence gratification. This will give the grain an increased addictive effect. They will have a tendency to crave it and this will mitigate a tendency to abandon the crop. Adding to this feature is the fact that humans already have relatively well-developed knowledge regarding the fermentation of foods. This includes the uses of their current inedible wheat grains for making alcohol, which they drink.

Their desire to obtain fermentation products is strong. They currently gather some grains, when in season, as they travel. Our scans revealed that they place the grain in a wet leather bag as they collect it, and eat it only if near starvation during a hunt after it has softened or sprouted as they travel. They prefer to save it and bring it back to camp where they contribute it to a communal animal hide that is tended by the sedentary. There it is fermented in water and herbs, and consumed by the tribe. This practice is common throughout the tribes, but is only seasonal when the grains are available. This limits their consumption due to the minimal supply. With the adoption of agriculture and the surpluses that will result, they will have access to their fermented drink year round. We have noticed that this drink tends to promote their reproductive activity, while decreasing their creativity and innovation. Again, this is in line with our desire to increase population while decreasing the technological innovations that accompany the more sedentary lifestyle of a curious organism. These factors have been accounted for in the Algorithm and exert a surprising 18 percent influential effect on the final outcome.

For those of you with a moral concern for the welfare of this species, I assure you that these modifications have been made with efficiency in mind, and with as little needless suffering as possible. This species, in their current state, maintains a tenuous existence that relies mostly on hunting and gathering with a small amount of superficial animal domestication in the form of rudimentary herding practices. Their lifespan, barring accident, infection, or infectious disease, is usually limited by accumulated parasite load, a condition completely alien to us. Their lives are extremely rigorous. Death occurs frequently due to infections from accidents in the course of their activities, or from starvation or predation when they become incapacitated and unable to hunt or locate food. All these forms of death are a terrible process, involving considerable prolonged suffering, or exceedingly abrupt brutality.

Once the adoption of agriculture is made, they will not be as afflicted by the exertions of a hunting/gathering life. Their mode of death, while not completely natural, will be, rather than abrupt and violent, peaceful and in the company of their kind, as a settled life would allow. A more sedentary life, while certainly leaving them open to more disease, will shelter them from the accidents that their current, more active life inflicts upon them. I should also emphasize, that while we are introducing wheat to numerous locations, not all of the populations will adopt it. Some will carry on in their current way for a long period. So while we expect agriculture to be fully established midterm for a minority of the population, the vast majority will not practice it for many thousands of years. Agriculture facilitates the organized exploration, settlement, and, if necessary, invasion of less developed regions that promote growing populations. But the process is slow. In fact, the Algorithm predicts that the majority of the population growth will occur only after approximately 8,000 years. This will result in the majority of the species being associated, some immediately, some secondarily, with agriculture for only two to three thousand years prior to our return. Agriculture will intensify in the last five hundred years before we arrive. Therefore, for the vast majority of our absence, agriculture will be mixed with other, more natural, methods of food provision. This is one reason why the deleterious effects will go largely unnoticed. During these last five hundred years most of their technological advances will be made, giving them only a brief time to scientifically observe, consider, and explore the deleterious effects. By then they will be the heirs of an agrarian culture that believes that at a certain age they are destined to become fat, feeble, and sick. It will be treated like the end of the day, with expectation and resignation.

Simultaneous to our arrival for harvest, as we begin phasing out of our Gravitational Dilation, we will send a team ahead to introduce an improvement on this crop that will allow it to be grown more efficiently and with even greater yield. This will result in wheat becoming so inexpensive it will render its universal use an economic imperative in almost all cultures. It will make wheat available as a feed for animals as well as promoting an increased use in human foods. With the technology they will have at this advanced stage, wheat is likely to be modified into all kinds of consumable products. We expect this process to circumvent some of the remaining cultural barriers that would have protected certain populations up to that point. Keep in mind these effects will initially hit some humans very hard, but the effects will taper off as those who suffer most are removed from the gene pool.

Starting from initial introduction, subsequent millennia will see the longer term negative effects that will reduce human progress by approximately 2.3 percent, year over year, effectively creating our desired limitations. The immediate effect in individual lives is therefore, over the long-term, extremely small. But in the larger sense, this makes for a significant impact.

There is one last element of the project which I need to cover, and that pertains to our recent scans. This project was conducted some twenty years ago and there must have been some inaccuracies in the initial surveys. It appears that a combination of weather activity and tidal influences imposed by the planet's small moon will influence settlement, in a negative manner, along some coastal areas. These settlements are vital to our plan, as coastal trade is vital to the spread of agriculture based civilizations across the planet. The Algorithm has analyzed all variables and has determined that removal of the small moon is required. This will be a simple matter. We've done similar things in the past with certain mining operations resulting in very little disruption to the surface. I've even thought of a way I can integrate the demolition with our appearance on the surface during our Contact Protocol. It will obviously be a demonstration of great power to these primitive beings, and will enhance our ability to introduce a few necessary cultural and religious activities.

Being a simple matter, and being consistent with the mandate under which I operate, I've unilaterally decided to include this action in the final proposal to this committee. If it is passed in this manner it will save us considerable expense to the alternative of getting Union approval.

In conclusion, I would like to submit this proposal, pending subsequent questions."

PAUSE

Listen and be heard, this twenty-fourth meeting of the 3-237 Perpetuant Cycle Project Planning Committee, all who have interest be here withheld of all selfish undoing, and maintain the good of the Nation for all and forever.

Break

QUESTION PERIOD

Project Minister:
Listen and be heard, this twenty-fourth meeting of the 3-237 Perpetuant Cycle Project Planning Committee, all who have questions be here withheld of all selfish undoing, and maintain the

good of the Nation for all and forever.

Synster:
"Consul Rydeo"

Consul Rydeo:
"What of the other species on the planet that will be, um, displaced? We, you know, have use for them. Will they not be obliterated by the proliferation of the subject species? I mean, ultimately?"

Synster:
"We do not anticipate this being a problem. The amount of land required for the subject species to successfully conduct agricultural activities will be minimal due to the productivity of the wheat grain. There will be considerable habitat to provide for all the other species, even at the projected maximum population upon our return. As you know, we have approval to harvest all large bestiary from land masses one, four and five. We will take full advantage of this."

Synster:
"Consul Wyriwort"

Consul Wyriwort
"Further explain why this species won't discover that this grain causes them physical decline as they get older. If they are as clever as we hear, they should be able to observe the correlations."

Synster:
"The poisonous effects of our wheat will initially be experienced rather violently by only a very small percentage of the population; approximately four percent. We know that this small percentage will find inclusion of wheat in their diet ultimately lethal. Our findings indicate that currently about five percent of the population becomes ill and sometimes even die, on a regular basis, from natural poisons in their food due to errors in identification, experimentation, emergency expedience, improper preparation and ongoing mishandling. Should the effects of wheat

increase this percentage dramatically for a short time, the change should not be noticed. With the long-term storage potential of wheat, if stores are in fact maintained, some of the above accidents won't happen. For instance, instead of trying to eat a carcass in questionable condition due to famine, the carnate will resort to its stores of wheat.

In addition, numerous types of parasites infect approximately seventy-five percent of the population by the time they reach their reproductive years. This parasite load starts in their youth and increases significantly as they age. As would be expected, they have natural defenses against them, the variety of their seasonal diet being one of these. Nevertheless, the critters ultimately have their impact. In fact, on an individual basis, the parasite load in their gut and elsewhere in the body is the largest single limiting factor to their lifespan. Parasites compete with the human's ability to efficiently absorb and allocate nutrients, aggravate their digestive process, open their tissues to a variety of unrelated secondary pathogens, and attack a variety of organs that limit a number of vital physiological functions. Without these parasites they would be incredibly healthy, but under their current level of technology, they aren't aware of them and so have not developed many strategies against them.

As part of their agricultural training, we will instruct them in various methods of hygiene that will be given religious significance. This will, to a great degree, minimize the onset of the parasite load that they currently have no recourse against. This, of course, can only serve to improve our end product. But beyond this, as the benefits of reduced parasitism are realized, the deleterious effects of a wheat-based diet will begin to emerge. The symptoms of disease that they experience from their wheat consumption will, in a great many ways, feel like symptoms from their usual parasite load: diarrhea, bloating, stomach pain, neuropathy, fatigue, skin problems, behavior changes, depression, sleep disturbances, weight problems, failure to thrive, stunted growth, muscle and joint pain. This is a list of symptoms from both parasite infestation as well as wheat sensitivities. Not so surprising when you consider that they both attack through the digestive system, permeate the intestines and propagate throughout the body, damaging organs. We have perfectly matched the deleterious effects of wheat to what they currently feel from their parasites. In fact, when you think about it, with regards to gut permeability and bacterial dis-biosis, having an intestinal tract full of wheat is very similar to having it full of parasites.

With their newly introduced hygienic customs preventing the usual parasite load, they will largely be trading the old symptoms for the new, without realizing the different source. In the past, as they grew older, they had a greater parasite load and felt more symptoms. As they grow older now, eating wheat, their autoimmune reaction will exhibit increasing symptoms, affecting them mostly, as I described, in their post-reproductive years, per our design. Aside from the additional autoimmune issues that wheat consumption will bring, they will appear to decline at approximately the same rate and in the same manner. Few will notice any difference. And, of course, this is all speaking in general terms, there will be exceptions"

General:
Applause. 7.2 scale

Synster:
"Consul Phyniki"

Consul Phyniki:
"Will these deleterious effects, as you call them, affect the quality of the product? If they should begin too early then we'll have no product. Or we'll have to harvest earlier resulting in lower weight."

Synster:
"Our projections do not anticipate that this will be a problem. The deleterious effects are engineered to begin immediately after their most efficient reproductive age as the body succumbs to the decades of irritation to the gut at about that age. This means it will not generally interrupt reproduction. There will always be exceptions, of course. The first effects on the body generally will

be inflammation and weight gain. This is what we are looking for during this optimal age for harvest. Only later, substantially after weight gain for most, will the other effects come into play. By themselves, they will only affect overall health, but not immediately the quality of the flesh or organs until some years before death. And during the harvest, we do not intend to gather from this older age group."

No further questions raised.
End Meeting

∞ SUBMITTED FOR RECORD ∞

■■■

ABOUT THE AUTHOR

Author Samuel Franklin has spent his life working and playing in extreme environments from alpine peaks to barren deserts, from high security prisons to the skies of the West Indies. As a United States Marine, educator, and member of the law enforcement and intelligence community he has developed a breadth of knowledge of the human condition. His work and diverse hobbies have led him on frequent adventures, the most recent of which nearly took his life. This didn't occur in the typical manner of nearly being killed, but rather through a progressive process of dying, perhaps the worst kind of dying. His life as he knew it was slowly but surely being eroded by an unidentified, unseen villain.

Franklin began his journey into the Primal Estate in a most unlikely place, a small aircraft flying over a tropical island. Part of a special operations group hunting a subject, he began to realize something had been hunting him. It was the Aedes aegypti mosquito from the island's steamy suburbs. It had given him dengue fever and the symptoms hit at thousands of feet while circling a target. From the time of his landing and for two weeks after, Sam was wracked with fever and bone-crushing pain. When it was all over, he was left with a debilitating, degenerative syndrome that doctors could neither identify nor understand, and yet it had a curious similarity to everything from fibromyalgia to multiple sclerosis.

What started as malaise and stiff muscles progressed to most of the autoimmune symptoms. During years of suffering, after giving up on doctors who only wanted to prescribe drugs, Sam took full responsibility for his condition and searched for the truth about autoimmunity. Using himself to experiment, he isolated the problem and recovered his health. He discovered that his immune system had lost its tolerance to eating common foods that were never meant for the human species. It was that simple. The science exists to explain it but the information is not getting out.

Sam dedicates his writing to a deeper understanding of the mind and body, and man's unique place in his environment.

www.ingramcontent.com/pod-product-compliance
Lightning Source LLC
Chambersburg PA
CBHW070408290526
45791CB00005B/1683